Handbook of Aromatic and Medicinal Plants

Handbook of Aromatic and Medicinal Plants

Editor: Cameron James

MURPHY & MOORE
www.murphy-moorepublishing.com

www.murphy-moorepublishing.com

MURPHY & MOORE

Cataloging-in-Publication Data

Handbook of aromatic and medicinal plants / edited by Cameron James.
p. cm.
Includes bibliographical references and index.
ISBN 978-1-63987-274-9
1. Aromatic plants--Therapeutic use. 2. Medicinal plants. 3. Botany, Medical. 4. Materia medica, Vegetable. I. James, Cameron.
RM666.A68 H36 2022
615.321--dc23

Murphy & Moore Publishing,
1 Rockefeller Plaza,
New York City, NY 10020, USA

ISBN 978-1-63987-274-9 (Hardback)

Contents

Preface

It is often said that books are a boon to mankind. They document every progress and pass on the knowledge from one generation to the other. They play a crucial role in our lives. Thus I was both excited and nervous while editing this book. I was pleased by the thought of being able to make a mark but I was also nervous to do it right because the future of students depends upon it. Hence, I took a few months to research further into the discipline, revise my knowledge and also explore some more aspects. Post this process, I begun with the editing of this book.

Aromatic plants are the type of plants that have a characteristic flavor and aroma. Medicinal plants are the plants that are used in traditional medicine practices. Plants synthesize many chemical compounds for functions such as defense against fungi, insects, herbivorous mammals and diseases. There are many plant compounds that have established biological activity. Pharmacologically active substances are discovered by drug research within the discipline of ethnobotany. Some of the common compounds that have medicinal properties and are derived from plants are opium, quinine, digoxin and aspirin. Most of the compounds belong to four biochemical classes. These are alkaloids, polyphenols, glycosides and terpenes. This book unfolds the innovative aspects of medicinal plants and aromatic plants which will be crucial for the progress of this field in the future. It includes some of the vital pieces of work being conducted across the world, on various topics related to aromatic and medicinal plants. This book is a vital tool for all researching or studying aromatic and medicinal plants as it gives incredible insights into emerging trends and concepts.

I thank my publisher with all my heart for considering me worthy of this unparalleled opportunity and for showing unwavering faith in my skills. I would also like to thank the editorial team who worked closely with me at every step and contributed immensely towards the successful completion of this book. Last but not the least, I wish to thank my friends and colleagues for their support.

Editor

1

Combinations of Extracts of Propolis and Other Compounds Against Methicillin-Resistant *Staphylococcus aureus*

Eduardo Lozano Guzmán and
Francisco Javier Moreno Cruz

Abstract

Staphylococcus aureus is a microorganism of great health risk because of its high resistance to antibiotics. Methicillin-resistant strains (MRSA) are most at risk, especially in hospital patients and children. In recent years, it has been shown that a combination therapy of two or more drugs is more effective than monotherapy traditional. Furthermore, it has also been seen that many natural substances and plant extracts can inhibit the MRSA growth and other microorganisms. However, little has been studied about the combinations of different extracts or extracts combination with other commonly used drugs. The purpose of this work was to evaluate of extracts of propolis with garlic, oregano and ciprofloxacin to inhibit growth of MRSA strains, using isobolographic method. The results showed that combinations of garlic with propolis inhibit the growth of MRSA, but only in small concentrations. High concentrations of these two extracts appear to have an antagonistic effect. Combinations of propolis and oregano show a synergistic effect at any concentration. Finally, the combination of propolis with ciprofloxacin has an antagonistic effect. The action of ciprofloxacin is decreased when was combined with propolis. Health professionals should know this to warn patients when they use a natural resource, especially if a drug is being administered.

Keywords: propolis, garlic, oregano, MRSA, isobolographic

1. Introduction

Staphylococcus aureus is a microorganism of great medical importance because it causes serious damage to health in children and hospital patients. In recent years, they have had a growing number of *S. aureus* infections having resistance to commonly used antibiotics. These resistant strains are known as "methicillin-resistant" and are identified as MRSA [1]. Between 1997 and 2003, MRSA was the third leading cause of serious infections in hospitals of which 5% were fatal [2]. In Mexico, the Hospital Epidemiological Surveillance Network reported that mortality rates among patients infected with *S. aureus* range from 5 to 70% and mortality rates attributable to MRSA can reach 50%. With data from general, pediatric, university and specialty hospitals, this network reported that in the period 1997–2003, *S. aureus* was third in morbidity and fourth in mortality [2].

They described three mechanisms that explain the resistance of *S. aureus* to β-lactams and others antibiotics:

1. Overproduction of β-lactamase or borderline resistance: Normal staphylococcal penicillinase hyperproduction mediated by plasmids. These strains produce high amounts of enzymes that degrade these antibiotics, resulting oxacillin and methicillin have no effect on them.
2. Modification of penicillin-binding proteins (PBP) corresponds to a minimum modification of PBPs 1, 2, 3 and 4. These proteins are normal molecular weight but have low affinity for β-lactam antibiotics, preventing these are set and fulfill its inhibitory action.
3. Intrinsic methicillin resistance is due to the incorporation into bacterial DNA of a gene mecA. This gene has two regulatory elements (mecR1 and mecI) that control the transcription of the mecA gene responsible for the induction of the synthesis of a binding protein supernumerary transpeptidase penicillin PBP capable of maintaining the integrity of the wall during the growth and division when the normal cellular enzymes are inhibited by antibiotics [3].

Because of this, they have studied various plant substances to inhibit and to control the growth of microorganisms, including propolis (propolis), oregano (*Lippia graveolens*) and garlic (*Allium sativum*). Propolis is a mixture of complex chemical composition containing balms, essential oils, pollen, vitamins, minerals and proteins, substances that confer a variety of biological properties of interest for therapeutic purposes [4]. The antimicrobial properties of garlic have been attributed to allicin that inhibits certain enzymes essential such as cysteine-proteinase and alcohol-dehydrogenase. Oregano has flavonoids, terpenes and phenylpropane derivatives which also confer antimicrobial properties. Each particular substance has proven to be a viable option to control MRSA. However, few studies have been devoted to the combination of these substances to evaluate the synergism in the antibacterial effect.

On the other hand, allopathic treatments used to fight MRSA include some fluoroquinolones such as ciprofloxacin (CPX) and levofloxacin (LVX), which act on DNA gyrase preventing replication. However, in recent years, it has detected an increasing resistance to these antibiotics in several microorganisms including MRSA. An alternative therapy could be the combination of natural extracts or the combination of these drugs such as ciprofloxacin with. There are few studies testing the efficacy of these drugs when combined with extracts commonly used as propolis.

This paper aims to evaluate combinations of extracts of propolis with garlic and oregano extracts and propolis combination with ciprofloxacin to inhibit MRSA in vitro. Microbial resistance tests were made by the macrodilution method, and combinations were evaluated by isobolographic analysis. The isobolographic analysis is a method based on determining the concentration of antimicrobial substance which has 50% of the inhibitory effect (EC50) and presents the advantage of having a greater statistical power than the traditional method to test dose subinhibitory, generally they are 90% of the minimum inhibitory dose (EC90). Furthermore, the isobolographic analysis reveals whether the effect of the combination is synergistic, simple additive or antagonistic.

2. Drugs and resistant strains

Infections due to *S. aureus* may be treated by a wide range of antibiotics. Among those are frequently reported in the literature penicillin, oxacillin, gentamicin, tobromicina, tetracycline, erytromicina, clindamycin, vancomycin, rifampin, ciprofloxacin and linezolid. The fluoroquinolones, such as ciprofloxacin and levofloxacin, have certain advantages over the others because they have very good effect to bacteria that are resistant to aminoglycosides such as penicillin, cephalosporin and tetracycline among others. It is general consensus that methicillin-resistant species such as MRSA are also resistant to aminoglycosides, so ciprofloxacin and levofloxacin are a good alternative. Both ciprofloxacin (CPX) and levofloxacin (LVX) are quinolones of second generation and are characterized by having a good antibacterial activity concentration dependent (or concentration-dependent) against most bacteria G− and against a broad range of bacteria G+. These antibiotics are widely used especially in intensive care units to combat bacteria such as Pseudomonas, Acinetobacter and *S. aureus*, among others [5]. Chemically, CPX is 1-cyclopropyl-6-fluoro-1,4-dihydro-4oxo-7-piperazin-1-alquinilin-3-carboxylic acid which is condensed formula C17H18FN3O3 and 331.35 with a molecular weight g/mol. CPX and LVX as other fluoroquinolones, act by inhibiting DNA gyrase bacteria (topoisomerase II).

Despite the good prospects offered by fluoroquinolones, since its inception, cases of resistance did not take long to appear. The data do not appear to be accurate, the early warning signs to microbial resistance generally occurred when some hospitals around the world announced that Vancomycin, a powerful antibiotic, was unable to fight *S. aureus*. Then, the same thing happened with penicillin in trying to fight *Streptococcus pneumoniae* [6]. After this came the quinolone resistance. Between 1997 and 1999 was conducted a study in six hospitals of Mexico, which were sampled. The incidence of MRSA was 15%, of these isolates showed 10% CPX resistance [7]. Another study indicates that the first case of complete resistance to CPX and norfloxacin was given in 2003 in the Andaman and Nicobar Islands (in the Indian Ocean) by a strain of *Shigella*. In 2007, it reported that the species of *Campylobacter* (commonly combated with CPX) showed a marked increase in the incidence of resistance to flurorquinolonas, whose cause was attributed to these antibiotics are regularly used in poultry regular consumption, such as chicken [8].

Reports of resistance to CPX and LVX in various species appear to have increased since 2010, *Escherichia coli, Salmonella* (which includes not only resistance but also CPX norfloxacin, ofloxacin) and *Clostridium difficile* (which has been particularly resist to LVX) are some examples [9]. As for *S. aureus* is concerned, the first reports of resistance to fluoroquinolones date from early 2000. In a study conducted in Cuba between 2000 and 2001, 284 healthy children hospitalized were sampled. Only 0.35% of healthy children and 2% of those hospitalized were identified as carriers of MRSA. All strains presented the mecA gene and showed marked resistance to tetracycline, penicillin and erythromycin but 7% of them already showed an intermediate sensitivity to ciprofloxacin. For 2005, it is reported in Colombia that of 131 patients diagnosed with conjunctivitis, 30% have confirmed to *S. aureus* as cause. 42% of the isolates showed multidrug resistance and 6% of them showed high resistance to CPX [10]. In other words, in just 5 years, the incidence of resistance to CPX MRSA strains grew alarmingly. For 2007, Callisaya et al. [11] in La Paz Bolivia reported an incidence of 3% CPX resistance in *S. aureus*. It was calculated that, in the past 5 years, 70% of hospital-acquired infections are due to multidrug-resistant strains and that most of them are due to MRSA.

It has been found that combination of two therapies is an excellent tool to combat MRSA. In recent years, these combinations have not only been carried out with various drugs, but is driving the study drugs and combinations of naturally substances as propolis, garlic or oregano and many others, it has been found that extracts of propolis, combined with various drugs have been successful in combating various kinds of pathogens, so research must continue in this direction.

3. Substances with antibacterial effect

It is known that many natural sources from traditional herbal medicine and ancient cultures have a strong inhibitory power against a large number of bacteria. The extracts of leaves, roots, stems or flowers have been used to great effect in this regard. Although only two decades ago they have begun seriously studying these remedies, they have found a large number of substances that are effective as antibiotic. The success of these effects has been attributed to the large number of compounds containing in plants that maybe have a synergistic effect per se. Several studies agree that it is precisely because of the presence of a large number and variety of compounds in such products that microorganisms can hardly get to develop resistance against them.

Propolis is a natural product that has attracted the attention of scientists because it has proven its effectiveness in combating a number of diseases such as cancer, respiratory tract infections, vaginal infections, skin, and promote the strengthening the immune system among others. One aspect that has begun to take in the past 5 years is the combination of these natural products with drugs commonly used in clinical practice or other plants, especially to combat *S. aureus*. Apparently, some of the mechanisms through which works propolis, as is the weakening of the cell wall and inhibition of gene expression, favor a synergism with these drugs reports tests propolis extract blends with antibiotics such as chloramphenicol, gentamicin, netilmicin, tetracycline and clindamycin with very good results have.

3.1. Propolis

Among the products that can be obtained from the hive are wax, honey, royal jelly and propolis. Propolis is a mixture of complex chemical composition containing balms, essential oils, pollen, vitamins, minerals and proteins, substances that confer antimicrobial activity, which is mainly attributable to flavonoids. It is characterized by having 55% aromatic resins and balsams, 30% waxes, 10% essential oils and 5% pollen grains. They have been reported around 38 flavones, 12 benzoic acid derivatives, 14 cinnamyl alcohol derivatives and cinnamic acid, 12 components from alcohols, ketones and phenols, seven terpenes, 11 steroids, few sugars and amino acids [4]. However, its components may vary due its origins, which are: exudates that bees collect from plants, substances secreted by the metabolism of bees or materials that may be added during the preparation of propolis [12]. However, all propolis have strong antimicrobial activity, which has been evaluated on Gram-positive bacteria and Gram-negative bacteria, being more effective on G+ [4].Cinnamic and flavone components of propolis alter membranes and inhibit the bacterial motility. It is believed that synergism can have so some other antibiotics [13]. Flavonoids (quercetin, apigenin, galangin, etc.) and phenolic acids (caffeic, isoferulic, cinnamic and benzoic acid), are toxic to bacteria and, in addition, inhibit the enzymatic activity of hyaluronidase and caffeic acid. The mechanisms of action of propolis depend mainly of flavonoids that bind to biological affinity to heavy metals and polymers, catalyze electron transport phenomena and are working to find free radicals. In order to process propolis, this is mixed with hot water to separate wax, dried by air and dissolved in ethyl alcohol 95% where it is eliminated wax residue, other insects and wood, finally is filtered [12].

3.2. Oregano

Oregano is mainly used to flavor food and as a medicinal plant for respiratory tract problems such as digestive and analgesic [14]. However, oregano was found other uses related to the treatment of more infections. It is known that the essential oil inhibits the growth of fungi, parasites and is an excellent bactericidal against streptococci and staphylococci [15]. In the essential oil of oregano, they have been detected numerous compounds such as flavonoids as apigenin and luteolin, aglycone, aliphatic alcohols, terpene compounds and derivatives of phenylpropane. Among the most common and high concentrations are limonene, caryophyllene, p-cymene, camphor, linalool, pinene, carvacrol and thymol. The antimicrobial activity depends on the chemical composition of the essential oil of oregano, which is related to the species of oregano, geographical conditions, periods of harvesting and extraction method, if however, its activity has been mainly attributed to carvacrol and thymol [16, 17]. Oregano essential oils have antimicrobial effect against certain Gram-positive bacteria and Gram-negative bacteria, such action is due to the effect on the phospholipids of the outer layer of the bacterial cell membrane, causing changes in the composition of fatty acids. Thymol and carvacrol have the high antimicrobial ability on Gram-positive bacteria and in particular on Gram-negative bacteria acting as disintegrators the outer cell wall and inhibit their growth. The hydroxyl group, which possesses both compounds, appears to be responsible for its antimicrobial capacity [18].

3.3. Garlic

Garlic is a plant that belongs to the monocot species of the Liliaceae family of Asian origin, whose medicinal properties have been known since antiquity. Contains an amino acid called alliin (S-allyl-L-cysteine sulfoxide) which is responsible for the characteristic odor and no antimicrobial activity in their natural state, but when garlic is crushed or fermented the aliinase enzyme is released. This enzyme transforms allin to 2-propene sulfonic acid. This compound presents itself antibiotic, antifungal, lipid-lowering, antioxidant and fibrinolytic [19]. Alliin is crystallized from ethanol or acetone dilutions and is stable in aqueous solutions and at high temperatures. When cells are broken, alliin is mixed with allinase and in about 10 seconds all exposed alliin becomes a new group of compounds: allicin and its closest relatives that emit the scent of fresh garlic. However, the importance of this reaction lies in the formation of allicin, which is the compound which has been mainly attributed to the antibacterial power of garlic. Recent studies conducted by numerous researchers have provided a large number of pharmacological evidence to justify its use as antihypertensives, antifungal, antimicrobial, antithrombotic and antihyperglycemic. It has been shown that allicin exhibits antimicrobial activity due to inhibition of RNA synthesis in bacteria [20].

4. Methodology

Twenty-five *S. aureus* strains were collected over a period of 3 months. Biochemical tests were applied to determine genus and species as established by Mac-Faddin [21]. To identify MRSA, strains were tested using oxacillin according to Clinical and Laboratory Standards Institute (CLSI) [22]. Strains spread massively in culture plate and handle samples were taken with the technique "snowball" which was suspended in an Eppendorf tube-containing medium skim milk. They were stored at −80°C until the time of study. *S. aureus* strain ATCC 29213 was used as a positive control, as established by the same CLSI.

4.1. Extraction and formulation of extracts of propolis

Propolis in beekeeper Canatlán region, Durango, Mex (24°35′N, 105°00′W) was collected. Propolis was cleaned manually, separating waxes, vegetable scraps or other insects; 20 g dry propolis was weighed and 100 mL of ethanol was added and allowed to stand for 8 days with occasional stirring, protected from light with aluminum foil covered at room temperature. Thus, the ethanol extract 20% of propolis was obtained (EEP20). Similarly, extract 30% (EEP30) was prepared by weighing 30 g of the same and adding the same amount of ethanol. Then the extracts were filtered through Whatman filter and aliquoted into 50-mL Corning conical tubes. The extracts were kept protected from light and cooling (5–7°C) until the time of the study.

4.2. Collection and formulation of extracts of garlic and oregano

Garlic and oregano were purchased in local supermarkets. The taxonomic classification and identification was carried out at the National Polytechnic Institute-Dgo by D Ph. Ma. Socorro Gonzalez Elizondo. Garlic was cut into cubes of about 1 mm, after 20 g was weighed and was added 100 mL of ethanol. It was allowed to stand for 8 days with occasional stirring, protected from light with aluminum foil covered at room temperature.

Thus, the ethanolic extract Garlic 20% was obtained (EEA20). Similarly, the extract 30% (EEA30) weighing 30 g thereof by adding the same amount of ethanol was prepared. Then, the extracts were filtered through Whatman filter and aliquoted into 50-mL Corning conical tubes. The extracts were kept protected from light and cooling (5–7°C) until the time of the study. Similarly, the extracts of oregano were obtained, which was cleaned of branches and flowers using only the leaves.

4.3. Isobolographic studies to evaluate synergism

Isobolographic analysis is one way to assess the interaction between two substances or two drugs resulting in the optimal combination of drugs. This method provides a safe way to assess whether substances are stronger by the combination that the application of each separately. This study is performed by a isobologram, which is a graph in rectangular coordinates of substances causing a certain level of effect when applied together. The line joining these two points it is known as "additivity line" and all points on this line, theoretically represent effective doses of the constituents administered jointly [23]. The interaction of the drug in the isobologram can be defined as additive, antagonistic or synergistic. Two drugs interact additively when the effect achieved after administration of both is equal to the sum of the effects that would be achieved if administered separately. When the effect achieved is less than that achieved if the same doses of both drugs were administered separately, it is a case of antagonism. When two drugs are administered and the effect achieved is significantly higher than would be achieved by the sum of doses from each interaction, it is defined as synergy [24]. Furthermore, the method includes a statistical evaluation and determination of the interaction index, as explained later.

The way it was carried out the study of synergism in the combinations was based on the methodology described by Tallarida [25, 26] which is known as isobolographic study. An inoculum of each strain of 105–106 CFU/mL was prepared. Each strain was exposed to seven different concentrations of each extract (25, 12.5, 6, 3, 1.5, 0.7, 0.3% extract v/v) cultivated in broth in tubes 13 × 100 by the macro dilution method [27]. An aliquot of each tube inoculated was also cultivated in Muller Hinton agar and incubated at 36°C for 24 h. After the growth of microorganisms, minimum inhibitory concentration (MIC) and minimum bactericidal concentration (MBC) was determinate as shown in **Figure 1**. The letters AB indicate the antibiotic and size of the bracket is indicative of the concentration of antibiotic.

Concentration of extract broth in which it is detected no turbidity into tubes was established as MIC. The concentration where no growth was detected in plates was established as MBC. An aliquot of the inoculum to be planted plaque was also taken. After appropriate incubation, the inoculum exact population was counted. This is necessary to set the following parameters:

a. Mortality: The difference between population in the inoculum and the populations in plate for each concentrations tested expressed as CFU/mL.

b. Percentage of inhibitory effect: mortality divided among the population of inoculum expressed as a percentage.

c. Dose-effect curve: The effect (%) was plotted (Y) vs. each concentration (dose X) as shown in **Figure 2**.

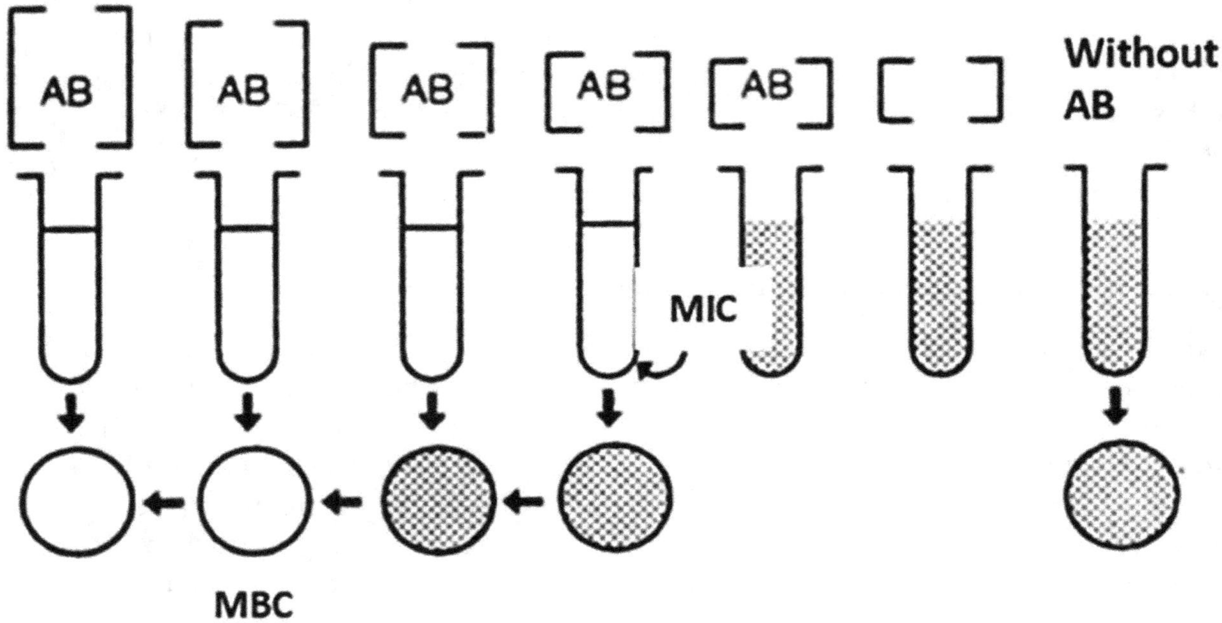

Figure 1. Determination of minimum inhibitory concentration (MIC) and minimum bactericidal concentration (MBC).

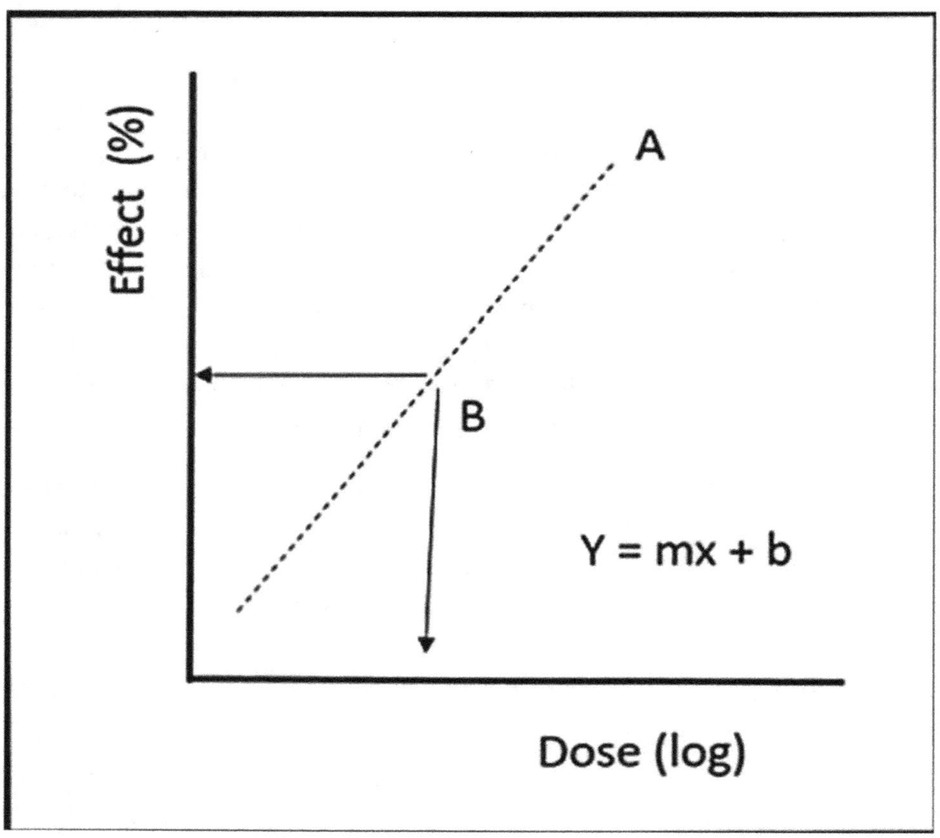

Figure 2. Graphical representation of % effect vs. log dose.

The dose-effect curve is defined by an equation (Y = mx + b) which allows us to calculate the effective concentration 50 (EC50). This is defined as the dose at which the 50% of effect is achieved, in this case, half of the population counted. Point A in **Figure 2** represents the maximum effect. Point B represents the dose at which 50% is obtained effect for a single drug.

The concentrations that produce a 50% effect is made the graph shown in **Figure 3**. The combinations of the two drugs A and B theoretically produce 50% effect (points a and b) is constructed. However, it may happen that lower concentrations of the drugs A and B combined have the same effect, for example, the point "c". This is a synergistic combination. The point "c" can also be placed above the line of additivity, indicating an antagonistic combination.

Additionally, the significance test or interaction index was performed by the Eq. (1):

$$g = \frac{a}{A} + \frac{b}{B} \quad (1)$$

where,

g = interaction index

A = individual concentration of A

B = individual concentration of B

a = concentration of A in the combination

b = concentration of B in the combination

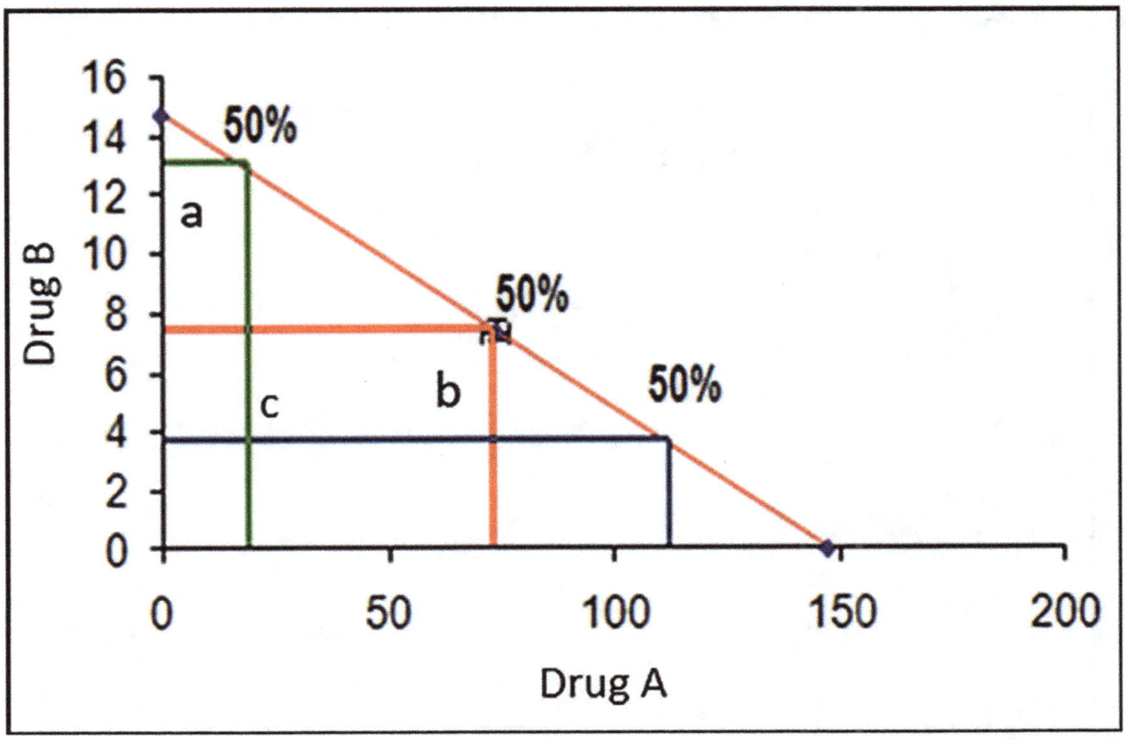

Figure 3. Isobologram.

When g = 1, we have an additive effect, if g < 1, the effect is synergistic, if g > 1, the effect is antagonistic.

Finally, the Student's t test was applied to identify differences between the effects of theoretical and experimental concentrations for each combination applied to five strains MRSA.

Three theoretical combinations for each pair of extracts were tested: propolis-garlic, propolis-oregano and propolis-ciprofloxacin. After that they were inoculated with MRSA strains and the experimental inhibitory effect was determined. With these results, the isobologram was made for each pair of extracts.

5. Results and discussions

5.1. Garlic-propolis combinations

Less inhibitory concentration of antimicrobial in the experimental stage in relation to the theoretical concentration was found. Average was determined as theoretical concentration of garlic and propolis a total concentration of 8.6 ± 0.0 mg/mL to obtain the EC50, however, experimentally a concentration of 5.95 ± 1.19 mg/mL was obtained for the same effect, in other words, a lower amount of extracts combined is required that each individually to obtain the same effect. The interaction index was <1. This indicates a synergistic effect. The statistical test ("t" Student) showed significant differences between the two groups ($p < 0.05$).

The corresponding isobologram is shown in **Figure 4**. The point A shows theoretical garlic and propolis concentrations necessary to obtain a 50% effect (EC50), point B shows the experimental concentration, which is visibly lower, which It indicates a strong synergistic effect.

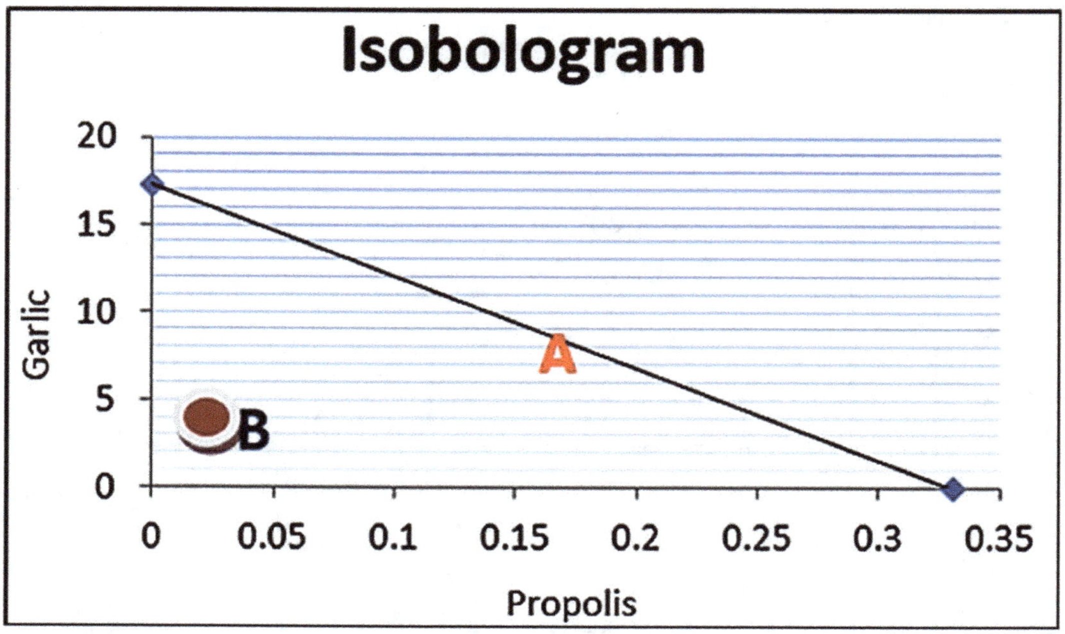

Figure 4. Isobologram combinations garlic-propolis percentage effect.

Figure 5 shows the colony forming units counted in concentrations EC50 (A) propolis, (B) garlic, (C) garlic + propolis (combination 1), (D) garlic + propolis (combination 2), where the combination 2 is half combination 1. Growth in (C) and (D) is less than that taken in the application of each extract separately, confirming the synergistic effect of the combinations.

In contrast to these results, other combinations tested garlic and propolis showed opposite results. Greater theoretical concentration (17 mg/mL) resulted in an experimental concentration of 60.07 ± 4.8 mg/mL to obtain the same effect. This was verified by determining the interaction rate, which was g = 3.5.

This suggests that increasing concentrations propolis and garlic, their compounds act antagonistically inhibited each other. The cause is not yet well defined but could be a saturation at the same site of action. This should be studied in future. In conclusion, it is recommended to use only diluted combinations of garlic and propolis extracts, for example extracts 20%.

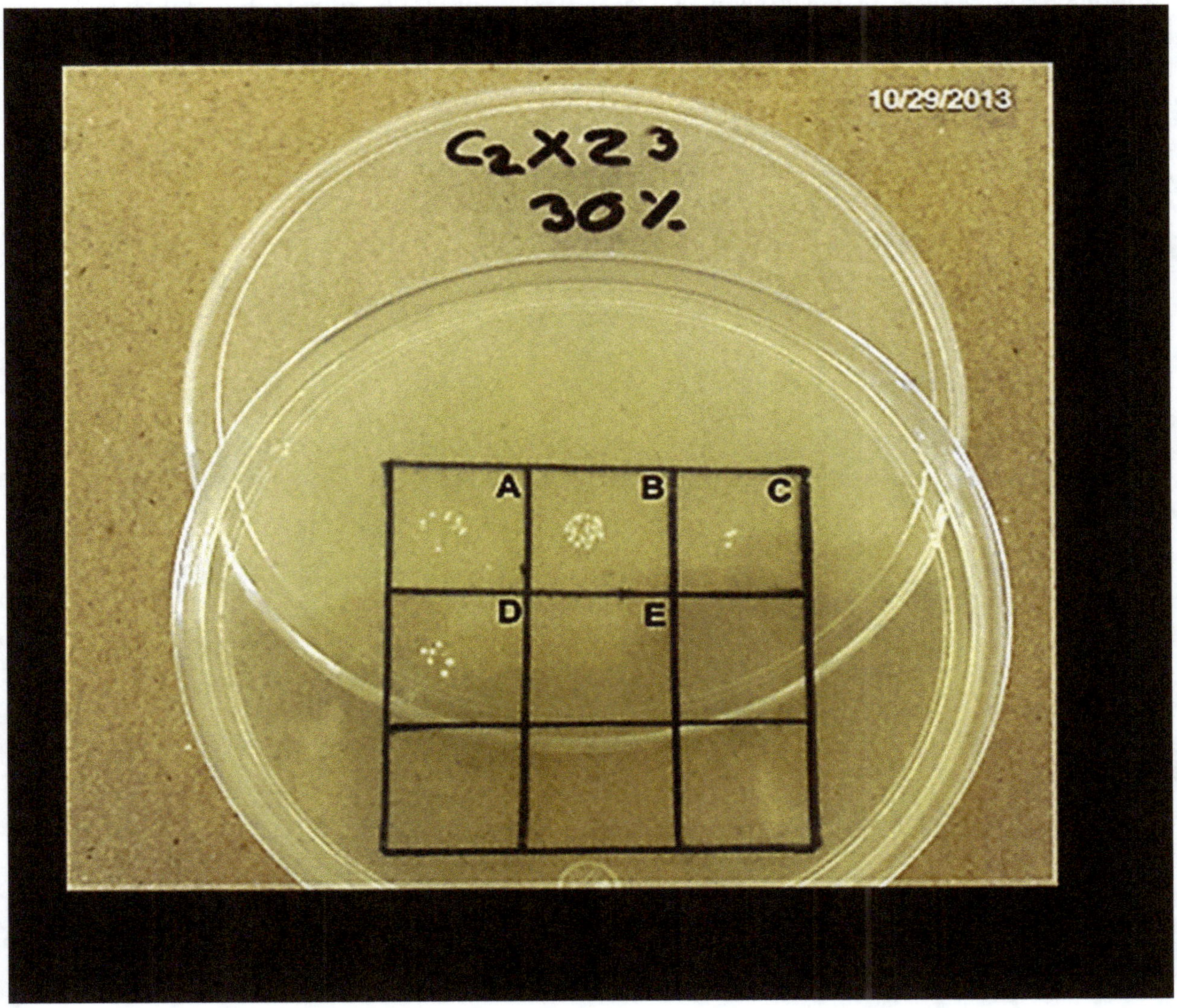

Figure 5. Population counted when grown with theoretical concentrations.

5.2. Oregano-propolis combination

In combination with propolis oregano, lower experimental concentration was also found that the theoretical: 4.9 mg/mL vs. 3.33 ± 0.86 mg/mL. **Figure 6** shows the corresponding isobologram. The interaction index was calculated 0.59 indicating a synergistic relationship. The corresponding Student's t test showed significant differences between treatments.

Unlike garlic, oregano in combinations with propolis shows a synergistic effect always. In fact, combinations of garlic extracts and propolis 30% were more synergistic than any other combination. Chavez et al. [28] had demonstrated the synergistic effect of oregano oil in combination with Gentamicin on E. coli isolates and had suggested that potentiates the effect of oregano other drugs when combined with them. No other reports found on combination of oregano and propolis, but we believe it is a combination that results in a good control of MRSA.

According to the research conducted by Waili et al. [29] on the synergistic effects of propolis extracts with ethyl alcohol on *S. aureus* and our studies agree that potentiates the effect of propolis another drug on *S. aureus* isolates; with the difference that Waili used as a second active substance honey; and this work highlighted the effects of propolis in combination with extracts of oregano.

Chavez et al. [28] showed a synergistic effect between essential oil of oregano and Gentamicin in E. coli isolates using the arithmetic mean of the halos of inhibition, however, we demonstrated a synergistic effect between propolis extracts and extracts of oregano in *S. aureus* applying an isobolographic analysis. In any case, it is shown that extracts of oregano in combination with other drugs or plants potentiates the effect against bacteria and could help fight serious infections in hospitalized patients and children [30, 31]

5.3. Propoleo-ciprofloxacin combination

The theoretical concentration established for ciprofloxacin (CPX) was 9 μg/mL. By combining this with propolis, the inhibitory effect of propolis disappeared. In other words, in 5 of the 7

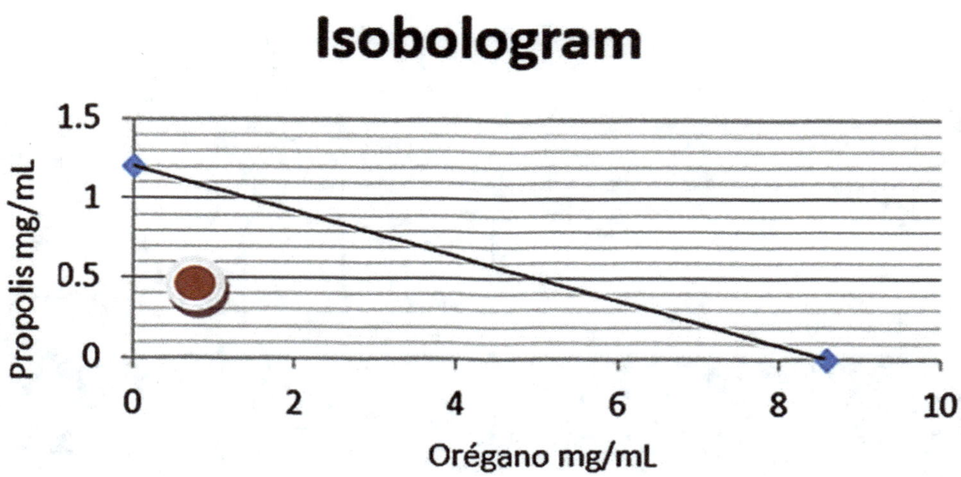

Figure 6. Isobologram oregano-propolis combinations.

strains studied further growth of MRSA was found in combinations in concentrations of each substance separately applied. This suggests that the propolis is an antagonist of CPX, so the combination of both substances is harmful. In a survey conducted in this study 821 people, 45% said propolis or their products are consumed in respiratory diseases, and 34% of them combined ciprofloxacin or levofloxacin with propolis.

Many studies have reported that *S. aureus* is susceptible to propolis, however, a work published by Wojtyczka et al. [32] showed that propolis has a synergism only when is used in combination with other antibiotics that act on the cell wall and ribosomal functions, but it seems not interact with antibiotics that act on DNA or folic acid biosynthesis. The lack of synergism could also be that both propolis and CPX compete for the same target action: genetic replication and mutually inhibiting effect. However, other studies have reported good results by combining propolis with other drugs: Fernandes et al. [33] reported synergism between extracts of propolis and Chloramphenicol, Gentamicin and Vancomycin among others, but claims to have obtained the same effect between them combined extracts with oxacillin, ampicillin and ofloxacin.

No reports on combinations of garlic-propolis or oregano-propolis were found, therefore, it is difficult to make a comparison and deeper discussion about our results. However, we must make it clear that the basis for further research on alternative medicine to combat MRSA, as our results provide a good foundation for further research feel.

Microbial inhibition studies showed that the presence of *S. aureus* acquired in the community has been increasing, especially in healthy carriers. Its high resistance to CPX and LVX makes potential public health risk. Traditional therapies such as the use of ethanol extracts of propolis are a good alternative combat with the restriction check whether the drug combinations strengthen or inhibit their control.

6. Conclusions

Natural products should be subject to further study and be equally controlled by the health professional to inform the population about the beneficial and nonbeneficial cases. Apparently, the combination of garlic-propolis and propolis extracts of oregano is very effective in combating MRSA in vitro.

Acknowledgements

The authors acknowledge the Faculty of Chemical Sciences received support.

Author details

Eduardo Lozano Guzmán* and Francisco Javier Moreno Cruz

*Address all correspondence to: elozano@ujed.mx

Faculty of Chemistry, Juarez University of the State of Durango, Durango, Dgo, Mexico

References

[1] Bustos J, Hamdan A, Gutierrez M. Staphylococcus aureus, the re-emergence of one pathogen into community. Biomed J. 2006;17:287–305.

[2] Velasquez-Meza ME. Staphylococcus aureus methicilin resistant. Salud Publica de Mexico. 2005;47:381–387.

[3] MONICA-GIL, D. M. *Staphyloccus aureus*: Microbiology and molecular features of methicillin resistant Staphylococcus aureus. Rev Chil Infect. 2000;17:145–152.

[4] Tolosa L, Cañizares E. Obtaining, characterization and evaluation of the antimicrobial activity of propolis extracts of Campeche. Ars Pharmaceutical. 2002;43(1–2):187–204.

[5] Khachman D, ColinJ, Georges B, Saivin S, Houin G, Toutain P. Optimizing ciprofloxacin dosing in intensive care unit patients trough the use of population pharmacokinetic-pharmacodynamic analysis and Monte Carlo simulations. J Antimicrob Chemother. 2011;66:1798–1809.

[6] Cabrera Y, Fadragas A, Guerrero L. Natural antibiotic; myth or reality. Rev Cubana Med Gen Integr. 2005;21:3–4.

[7] Sifuentes O, Donis H, Arredondo G, Escalante R, Macias A, Muñoz J. Report on bacterial resistance: a pilot study. Revista Panamericana de Infectologia. 1999;s545–s547.

[8] Roy S, Debbuta B, Ghosh A, Sathya P, Bharadwaj A, Singhania M. Emergence of fluoroquinilone resistance in Shigella isolated from Andam and Nicobar Islands, India. Indian J Med Res. 2010;131:720–722.

[9] Henning N, Witte W, Nübel U. Fluoroquinolone resistence and Clostridium difficile, Germany. Emerg Infec Dis. 2010;16(4):675–677.

[10] Hernandez I, Toraño G, Gonzalez M, Gonzalez I. Meticilin resistant Staphylococcus aureus: carrier screening children in hospital and community. Revista Cubana de Medicina Tropical. 2003;55(3):153–161.

[11] Callisaya H, Sarmiento Z, Choque C. Prevalence of nasal carriers of Staphylococcus aureus in cleaning staff of hospital Obrero. Biofarbo. 2007;15(1):55–61.

[12] Gutierrez C, Suarez M. Antimicrobial activity of propolis and its effect on the physiocechemical and sensoral characteristics in sausages. Vitae, Revista de la Facultad de Química Faraceutica, UNC. 2014;21(2):90–96.

[13] Farre R, Frasquet I, Sanchez A. Propolis and health. Ars Pharmaceutica. 2004;45(1):21–43.

[14] Huerta C. Mexican oregano, cegetable gold. Biodiversitas. 1997;15(1):8–13.

[15] Villavicencio G. Oregano, resource with high potential. Revista Ciencia y Desarrollo - CONACYT. 2007;33(211):60–66.

[16] Amador-Martinez. Secondary metabolites of Lippia graveolens [thesis]. Mexico; 2007.

[17] De la Cruz M, Gastelum M. Micobrial effect of mexican oregano and essential oil in five strains of Vibro. Revista Fitotecnia Mexicana. 2007;261–267.

[18] Nuñez M. Preliminary assessment of bacterial populations associated with the intestinal tract of Tilapia (Oreochromis niloticus) exposed to oregano essenctial oils in the diet [thesis]. Mexico; 2011.

[19] Ramirez-Medina H. Identification and cloning of genes involved in the pathogenesis of Sclerotium cepivorum in garlic (Allium sativum) [thesis]. 2004.

[20] Hughes BG, Lawson LD. Antimicrobial effects of Allium sativum (garlic), Allium ampeloprasum (elephant garlic) and Allium cepa (onion), garlic compunds and commercial garlic supplement products. Phytother Res. 1991;5:154–158.

[21] Mac-Faddin J. Panamerican Medical Ed, editor. Biochemical test for identificaction of bacteria clinical significance. 2003, 3rd ed. Mexico; 45–47.

[22] Clinical and Laboratory Standards Institute. Performance Standards for Antimicrobial Susceptibility Testing. CLSI. 2010;30(1).

[23] Navarrete A, Flores A, Sixtos C, Reyes B. isobolographic analysis of the interaction between sesamia, asarinia, fagaramida y piperin over Culex quinquefasciatus larves. J Mexican Chem Soc. 2003;47(2).

[24] Gambus PL, Troconiz IF. Pharmacokinetic-pharmacodynamic modeling in anesthesia. International Congress Series. 2001;1220:89–97.

[25] Tallarida R. Drug Synergism: its detection and applications. J Pharm Exp Ther. 2001;298 (3):865–893.

[26] Tallarida R. Interactions between drugs and occupied receptors. Pharmacol Ther. 2007; 113(1):197–209.

[27] Taroco R, Seija R, Vignoli R. methods of antibiotic sensitivity studies [Internet]. 2008 [Updated: 2010]. Available from: htpp://higiene.edu.uy/cefa/2008/BacteCEFA36.tif [Accessed: 2013/10/08]

[28] Chavez L, Castañeda F, Rosario G, Estrada E. Synergistic effect of oil essence of Origanum vulgare and Gentamicin on strains of Escherichia coli. CIMEL. 2008;13(2).

[29] Waili N, Ghamdi A, Ansari M, Al-Attal Y, Salom K. Synergistic effects of honey and propolis toward drug multi-resistantan Staphilococcus aureus, Escherichia coli and Candida albicans. Int J Med Sci. 2012;9(9):783–800.

[30] Salgado C. Meta-analysis of natural substances to children's health. Natura Solutions. 2011;18(2).

[31] Pacual ME, Slowing K, Carretero E, Sanchez M, Villar A. Lippia, traditional uses, chemistry and pharmacology. J Pharmacol. 2001;76:201–214.

[32] Wojtyczka R, Dziedzic A, Idzik D, Kepa M, Kubina R, Kabala-Dzik A, et al. Susceptibility of Staphylococcus aureus clinicla isolates to propolis extract alone or in combination with antimicrobial drugs. Molecules. 2013;18:9623–9640.

[33] Fernandes JA, Balestrin EC, Betoni JE, Orsi Rdo O, Cunha Mde L, Montelli AC. Propolis: anti Staphylococcus aureus activity and synergism with antimicrobial drugs. Mem Inst Oswaldo Cruz. 2005;100(5):563–566.

2

Aromatic Plants from Western Balkans: A Potential Source of Bioactive Natural Compounds

Ana M. Džamić and Jelena S. Matejić

Abstract

Documentation of traditionally used aromatic and medical plants has been carried out in many European countries over the last several years. Over the last decade, the Western Balkans has become the area of a huge number of ethnobiological field studies. Many of those focused on Balkans ethnobotany are linked to the long and ongoing history of gathering and trading local wild aromatic and medicinal plants from this territory into Western European markets. But only less than a half percent of these have been studied for their chemical composition and medicinal value. The most investigated aromatic species in this area belongs to the few biggest families: Asteraceae, Apiaceae, Lamiaceae and Rosaceae. Medicinal value of plants lies in some chemical substances that produce physiological action on the human body, which leads to positive effect on health. Essential oils are secondary metabolites which are the most examined, as well as various plant extracts. Isolation and identification of the compounds in combination with its biological screening can considerably contribute to plant studies. Also, application of new activities and novel techniques for susceptibility testing provide better knowledge of wild growing medicinal plants as potential sources of biological agents and justified their traditional uses.

Keywords: Western Balkans, ethnobiological studies, wild growing plants, essential oil, extract

1. Introduction

World is endowed with wealth of medicinal and aromatic plants. Plants have always been the principal form of traditional medicine in many undeveloped countries, and presently, they are becoming popular throughout the developed world, where people strive to stay healthy because of influence of chronic stress and pollution. One definition says that aromatic plants are the local heritage of global importance [1]. In many countries of Balkans, people practiced traditional medicine which is based on the use of plants. The way of use is determined with culture, philosophy and personal attitude. This practice is usually different than conventional medicine. Long period of using traditional medicine has demonstrated that it is safe and effective [2]. Medicinal plants also play an important role in the lives of rural people, particularly in remote parts of developing countries with a few health facilities. It is estimated that around 70,000 plant species have been used at one time or another for medicinal purposes. At the present time, when there is a tendency to respect nature and natural processes more and more, the value of local knowledge on the stability of ecosystem dynamics *in sensu lato* deserves the most attention of scientists [3]. Various pathological conditions of humans that could not be fully treated by conventional pharmaceutical agents are numerous [4]. For this reason, there is a growing tendency in use of herbal preparations. However, scientific researches need to provide additional evidence of their safety and efficacy. Medicinal plants contain active substances which may have active effects on human body and its health. Different diseases could be treated with different plants, which may have 2–3 up to 30–40, sometimes even more, different active substances. Any wrong use can cause various complications, due to the established cytotoxicity for many plant compounds [5]. For all these reasons, medicinal and aromatic plants are in focus of many scientific groups which doing experiments and trying to find new useful compounds.

2. Plant diversity of Western Balkans countries

It is estimated that at least 265,000 species of seed plants [6] exist on earth. Only less than a half percent of these have been studied exhaustively for their chemical composition and medicinal value [7]. With about 6340 different vascular plant species reported, the Balkans, compared to 10,500 species accepted in the Flora Europaea, is one of the most important biodiversity centres of Europe [8]. Region of Serbia is rich in medicinal herbs; about 700 species exist on its territory which is 10.7% of total flora with 3662 taxa. Abundance of medicinal herbs placed Serbia in 158 centres of biodiversity in the world [9]. Despite the inconspicuous extension of the territory of Bosnia and Herzegovina (Western Balkan Peninsula; Southeast Europe), the country holds about 3600 species of vascular plants [10]. In Flora Croatica, around 5000 species and subspecies are registered. Among them, 1144 species and subspecies (21% of total flora) are used for different purpose. The greatest number (25%) of these plants is used in traditional as well in official medicine [11]. Croatia is also one of the centres of endemism in south-eastern Europe. No less than 5.65% of the total numbers of known plant species are endemic. Flora of Montenegro consists about 2632 species of vascular plants, as well as of numerous lower infraspecies taxa as varieties and forms [12]. New data suggest 104 taxa more in second supplement to Rohlena`s Conspectus [13]. The flora of the Republic of Macedonia is among the richest floras not only in respect to the Balkan Peninsula, but also in the context of the whole European continent. According to recent data, 210 families, 920 genera and 3700 species comprise the flora of higher plants, angiosperms being the richest group with about 3200 species. Endemic taxons represent a special characteristic and value of the Macedonian flora. Among them, 114 flowering plant species are Macedonian endemics [14].

3. Ethnobotanical studies

The knowledge of plants, which are used by local people in different geographical areas, is documented in ethnobotanical studies. People in rural areas with traditional knowledge about plants, which are used as a food, spices, flavouring and for medicinal purposes, transmitted that information from one generation to the next. This knowledge is associated to plant identification, conservation and uses. An extensive ethnobotanical work yielded interesting results that confirmed many assumptions and estimates about plant uses [15].

A group of scientists investigated the local traditions of using wild food plants around Lake Vrana (northern Dalmatia, Zadar region) [16]. This research includes studies and interviews of 43 inhabitants of six traditional villages north of Lake Vrana. On average, 12 species were listed, which in total produced an inventory of 55 food plants. The most common medicinal species were *Rosa canina* L., *Salvia officinalis* L., *Achillea millefolium* L., *Helichrysum italicum* (Roth) G. Don and *Mentha* spp.

Ethnobotanical study on medicinal use of wild and cultivated plants in middle, south and west Bosnia and Herzegovina was presented with 228 wild and cultivated species (belonged to 50 families and 124 genera) and 730 different preparations for the use in human therapy. Species of the genus *Achillea* L., *Hypericum* L., *Mentha* L., *Teucrium* L., *Thymus* L. and *Urtica* L. were particularly highly recommended, by almost 90% of the informants that used these species in preparations. Medicinal plants are often used for treatment of different illness such as urogenital tract—16.0%, respiratory system—16.0%, gastrointestinal tract—14.4%, skin ailments—11.5%, blood system—8.8%, nervous system—7.1%, cardiovascular system—6.6%, rheumatism—5.9%; metabolism disorders—3.8%, senses disorders—2.1%, influenzal infections—2.1%, lever and gall disorders—1.9%, parasitic induced ailments—1.6%, inflammations—1.0%, musculoskeletal system—0.8%, endocrinological—0.3% [10].

Usually used plants from the region of Suva Planina Mountain are from families of Lamiaceae —20, Asteraceae—17, Rosaceae—16, Brassicaceae—5, Alliaceae—4 and Apiaceae—4. On this region were identified 128 plants and 2 fungi. Most of them are used in ethnomedicine but some of them in ethnoveterinary medicine. Some plants have 'other' purposes. While the most common conditions treated with medicinal plants are respiratory (79), urogenital (53), gastrointestinal (51), skin (43) and those relating to the circulatory system (35) [17]. On Kopaonik Mountain (the central part of Serbia), 83 wild plant species reported by informants to have medicinal properties have been recorded. The most often used plants belong to six families: Asteraceae—15.8%, Lamiaceae—15.8%, Rosaceae—7.3%, Malvaceae—3.7%, Apiaceae—3.7% and Plantaginaceae—3.7%, within 69 genera and 41 families. In all other families, authors detected the uses of only two or one species (2.4 and 1.2%). Based on investigations, they concluded that tested plants had the highest influence on gastrointestinal ailments—50%, skin injures and problems—25.6%, respiratory—20.5%, urinary-genital—20.5%, cardiovascular problems—19.2%, antiseptic—15.4% and anti-infective effect—14.1% [18]. Botanical remedies in the South-western Serbia (Zlatibor district) comprise 69 species belonging to 36 families. The predominant botanical families were Rosaceae (16%), Lamiaceae (13%) and Asteraceae (12%). From 69 mentioned species, 23 species are included in European Pharmacopoeia 7.0 [19].

Those plants are used for treatment of gastrointestinal—33.1%, respiratory diseases—29.6%, dermatologic diseases—14.8%, urinary tract ailments—6.1%, circulatory system—5.1%, nervous system and psyche—5.1%, nutritional endocrine glands and metabolism—4.3%, skeletal, muscle and connective tissues problems—1.0%, gynecological complications—0.5%, disease of the sensorial system—0.3% [20].

On Prokletije Mountains (Montenegro), the most often used are Rosaceae—11 species which

Ninety-four species are reported, 35 species in Ph. Eur. 6.0, which makes 37.2%, 12 species in national pharmacopoeias or 12.8%. In most cases, aerial parts were used—43.6%. People usually used those plants for treating gastrointestinal—57.4% and respiratory diseases—41.5% [21].

In one of the most remote and poorest areas of Europe, the village of Theth, which is located in the upper Shala Valley in the Northern Albanian Alps, 79 botanical taxa known and used by the local population. This area is characterised by total absence of medical assistance, but villagers of Theth used a small number of medicinal herbs for minor ailments. They usually used aerial parts of *Origanum vulgare* L., also *Hypericum maculatum* Crantz, as well as aerial part of *Agrimonia eupatoria* L., and they used roots of *Gentiana lutea* L. [22]. Among of ethnobiological study of Pešter plateau (South-western Serbia), where two communities of Serbians and Albanians have been lived together from three centuries ago when they immigrated to the area, 62 taxa in 129 plant-based remedies recorded as well as 204 plant uses. *Chenopodium-bonus hendricus* (L.)Rchb., *Gentiana lutea* L., *O. vulgare* L., *Hypericum* spp., *R. canina* L., *Urtica dioica* L., which are mostly used in the same way and for the same folk medical purposes, may be viewed as the medicinal plants whose cultural salience, measured through the lens of quotations elicited during the free listing exercises, appears remarkable in both communities [23].

A medico-ethnobotanical study was conducted among Albanians, Macedonians and Gorani in 41 villages located in the Sharr Mountains in Western Macedonia. Seventy-six mainly wild taxa (belonging to 34 families) were found to represent the remaining folk medical heritage of the area. The most frequently cited families were Lamiaceae (15.7%), Asteraceae (14.4%), Rosaceae (5.2%), Malvaceae (5.2%) and Fabaceae (5.2%). The large majority of the recorded plants are used in form of teas, and mainly for minor dysfunctions of the respiratory system (46%). According to results of investigations, leaves of *Ballota nigra* L. as a tea is used as a digestive, leaves and fruits of *Cornus sanguine* L. as a tea against stomachaches, topically applied leaves of *Chenopodium urbicum* L. for treating hemorrhoids, aerial parts of *Convolvulus arvensis* L. as a tea against hypertension. This could be interesting for further phytopharmacological investigations. Similar uses were reported by Gorani and Albanians, because those two communities lived together over the century in the same area shared faith, while Orthodox Macedonians reported different uses of these ethnic groups [24].

Comparison with traditional therapy in neighbouring countries showed that there exists considerable similarity with respect to plants used and the way of usage [25, 18, 26]. Results obtained in the area of Suva Planina Mountain comparing with results from other investigated areas of the Western Balkans showed similarities with Zlatibor region—37.2% and Kopaonik Mountain—32.3%. Compare the wider regions showed similarities with Bosnia and Herzegovina—40.9% and Bulgaria—40.6% [17]. It has also been observed that the inhabitants of mountain regions have longer traditional therapeutic tradition (more than six generations) compared to the rest of the population [10].

An important point in research is paying attention on analysis of endemic and rare species, because they are potential source of new active compounds. However, strict rule and regulations for protection of its localities are necessary because of threat of its extermination. If phytochemical analyses show that those plants represent valuable sources of new compounds, it could be necessary to find adequate way to its cultivations and preservation. The new activities and novel techniques for susceptibility testing provide field for research of well-known medicinal plants as well as unknown plants.

4. Composition and biological activity of essential oils and extracts of wild growing Lamiaceae species

The knowledge of plants which in ethnobotanical studies of Western Balkans countries *O. vulgare* is recognised as a plant with a range of health benefits. This uses are confirmed by scientific research. Essential oil of this, well-known species, was characterised with dominance of carvacrol (64.1%) and linalool (17.6%) and possesses strong antifungal activity against wild-type strains [27]. The cytotoxic, antioxidant and antibacterial activities are attributed mostly to the presence of the isomeric phenolic constituents, carvacrol and thymol [28]. The dominance of 1.8-cineole (44.3%) was found in essential oils of *Rosmarinus officinalis* L. as well as in sample of wild growing *Hyssopus officinalis* L. subsp. *pilifer* (Pant.) Murb (36.4%) (**Table 1**) [27, 29]. The results showed that antifungal activity offered by 1.8-cineole was incomplete and exhibited moderate activity at the highest concentration tested. Otherwise, this compound was arguably the most effective compounds regarding fumigant activities against storage pest *Cryptolestes ferrugineus* Stephens followed by camphor and carvacrol [30]. Phenolic acids were identified in post-distillation waste extract of *H. officinalis* subsp. *pilifer* which possessed valuable radical scavenging activities (**Table 1**). The antioxidant activity of phenolic acids is related to the number and position of hydroxyl groups [29]. *Stachys anisochila* Vis. et Panč. is Balkans endemic species, distributed in Bulgaria, Serbia and Albania. Essential oil composition of *S. anisochila* collected from Stara Planina, Serbia, shows α-pinene (7.6%), α-copaene (6.2%), β-pinene (5.3%) and β-caryophyllene (4.5%) as the main compounds. Many species of genus *Stachys* L. possess strong antioxidant and antimicrobial activity [31].

Nine species of genus *Satureja* L. have been registered in the area of the Central and Western Balkans. The essential oils isolated from various *Satureja* species have shown antibacterial, fungicidal, antiviral and antioxidant activities. Essential oil of *Satureja horvatii* Šilić (**Table 1**) shows significant antimicrobial effect, and this oil successfully inhibited the development of *Lysteria monocytogenes* in pork meat and also can be a useful source of natural antioxidants [32]. Oxygenated monoterpene hydrocarbons were the major compounds: carvacrol, thymol, carvacrol methyl ether and β-linalool in essential oil of *S. montana* L. subsp. *pisidica* (Wettst.) Silic from two localities (mountains Korab and Galičica, Macedonia). Both oils showed excellent antimicrobial activity and good cytotoxic potential [33]. Antioxidant activity of essential oils and water wastes after distillation process of *S. montana* L. and *S. cuneifolia* Ten. was demonstrated

Plant	Origin	Essential oil/main compounds	Activity	References
Hyssopus officinalis L. subsp. *pilifer* (Pant.) Murb	Sicevo gorge (Serbia)	1.8-cineole (36.43%), β-pinene (19.55%), isopinocamphone (15.32%) pinocamphone (6.39%)	Antifungal, antioxidant	[29]
Micromeria dalmatica Benth.	Mt. Lovcen (Montenegro)	piperitenone (41.46%), pulegone (19.02%), piperitenone oxide (14.49%), D-limonene (6.23%) and p-menthone (5.06%)	Antimicrobial	[35]
Satureja montana L.	Mt Biokovo (Croatia)	Carvacrol (63.4%), thymol (19.4%)	Antioxidant	[34]
Satureja montana L. ssp. *montana*	Budva Cetinje MtOrijen (Montenegro)	Thymol (24.7%), carvacrol (15.2%), linalool (15.4%). Carvacrol (24.5%), linalool (17.9%), cis-sabinene hydrate (14.61%), terpinen-4-ol (10.6%). Linalool (32.6%), cis-sabinene hydrate (23.0%), terpinen-4-ol (11%), nerolidol (9.4%)	Antimicrobial, antioxidant, anticholinesterase activity	[39]
Satureja horvatii Šilić	Mt Orijen (Montenegro)	p-cymene (33.1%), thymol (26.1%) and thymol methyl ether (15.1%)	Antimicrobial	[32]
Satureja cuneifolia Ten.	Mt Biokovo (Croatia)	Carvacrol (17.7%), spathulenol(13.2%), caryophyllene oxide (9.5%), α-cadinol (7.1%), amorpha-4,9-dien-2-ol (6.7%)	Antioxidant	[34]
Thymus praecox Opiz ssp. *polytrichus*	Mt Pasjača (Serbia)	trans-nerolidol (24.2%), germacrene-D (16.0%), thymol (9.6%)	Antimicrobial, antioxidant	[38, 40]
Thymus longicaulis C. Presl	Jasenice (Croatia)	Thymol (46.3%), γ-terpinene (16.2%), thymyl methyl ether (11.4%) and p-cymene (9.4%)	Antimicrobial	[41]

Table 1. Main components and biological activity of essential oils from wild growing plants from Western Balkans—Lamiaceae family.

(**Table 1**). The extract from waste water after hydrodistillation of these plant species was rich in thymoquinone (38.7%) and (E)-coniferyl alcohol (18.1%), respectively [34]. *Micromeria dalmatica* Benth. is an endemic species of Balkan Peninsula. In essential oil of *M. dalmatica*, the dominant compounds were piperitenone, pulegone and piperitenone oxide (**Table 1**). This oil possess high antimicrobial efficacy against food spoilage microorganisms, and significant activity of this oil in pork meat against *Salmonella typhimurium* enhances the possibility to use it in food preservation. Also, the essential oil of *S. horvatii* and oregano has been shown to be more or less effective against spoilage microbiota in meat products [35].

Collection of *Sideritis raeseri* Boiss & Heldr. subsp. *raeseri* has a long tradition in local communities in the Ohrid-Prespa region. Recently, identified 17 compounds could be classified into flavonoid glycosides or hydroxycynnamic acid derivatives [36]. They found that hypolaetin derivatives, known for their anti-inflammatory activity, were more abundant in *S. raeseri* subsp. *raeseri* grown in National Park Galičica (Macedonia) in comparison with *S. scardica* Griseb grown near Galičica.

Since ancient times, plants from the genus *Thymus* L. are known according to their therapeutic benefit. Recently, scientists discovered its new medicinal properties. They reported their chemical composition, biological activities and occurrence of *Thymus* species from Balkans [37]. Essential oil of wild growing *T. praecox* Opiz showed high radical scavenging and antimicrobial activities (**Table 1**). The major component, which is identified in supercritical extracts, was thymol, with the strongest antimicrobial activity. Hexane/ethanol extract possessed strongest antibacterial potential, while supercritical extracts were more efficient antifungal agents. In 1,1-diphenyl-2-picrylhydrazyl (DPPH), radical scavenging assay hexane/ethanol extract of *T. praecox* showed the best antioxidant activity, which is connected with the high level of phenolics antioxidants [38].

5. Composition and biological activity of essential oils and extracts of wild growing Apiaceae species

Many plants from "spices" family, Apiaceae, are phytochemicaly characterised, and they are used in official medicine, but for much of them data are still missing or scant. *Eryngium palmatum* Vis. et Pancic is an endemic perennial herb, distributed in the central part of the Balkan Peninsula (Serbia, Bulgaria, Macedonia and Albania). Essential oil of *E. palmatum*, collected from Ozren Mountain (Serbia), was characterised by high presence of sesquicineole (21.3%), caryophyllene oxide (16.0%), spathulenol (16.0%) and sabinene (5.5%). Related species, *Eryngium serbicum* Pancic, endemic in Serbia, in essential oil of aerial parts contains germacrene D (19.7%), β-elemene (10.0%) and spathulenol (6.9%). The main compounds in both studied species consisted of sesquiterpenes [42]. In general, sesquiterpenes possess promising anti-inflammatory, antiparasitic and anticarcinogenic activities, but some of them can cause serious toxicity. The essential oils of different *Seseli* L. species show antimicrobial and antifungal activity, while extracts exhibit anti-inflammatory and antinociceptive properties. Essential oil from aerial parts in the flowering stage and rosette in the vegetative stage of *Seseli annum* L. collected on mountain Rtanj (Serbia), as dominant compounds contain sesquiterpenes β-selinene, germacrene D, caryophyllene oxide, germacrene A (0–21.4, 3.4–19.1, 1.2–18.1,0–14.6%, respectively) and in lowest percentage α-selinene, β-elemene, E-caryophyllene, α-pinene, vetiselinenol, isodaucene (0–12.4, 0–11.4, 3.2–10.3, 0.6–7.5, 0–6.3, 0–5.4%, respectively) [43]. Also, different extracts from three *Seseli* taxa (*Seseli pallasii* Besser, *S. libanotis* (L.) Koch ssp. *libanotis* and *S. libanotis* (L.) Koch ssp. *intermedium* (Rupr.) P. W. Ball, growing wild in Serbia) possessed antioxidant and antimicrobial activity [44]. Correlation from the total phenolic and flavonoid content and in vitro antioxidant and antimicrobial activity of methanol and water extracts was presented from *Tordylium maximum* L. (Ozren Mountain, Serbia) [45]. Essential oil isolated from the aerial parts and fruits of *Cachrys cristata* DC., a rare and critically endangered species in the flora of Serbia (**Table 2**), were rich in sesquiterpenes (45.7%) and oxygenated sesquiterpenes (32.9%), while fruit oil consisted of a higher percentage of sesquiterpenes (48.3%) and oxygenated sesquiterpenes (36.7%) [46]. In fruit and aerial part was found germacrene D which is known for its effect on insects and present a potential source of antibacterial and antifungal agents. It cannot be said that only germacrene D is responsible for high activity because essential oils present mixture of different components which have synergetic effect. Various extracts of traditionally used medicinal plants prepared with different extraction method and solvent of different polarity possessed valuable antimicrobial and antioxidant activity. Good activity is related to high concentration of total phenolic and total

Plant	Origin	Essential oil/Main compounds	Activity	References
Cachrys cristata DC.	Mt Rujan (Serbia)	Aerial parts: phytol (13.1%), germacrene D (12.9%), β-caryophyllene (9.7%), β-bourbonene (8.5%) Fruit: suberosin (19.7%), germacrene D (12.3%), germacrene B (10.0%)	Antimicrobial, antioxidant	[46, 50]
Echinophora sibthorpiana Guss.	Stip (Macedonia)	Aerial parts: methyl eugenol (60.4%), p-cymene (11.2%), α-phellandrene (10.2%). α-Phellandrene epoxide (6.9%)	Antimicrobial, antioxidant	[51]
Ferulago macedonica Micevski & E. Mayer	Negotino city (Macedonia)	Inflorescence: α-pinene (43.1%) and sabinene (26.7%), limonene (6.5%) Aerial part: α-pinene (22.8%), sabinene (15.5%), terpinen-4-ol (9.6%), cis-chrysanthenyl acetate (9.5%) and p-cymene (9.1%)	Antimicrobial, antioxidant	[52]
Heracleum orphanidis Boiss.	Mt Pelister (Macedonia)	n-octanol (39.6), octylhexanoate (17.6%), n-octyl acetate (14.1%).	Antimicrobial, antioxidant, antiquorum sensing	[47]
Heracleum sphondylium L.	Mt Kopaonik (Serbia)	ar-curcumene (13.4%), β-sesquiphellandrene (11.9%), caryophyllene oxide (9.2%)	Antimicrobial, antioxidant	[48]
Laserpitium latifolium L.	Mt Staraplanina (Serbia)	Sabinene (47.8%), α-pinene (24.9%), β-pinene (7.1%), terpinen-4-ol (5.4%)	Antimicrobial, antioxidant	[53]

Table 2. Main components and biological activity of essential oils from wild growing plants from Western Balkans—Apiaceae family.

flavonoid content. Recently, in the study of four *Peucedanum* L. species (*P. officinale* L., *P. longifolium* W. et K., *P. aegopodioides* (Boiss.) Vandas and *P. alsaticum* L. from Serbia), their various extracts were found significant correlation coefficient between radical scavenging DPPH and 2,2-azino-bis(3-ethylbenz-thiazoline-6-sulfonic acid) (ABTS) radical scavenging activities with the total phenolic content/total flavonoids content. Therefore, total phenolic components can be used as an indicator in assessing the antioxidant activity of fruits and vegetables, including *Peucedanum* species [47]. Many *Heracleum* L. species are edible, and medicinal plants *Heracleum sphondylium* L. are used as food or food additive in many countries. Essential oil and extracts of these plants were presented in **Table 2**. Aerial parts of *H. sphondylium* showed antioxidant and antimicrobial effects [48]. Essential oil of *Heracleum orphanidis* Boiss consisted mainly of fatty acid derivate (80.8%) was effective antimicrobial agent (**Table 2**). The methanol extracts from aerial parts and roots of *H. orphanidis* were characterised by furanocoumarins, but stronger antioxidant potential was detected by extracts from aerial parts. *H. orphanidis* showed considerable biological potential considering free radical and various pathogenic strains, including wild type of *Pseudomonas aeruginosa*. One of a new strategy for the treatment of bacterial infections is inhibition of bacterial quorum sensing activity. The higher plants represent native source rich in anti-quorum compounds as novel virulence inhibitors [49].

6. Composition and biological activity of essential oils and extracts of wild growing Asteraceae species

Considering chemical composition of *Artemisia absinthium* L. essential oil, different chemotypes have been established in Croatia β-thujone/(Z)-epoxy ocimene chemotype, while in samples of *A. absinthium* from Serbia, pure β-thujone chemotype and β-thujone/cis-epoxy ocimen chemotype and sabinene/α-phellandrene/sabinyl acetate chemotype were found. In previous study were analysed chemical composition and biological activity of the essential oil of *A. absinthium* (**Table 3**) [54]. This oil showed high antimicrobial and significant antioxidant activity. Undiluted *A. absinthium* essential oil shown negative skin irritant reaction on all 30 tested volunteers.Essential oil in oral application did not cause mortality in the treated mice. Negative effects were neurological, muscle and gastrointestinal problems. In examinations with *Drosophila melanogaster*, the result showed that the essential oil was toxic for insect larvae in development.

The chemical analysis of essential oils of *Tanacetum parthenium* (L.) Sch. Bip., *Achillea grandifolia* Friv. and *Achillea crithmifolia* Waldst. & Kit. (collected on the territory of Southeast Serbia) was contained the monoterpenes. The major class of components showed camphor in *T. parthenium*, *A. grandifolia* and *A. crithmifolia* and 1,8—cineole in *A. grandifolia* and *A. crithmifolia* (**Table 3**). The antiradical and antioxidant activities were determined using ABTS and DPPH radical scavenging methods. The essential oil of *A. grandifolia* showed the highest antioxidant activity. The antimicrobial activity was tested against 16 multi-resistant pathogenic bacteria isolated from human source material. The essential oils of plant species used in the present study can be considered as potential source of antimicrobial substances and may contribute to solution of bacterial multiresistance [53].

Pant	Origin	Essential oil/Main compounds	Activity	References
Artemisia absinthium L.	Near the city of Niš (Srbia)	Sabinene (24.5%), sabinyl acetate (13.6%), α-phellandrene (10.3%)	Antimicrobial, antioxidant, insect repellent	[54]
Tanacetum parthenium (L.) Sch.Bip.	Mt Staraplanina (Serbia)	Camphor (51.4%), camphene (7.3%)	Antimicrobial, antioxidant	[53]
Achillea grandifolia Friv.	Jerma Gorge (Serbia)	Camphor (45.4%), 1,8-cineole (16.4%), α-thujone (15.1%), borneol (8.1%)	Antimicrobial, antioxidant	[53]
Achilea crithmifolia Waldst. & Kit.	Mt Staraplanina (Serbia)	Artemisia ketone (31.7%), camphor (25.4%), 1,8-cineole (14.8%)	Antimicrobial, antioxidant	[53]
Helichrysum italicum (Roth) G. Don	Bar (Montenegro)	γ-curcumene (22.5%), α-pinene (15.9%) and neryl acetate (7.8%), β-selinene (6.9%)	Antifungal	[55]

Table 3. Main components and biological activity of essential oils from wild growing plants from Western Balkans—Asteraceae family.

7. Composition and biological activity of essential oils and extracts of wild growing Rosaceae species

Investigation was carried out on air-dried flowers, leaves, stem-bark and wood of *Prunus mahaleb* L. (wild growing trees near Sinj, sout Croatia). The main component that was isolated from bark volatiles is coumarin with 34.1%, while in the wood is hexadecanoic acid with 46.0%. In the wood, eicosane was also detected with 12.9%. Hexadecanoic acid was isolated in the leaves and bark (17.8 and 9.3%, respectively). As the main compound in the flowers are isolated n-alkanes, heneicosane with 22.1% and octacosane with 13.0%. Phytol was isolated in the leaves with 5.1%. In addition to the main components, three fatty acids—dodecanoic, tetradecanoic and linoleic acids—were presented in all samples [56].

Geum rhodopeum Stoj. & Stef. is representative of the East Moesian endemic taxa of the Balkans floristic subregion. Aerial parts of *G. rhodopeum* were collected at Prestojceva mahala (Cemernik Mountain, Serbia). The major component of aerial parts from this essential oil was α-bisabolol with 12.7% constituting of the oil. It is documented that α-bisabolol may be a useful therapeutic candidate for the treatment of skin inflammation. Significant compounds were also myrtenal (9.5%), 1-isopropyl-4,8-dimethylspiro[4.5]dec-8-en-7-one (7.7%), palmitic acid (6.4%), myrtanal (5.8%) and 1-octen-3-ol (5.3%) [57]. The major component of aerial part from *G. coccineum* Sibth. et Sm. essential oil (collected from natural populations of Jablanica Mountain, Macedonia) was phytol constituting 24.3% of the oil [58]. According to the literature data, dewberry (*Rubus caesius* var. *aquáticus* Weihe. & Nees.) leaves have been used in traditional medicine due to their anti-inflammatory, antiviral and antimicrobial, antiproliferative activity against cancer cells and antitumor and wound-healing properties. Leaf methanol, ethanol, acetone and water extracts from dewberry collected near city of Zaječar (Serbia) were examined for its antioxidant activity using DPPH, ABTS, ferric reducing power (FRAP) assay, total reducing power (TRP) methods. Acetone extract was with the highest antioxidant activity against DPPH and ABTS•+ radicals as well as for total reducing capacity. Obtained results showed that phenolic compounds are major contributors to the antioxidant properties of *R. caesius* var. *aquaticus*) leaves [59].

8. Conclusion

According to numerous references, many aromatic plants from Western Balkans represented valuable sources of potential new bioactive compounds. Considerable efforts were made for investigation of essential oils and extracts and discovering new, natural antimicrobials, antioxidants or cytotoxic agents. The results encourage the application of the plants for further evaluations of other possible bioactivities and detection of active pure compounds as constituents of the essential oils and extracts. Studies to date have identified a number of plant compounds and explained its mechanism of action in organisms. All presented data additionally validate the use of well-known aromatic plants in new treatments, as well as endemic or rare plants which could be only scientifically investigated. High protection of their natural localities is necessary, and new potential active compounds from those plants could be used only with their possible cultivation. The beneficial effect of the aromatic plants from Western Balkans that are recognised in traditional knowledge could be useful for conventional medicine or other aspects for improving life quality.

Acknowledgements

The authors are grateful to the Ministry of Education, Science and Technological Development of the Republic of Serbia for financial support (Grant No. 173029).

Author details

Ana M. Džamić[1]* and Jelena S. Matejić[2]

*Address all correspondence to: simicana@bio.bg.ac.rs

1 Faculty of Biology, Institute of Botany and Botanical Garden "Jevremovac", University of Belgrade, Belgrade, Serbia

2 Faculty of Medicine, University of Niš, Niš, Serbia

References

[1] Thirumagal A, Sivasubramanian S. Bibliometric analysis medicinal and aromatic plants research. Library Philosophy and Practice. Academic OneFile; 2014. http://digitalcommons.unl.edu/libphilprac/1129

[2] World Health Organization (WHO). General guidelines for methodologies on research and evaluation of traditional medicine. World Health Organization: Geneva; 2000. 1 p. (document reference WHO/EDM/TRM/2000.1)

[3] Cunningham AB. Applied ethnobotany: people, wild plant use and conservation. Earthscan: London; 2001.

[4] Redzić S. The ecological aspect of ethnobotany and ethnopharmacology of population in Bosnia and Herzegovina. Collegium Antropologicum. 2007;**31**:869–890.

[5] Miler D. Natural medicine. 1st ed. Metaphysica: Belgrade; 2009.

[6] Stevens PF. (2001 onwards). Angiosperm Phylogeny Website [Internet]. 2012. Available from: http://www.mobot.org/MOBOT/research/APweb/. [Accessed: 2016-15-09]

[7] Cox PA, Balick MJ. The ethnobotanical approach to drug discovery. Scientific American. 1994;**270**(6):82–87.

[8] Turrill WB. The plant-life of the Balkan Peninsula. Oxford: Leipzig; 1929.

[9] Sarić M. The medicinal plants of the Federal Republic of Serbia. SAAS: Belgrade; 1989.

[10] Sarić-Kundalić B, Dobes C, Klatte-Asselmeyer V, Saukel J. Ethnobotanical study on medicinal use of wild and cultivated plants in middle, south and west Bosnia and Herzegovina. Journal of Ethnopharmacology. 2010;**131**:33–55. doi:10.1016/j.jep.2010.05.061

[11] Nikolić T. Sistematska botanika: Raznolikost i evolucija biljnog svijeta. [Systematic botany: Diversity and evolution of plant life]. 1th ed. Alfa d.d: Zagreb; 2013. 20 p.

[12] Rohlena J. Conspectus Florae Montenegrinae. Preslia; 1942. 20p.

[13] Stešević D, Petrović D, Bubanja N, Vuksanović S, Biberdžić V. Contribution to the flora of Montenegro (Supplementum to the material for Vascular flora of Montenegro). Natura Montenegrina. 2008;**7**(3):463–480.

[14] Niketić M, Tomović G, Melovski L, Stevanović V, Matevski V. New species for the vascular flora of Republic of Macedonia and their distribution in the Balkan Peninsula. Botanica Serbica. 2014;**38**(1):57–67.

[15] Barata AM, Rocha F, Lopes V, Bettencourt E, Figueiredo AC. Medicinal and Aromatic Plants—Portugal. Eolss Publishers: Oxford; 2014. doi:10.13140/2.1.1456.0326

[16] Łuczaj Ł, Fressel N, Perković S. Wild food plants used in the villages of the Lake Vrana Nature Park (northern Dalmatia, Croatia). Acta Societatis Botanicorum Poloniae. 2013;**82**(4):275–281. doi:10.5586/asbp.2013.036

[17] Jarić S, Mačukanović-Jocić M, Djurdjević L, Mitrović M, Kostić O, Karadžić B, Pavlović P. An ethnobotanical survey of traditionally used plants on Suva planina mountain (south-eastern Serbia). Journal of Ethnopharmacology. 2015;**175**:93–108. doi:10.1016/j.jep.2015.09.002

[18] Jarić S, Popović Z, Mačukanović-Jocić M, Djurdjević L, Mijatović M, Karadžić B, Mitrović M, Pavlović P. An ethnobotanical study on the usage of wild medicinal herbs from Kopaonik Mountain (Central Serbia). Journal of Ethnopharmacology. 2007;**111**:160–175. doi:10.1016/j.jep.2006.11.007

[19] European Pharmacopoeia 7.0. European directorate for the quality of medicines and healthcare. Council of Europe EDQM: Strasbourg, France; 2011.

[20] Šavikin K, Zdunić G, Menković N, Živković J, Ćujić N, Tereščenko M, Bigović D. Ethnobotanical study on traditional use of medicinal plants in South-Western Serbia, Zlatibor district. Journal of Ethnopharmacology. 2013;**146**:803–810. doi:10.1016/j.jep.2013.02.006

[21] Menković N, Šavikin K, Tasić S, Zdunić G, Stešević D, Milosavljević S, Vincek, D. Ethnobotanical study on traditional uses of wild medicinal plants in Prokletije Mountains (Montenegro). Journal of Ethnopharmacology. 2011;**133**(1):97–107. doi:10.1016/j.jep.2010.09.008

[22] Pieroni A. Local plant resources in the ethnobotany of Theth, a village in the Northern Albanian Alps. Genetic Resources and Crop Evolution. 2008;**55**:1197–1214. doi:10.1007/s10722-008-9320-3

[23] Pieroni A, Giusti MA, Quave CL. Cross-cultural ethnobiology in the Western Balkans: medical ethnobotany and ethnozoology among Albanians and Serbs in the Pešter Plateau, Sandžak, South-Western Serbia. Human Ecology: An Interdisciplinary Journal. 2011:**39**(3):333–349. doi:10.1007/s10745-011-9401-3

[24] Rexhepi B, Mustafa B, Hajdari A, Rushidi-Rexhepi J, Quave CL, Pieroni A. Traditional medicinal plant knowledge among Albanians, Macedonians and Gorani in the Sharr Mountains (Republic of Macedonia). Genetic Resources and Crop Evolution. 2013;**60**:2055–2080. doi:10.1007/s10722-013-9974-3

[25] Gursky Z. Zlatna knjiga ljekovitog bilja. Nakladni zavod matice Hrvatske: Zagreb; 1978.

[26] Pieroni A, Giusti ME. The remedies of the folk medicine of the Croatians living in Ćićarija, northern Istria. Collegium Antropologicum. 2008;**32**:623–627.

[27] Stupar M, Ljaljević-Grbić M, Džamić A, Unković N, Ristić M, Jelikić A, Vukojević J. Antifungal activity of selected essential oils and biocide benzalkonium chloride against the fungi isolated from cultural heritage object. South African Journal of Botany. 2014;**93**:118–124. doi:10.1016/j.sajb.2014.03.016

[28] Coccimiglio J, Alipour M, Jiang Z-H, Gottardo C, Suntres Z. Antioxidant, antibacterial, and cytotoxic activities of the ethanolic *Origanum vulgare* extract and its major constituents. Oxidative Medicine and Cellular Longevity. 2016;**2016**:1–8. doi:10.1155/2016/1404505

[29] Džamić AM, Soković MD, Novaković M, Jadranin M, Ristić MS, Tešević V, Marin PD. Composition, antifungal and antioxidant properties of *Hyssopus officinalis* L. subsp. *pilifer* (Pant.) Murb.essential oil and deodorized extracts. Industrial Crops and Products. 2013;**51**:401–407. doi:10.1016/j.indcrop.2013.09.038

[30] Rozman V, Kalinovic I, Liška A. Bioactivity of 1,8-cineole, camphor and carvacrol against rusty grain beetle (*Cryptolestes ferrugineus* Steph.) on stored wheat. Proceedings of the 9th International Working Conference on Stored Product Protection; 15–18 October 2006; Campinas, São Paulo, Brazil. Brazilian Post-harvest Association—ABRAPOS, Passo Fundo, RS, Brazil, 2006. pp. 688–694.

[31] Grujic-Jovanovic S, Dzamic A, Ristic MS, Marin PD. Essential oil composition of *Stachys anisochila*. Chemistry of Natural Compounds. 2011;**47**(5):823–825. doi:10.1007/s10600-011-0074-3

[32] Bukvički D, Stojković D, Soković M, Vannini L, Montanari C, Pejin B, Savić A, Veljić M, Grujić S, Marin PD. *Satureja horvatii* essential oil: in vitro antimicrobial and antiradical properties and in situ control of *Listeria monocytogenes* in pork meat. Meat Science.2014;**96**(3):1355–1360. doi:10.1016/j.meatsci.2013.11.024

[33] Kundaković T, Stanojković T, Kolundzija B, Marković S, Sukilović B, Milenković M, Lakušić B. Cytotoxicity and antimicrobial activity of the essential oil from *Satureja montana* subsp. *pisidica* (Lamiceae). Natural Product Communications. 2014;**9**(4):569–572.

[34] Ćavar S, Šolić EM, Maksimović M. Chemical composition and antioxidant activity of two *Satureja* species from Mt. Biokovo. Botanica Serbica. 2013;**37**(2):159–165.

[35] Bukvicki D, Stojkovic D, Sokovic M, Nikolic M, Vannini L, Montanari C, Marin PD. Potential application of *Micromeria dalmatica* essential oil as a protective agent in a food system. LWT-Food Science and Technology. 2015;**63**:262–267. doi:10.1016/J.LWT.2015.03.053

[36] Menković N, Gođevac D, Šavikin K, Zdunić G, Milosavljević S, Bojadži A, Avramoski O. Bioactive compounds of endemic species *Sideritis raeseri* subsp. *raeseri* grown in National Park Galičica. Records of Natural Products. 2013;**7**(3):161–168.

[37] Zeljković ČS, Maksimović M. Chemical composition and bioactivity of essential oil from *Thymus* species in Balkan Peninsula. Phytochemical Review. 2015;**14**:335–352. doi:10.1007/s11101-014-9378-9

[38] Petrović NV, Petrović SS, Ristić MS, Džamić AM, Ćirić AD. Chemical composition and antimicrobial activity of *Thymus praecox* Opiz ssp. *plytrychus* essential oil from Serbia. Records of Natural Products. 2016;**10**(5):633–638.

[39] Capetanos C, Saroglou V, Marin P, Simić A, Skaltsa H. Essential oil analyses of two endemic *Eryngium* species from Serbia. Journal of Serbian Chemical Society. 2007;**72**:961–965. doi:10.2298/JSC0710961C

[40] Kovacevic NN, Marcetic MD, Lakusic DV, Lakusic BS. Composition of the essential oils of different parts of *Seseli annuum* L. (Apiaceae). Journal of Essential Oil Bearing Plants. 2016;**19**(3):671–677. doi:10.1080/0972060X.2014.901604

[41] Matejić J, Džamić A, Mihajilov-Krstev T, Ranđelović V, Krivošej Z, Marin PD. Total phenolic content, flavonoid concentration, antioxidant and antimicrobial activity of methanol extracts from three *Seseli* L. taxa. Central European Journal of Biology. 2012;**7**(6):1116–1122. doi:10.2478/s11535-012-0094-4

[42] Matejić J, Džamić A, Mihajilov-Krstev T, Ranđelović V, Krivošej Z, Marin PD. Total phenolic and flavonoid content, antioxidant and antimicrobial activity of extracts from *Tordylium maximum*. Journal of Applied Pharmaceutical Science. 2013;**3**(1):055–059. doi:10.7324/JAPS.2013.30110

[43] Matejić J, Džamić A, Ristić M, Ranđelović V, Marin P. Essential oil composition of *Cachrys cristata*—a rare and endangered species in the flora of Serbia. Natural Products Communications. 2012;**7**:1–2.

[44] Matejić J, Džamić A, Ćirić A, Ranđelović V, Krivošej Z, Marin P. Antioxidant and antimicrobial activities of extracts of four *Peucedanum* L. species. Digest Journal of Nanomaterials and Biostructures. 2013;**8**(2):655–665.

[45] Matejic JS, Dzamic AM, Mihajilov-Krstev T, Ristic MS, Randjelovic VN, Krivošej ZĐ, Marin PD. Chemical composition, antioxidant and antimicrobial properties of essential oil and extracts from *Heracleum sphondylium* L. Journal of Essential Oil Bearing Plants. 2016;**19**(4):944–953. doi:10.1080/0972060X.2014.986538

[46] Mileski KS, Ćirić AD, Trifunović SS, Ristić MS, Soković MD, Matevski VS, Tešević VV, Jadranin MB, Marin PD, Džamić AM. *Heracleum orphanidis*: chemical characterisation, and comparative evaluation of antioxidant and antimicrobial activities with specific interest in the influence on *Pseudomonas aeruginosa* PAO1. Food and Function. 2016;**7**:4061–4074. doi:10.1039/c6fo01018k

[47] Mihajilov-Krstev TM, Jovanović B, Jović JL, Ilić BS, Miladinović DL, Matejić JS, Rajković JS, Djordjević L, Cvetković VJ, Zlatković BK. Antimicrobial, antioxidative, and insect repellent effects of *Artemisia absinthium* essential oil. Planta Medica. 2014;**80**(18):1698–1705. doi:10.1055/s-0034-1383182

[48] Stanković N, Mihajilov-Krstev T, Zlatković B, Matejić J, StankovJovanović V, Kocić B, Čomić L. Comparative study of composition and antioxidant and antimicrobial activities of essential oils of selected aromatic plants from Balkan Peninsula. PlantaMedica. 2016;**82**(7):650–661. doi:10.1055/s-0042-101942

[49] Mastelić J, Jerković I, Mesić M. Volatile constituents from flowers, leaves, bark and wood of *Prunus mahaleb* L. Flavour and Fragrance Journal. 2006;**21**:306–313.doi:10.1002/ffj.1596

[50] Miladinovic DL, Ilic BS, Matejic JS, Randjelovic VN, Nikolic DM, Mihajilov-Krstev TM, Mladenovic IO. Chemical composition of the essential oil of *Geum rhodopeum*. Chemistry of Natural Compounds. 2014;**50**(5): 926–928. doi:10.1007/s10600-014-1120-8

[51] Miladinovic DL, Ilic BS, Matejic JS, Randjelovic VN, Nikolic DM. Chemical composition of the essential oil of *Geum coccineum*. Chemistry of Natural Compounds. 2015;**51**(4): 785–786. doi:10.1007/s10600-015-1412-7

[52] Veličković I, Grujić S, Džamić A, Krivošej Z, Marin PD. *In vitro* antioxidant activity of dewberry (*Rubus caesius* L. var. *aquáticus*Weihe. and Nees.) leaf extracts. Archives of Biological Sciences. 2015;**67**(4):1323–1330. doi:10.2298/ABS150414109V

[53] Matejić JS, Džamić AM, Mihajilov-Krstev TM, Ranđelović VN, Mileski KS, Marin PD. Total phenolic and flavonoid contents and biological activities of *Cachrys cristata* Dc. extracts. Archives of Biological Science. 2014;**66**(3):1117–1123. doi:10.2298/ABS1403117M

[54] Mileski K, Džamić A, Ćirić A, Grujić S, Ristić M, Matevski V, Marin PD. Radical scavenging and antimicrobial activity of essential oil and extracts of *Echinophora sibthorpiana* Guss. from Macedonia. Archives of Biological Sciences. 2014;**66**(1):401–413. doi:10.2298/ABS1401401M

[55] Mileski K, Džamić A, Ćirić A, Ristić M, Grujić S, Matevski V, Marin PD. Composition, antimicrobial and antioxidant properties of endemic species *Ferulago macedonica* Micevski and E. Mayer. Records of Natural Products. 2015;**9**(2):208–223.

[56] Mihajilov-Krstev T, Radnović D, Kitić D, Stankov-Jovanović V, Mitić V, Stojanović-Radić Z, Zlatković B. Chemical composition, antimicrobial, antioxidative and anticholinesterase activity of *Satureja montana* L. ssp *montana* essential oil. Central European Journal of Biology. 2014;**9**(7):668–677. doi:10.2478/s11535-014-0298-x

[57] Petrović NV, Petrović SS, Džamić AM, Ćirić AD, Ristić MS, Milovanović SL, Petrović SD. Chemical composition, antioxidant and antimicrobial activity of *Thymus praecox* supercritical extracts. Journal of Supercritical Fluids. 2016;**110**:117–125. doi:10.1016/j.supflu.2016.01.001

[58] Vladimir-Knežević S, Kosalec I, Babac M, Petrović M, Ralić J, Matica B, Blažeković B. Antimicrobial activity of *Thymus longicaulis* C. Presl essential oil against respiratory pathogens. Central European Journal of Biology. 2012;**7**(6):1109–1115. doi:10.2478/s11535-012-0088-2

[59] Stupar M, Ljaljević-Grbić M, Džamić A, Unković N, Ristić M, Vukojević J. Antifungal activity *Helichrysum italicum* (Roth) G. Don (Asteraceae) essential oil against the fungi isolated from cultural heritage objects. Archives of Biological Sciences.2014;**66**(4):1539–1545. doi:10.2298/ABS1404539S

3

Fenugreek (*Trigonella foenum-graecum* L.): An Important Medicinal and Aromatic Crop

Peiman Zandi, Saikat Kumar Basu, William Cetzal-Ix,
Mojtaba Kordrostami,
Shahram Khademi Chalaras and
Leila Bazrkar Khatibai

Abstract

Fenugreek (*Trigonella foenum-graecum* L.) is an annual forage legume and a traditional spice and aromatic crop that has been grown for centuries across the Indian subcontinent. In addition to South Asia, the crop is also grown in some parts of North Africa, Middle East, Mediterranean Europe, China, South East (SE) Asia, Australia, the USA, Argentina and Canada. The plant has been used traditionally in Indian Ayurvedic medicines as well as in traditional Tibetan and Chinese medication for several centuries. Modern research has also demonstrated that fenugreek seed and leaves are useful in the treatment of a number of diseases including successfully reducing blood sugar and blood cholesterol levels in both animals and humans. The plant has recently attracted great interest in the pharmaceutical, nutraceutical and functional food industries due to its rich medicinal properties.

Keywords: fenugreek, *Trigonella foenum-graecum*, spice, medicinal, aromatic, legume, crop

1. Introduction

Fenugreek (*Trigonella foenum-graecum* L.) is an annual forage legume and a traditional spice crop that has been grown for centuries across the Indian subcontinent [1–3]. In addition to South Asia the crop is also grown in some parts of North Africa, Middle East, Mediterranean Europe, China, South East (SE) Asia, Australia, the USA, Argentina and Canada. India is the largest fenugreek producer in the world but due to high internal consumption do not have a major share of the global fenugreek trade [1–3]. The crop has been recommended for the dry and semiarid regions of Asia, Africa and Latin America [4]. The plant has been used traditionally in Indian Ayurvedic medicines as well as in traditional Tibetan and Chinese medication for several centuries. Modern research has also demonstrated that fenugreek seed and leaves are useful in the treatment of a number of diseases including successfully reducing blood sugar and blood cholesterol levels in both animals and human subjects in experimental trials [5]. The crop has the potential to act as a panacea in treatment of diabetic, microbial and cancer disease. The reason behind the rich medicinal properties of fenugreek is due to the presence of a wide diversity of important phytochemicals (diosgenin, trigonelline, fenugreekine, galactomannan and 4-hydroxy isoleucine [4]. Hence, the crop has huge international demand in the associated pharmaceutical, nutraceutical and functional food industries. Being known as a chemurgic crop, fenugreek has a widespread adoption in industrial sectors. Its seeds contain a reliable source of steroid diosgenin, which acts as a supplement in pharmaceutical industry [6].

Furthermore, being a forage legume and a natural nitrogen fixer, it could be easily incorporated in the local crop cycles (short-term rotation) for natural replenishment of soil, for fixation of nitrogen and for feeding the livestock as hay or silage (**Figure 1**). The crop grows well under rainfed conditions and hence cost of production is lower compared to other commercial crops suitable for semiarid regions.

Fenugreek is also well known as a global spice crop grown in all the major continents (depending on soil and climatic conditions) across the globe including parts of North Africa, Mediterranean Europe, Russia, Middle East, China, India, Pakistan, Iran, Afghanistan, parts of Far East and SE Asia, Australia, the USA, Canada and Argentina [7, 8]. India once maintained and still holds the largest fenugreek harvested area in the world [5].

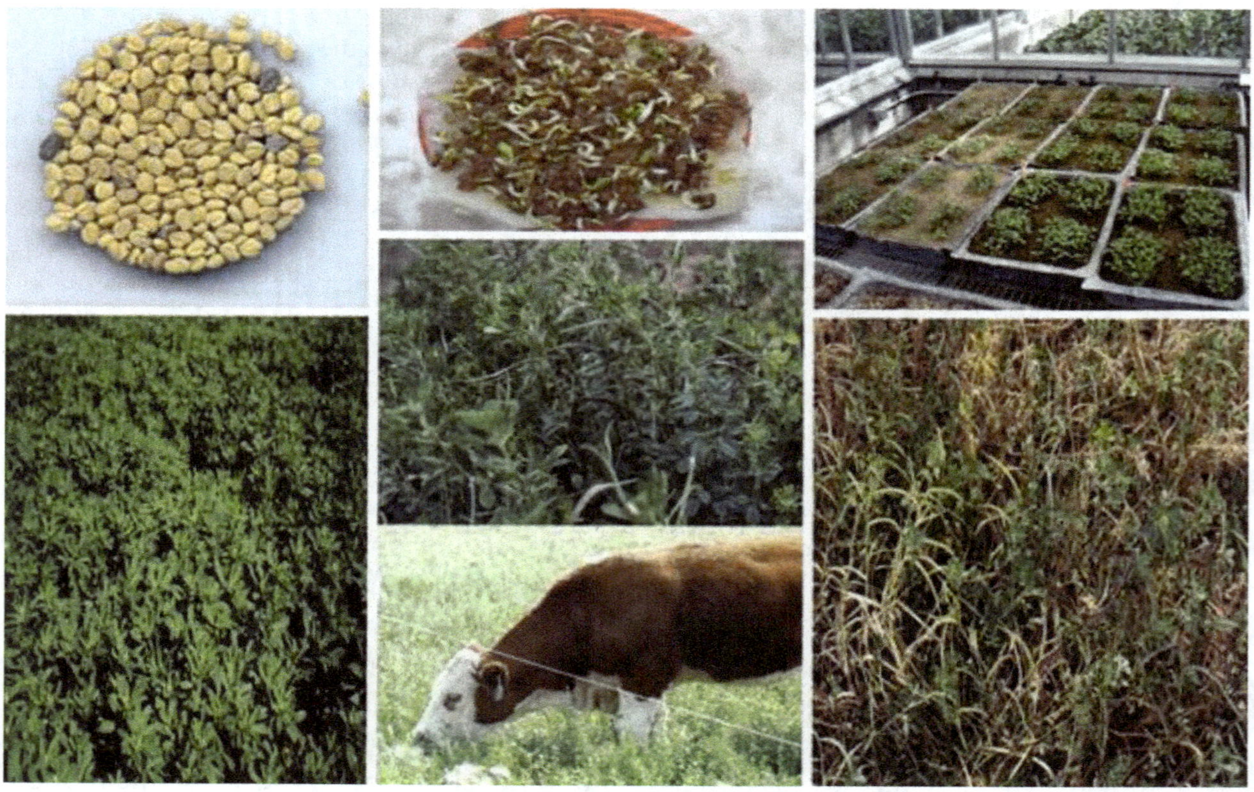

Figure 1. Fenugreek crop in different growth stages (fenugreek seed, seed germination, seedling growth, vegetative-immature and reproductive growth stages of stem formation, podding and physiological ripeness-mature (Image credit: S.K. Basu).

The crop has been recommended for agricultural production in the dry and semiarid localities of the continents of Asia, Africa and Latin America [3 4, 9, 10]. The plant has been used extensively for centuries as a traditional forage crop in several ancient civilizations across Eurasia. Fenugreek has been reported to be used as an important medicinal herb in Indian Ayurvedic medicinal practices as well in traditional Chinese medication and Tibetan medicines for the treatment of several diseases in humans and also in animals. Ancient Islamic scholars and physicians have also recorded the use of fenugreek in traditional Islamic medicinal practices in ancient texts and scriptures [9]. Modern clinical trials have also established without doubt the efficacy of this medicinal herb in the treatment of several human and animal diseases [5, 8, 11]. Relative frequencies of the major well-known accessions of fenugreek which are produced all over the world are listed out in **Table 1** [1].

Origin	**Number of reported fenugreek accessions**	***Relative* frequency (%)**	**Average forage production 1961–2013 (tone/acre) per country**
Afghanistan	27	2.48	>550,682
Algeria	2	0.18	3,835,860
Australia	7	0.64	2,868,759
Austria	1	0.09	1,539,297
Azerbaijan	1	0.09	624,045
Canada	54	4.95	>550,682
China	44	4.04	51,489,483
Egypt	16	1.47	>550,682
England	17	1.56	>550,682
Eritrea	1	0.09	>550,682
Ethiopia	152	13.94	>550,682
France	3	0.28	>550,682
Germany	4	0.37	7,445,345
Greece	6	0.55	>550,682
Hungary	3	0.28	>550,682
India	401	36.79	91,881,132
Iran	46	4.22	2,653,431
Iraq	7	0.64	230,685
Israel	3	0.28	>550,682
Italy	4	0.37	9,906,660
Jordan	5	0.46	30,439
Kenya	1	0.09	>550,682
Libya	5	0.46	573,678
Morocco	5	0.46	1,694,057
Nepal	2	0.18	>550,682

Origin	Number of reported fenugreek accessions	*Relative* frequency (%)	Average forage production 1961–2013 (tone/acre) per country
Oman	77	7.06	>550,682
Pakistan	41	3.76	13,819
Poland	2	0.18	7,142,332
Portugal	1	0.09	6,894,828
Romania	15	1.38	694,961
Russia	3	0.28	10,701,727
Slovenia	4	0.37	86,966
South Africa	1	0.09	>550,682
Spain	8	0.73	163,784
Sudan	10	0.92	1,187,407
Sweden	3	0.28	>550,682
Switzerland	2	0.18	3,218,208
Syria	15	1.38	33,113
Taiwan	1	0.09	>550,682
Tunisia	42	3.85	>550,682
Turkey	40	3.67	>550,682
Turkmenistan	1	0.09	>550,682
U.S.A.	3	0.28	>550,682
Ukraine	1	0.09	475,316
Yemen	3	0.28	92,026

Table 1. Origin, number of registered and relative frequency of fenugreek crop distributed across the given countries.

2. Medicinal properties and chemical constituents

Fenugreek leaves and seed are known to have major medicinal properties and have been reported to significantly reduce both blood glucose and cholesterol levels in human and animal subjects in clinical trials around the world [1]. Fenugreek is therefore highly sought after as a chemurgic crop in the local, regional and international pharmaceutical, nutraceutical and functional food industries and markets as a medicinal herb [12]. Fenugreek seed and leaves are a rich source of a wide diversity of medicinally rich phytochemicals like steroidal saponins (diosgenin), fenugreekine (alkaloid), galactomannan (carbohydrate), 4-hydroxy isoleucine (amino acid) among several others [4, 7, 11, 12]. More specifically, fenugreek seed itself contain carbohydrates (45–60%) as in mucilaginous fiber (galactomannans), proteins (20–30%) enriched in tryptophan and lysine, lipids (5–10%) or fixed oil, alkaloids of pyridine type (0.2–0.38%) as in trigonelline; choline (0.5%), and other materials including carpaine and gentianine, flavonoids (apigenin, luteolin, orientin, quercetin, vitexin and isovitexin) and 4-hydroxyisoleucine (0.09%), lysine and histidine, arginine, calcium and iron, saponins

(0.6–1.7%), glycosides such as, yamogenin, tigogenin, neotigogenin and diosgenin (generating steroidal sapogenins on hydrolysis); and sitosterol and cholesterol, vitamins (A, B1, C) and nicotinic acid; n-alkanes and sesquiterpenes (0.015%) known as volatile oils [6]. Fenugreek has been also reported to be rich in antioxidant [13] and antimicrobial properties [14].

3. Agronomy

Agronomic production of fenugreek crop has been well studied and reported in arid and semiarid regions of the world and has been well documented in primary literature [15–17]. Climatic and edaphic environmental (external condition) factors as well as genetic makeup (internal condition) are greatly accounted for metabolic processes in fenugreek crop [18]. It is also believed that the regulation of yield potential in fenugreek is feasible through either breeding programs or modification of cultural treatments [18, 19]. Fenugreek crop growth has been found to be significantly increased by the application of phosphate fertilizer [20]. The plant has indeterminate growth habit and hence mutant population generated through physical and chemical mutating agents have been reported to be successful in generating plants with determinate and fast growing habits [11, 21]. The crop has been found to be attacked by several biological agents like insects, fungi, bacteria and non-biological diseases like micronutrient deficiency, flooding, salinity, stagnant water [22–24].

4. Species, names, origin and distribution

There are noticeable discrepancies in the range of reported species of fenugreek (around 70–97) in the literature [25–29]; however, older taxonomies like Linnaeus have explicitly accentuated on the existence of 260 species [1]. Across the mentioned species of fenugreek, the following are mostly celebrated as for their medicinal and pharmaceutical properties [1]: *T. foenum-graecum, T. balansae, T. corniculata, T. maritima, T. spicata, T. occulta, T. polycerata, T. calliceras, T. cretica, T. caerulea, T. lilacina, T. radiata, T. spinosa*. Among which *T. foenum-graecum* is widely cultivated throughout the world [30]. The genus name, *Trigonella* meaning 'little triangle' resemble the triangular shape of its small yellowish-white flowers. The species name *foenum-graecum* meaning 'Greek hay' in reference to its initial introgression from Greece [1]. To date different indigenous names have been ascribing to the plant depending on the nations, local language and culture on which the crop is grown and/or consumed. For instance, fenugreek in Arabic is called Hulba; in Persian called Shanbalilae; in Greek called Tili, Tipilina, Trigoniskos, Tintelis, Tsimeni and Moschositaro; in Uzbekistani called Boidana, Ul'ba and Khul'ba; in Armenian called Shambala; in Chinese called K'u-Tou; in Ethiopian called Abish; in Japanese called Koroba; in England called fenugreek or Fenigrec; in Pakistani and Indian called Methi; in Italian called Fieno Greco; in Russian called Pazhitnik; and in French called Senegre [30, 31].

Fenugreek is an ancient and multipurpose crop in various geographical latitudes. Species of fenugreek have been identified in the five continents of Asia, Africa, Europa and Australia; being cultivated mostly in North America, West and South Asia, Australia, Russia, Meddle East, North West of Africa. Potential areas for fenugreek production are parts of South East Asia, Japan, Central Asia (Mongolia), wide parts of Africa and South America (**Figure 2**).

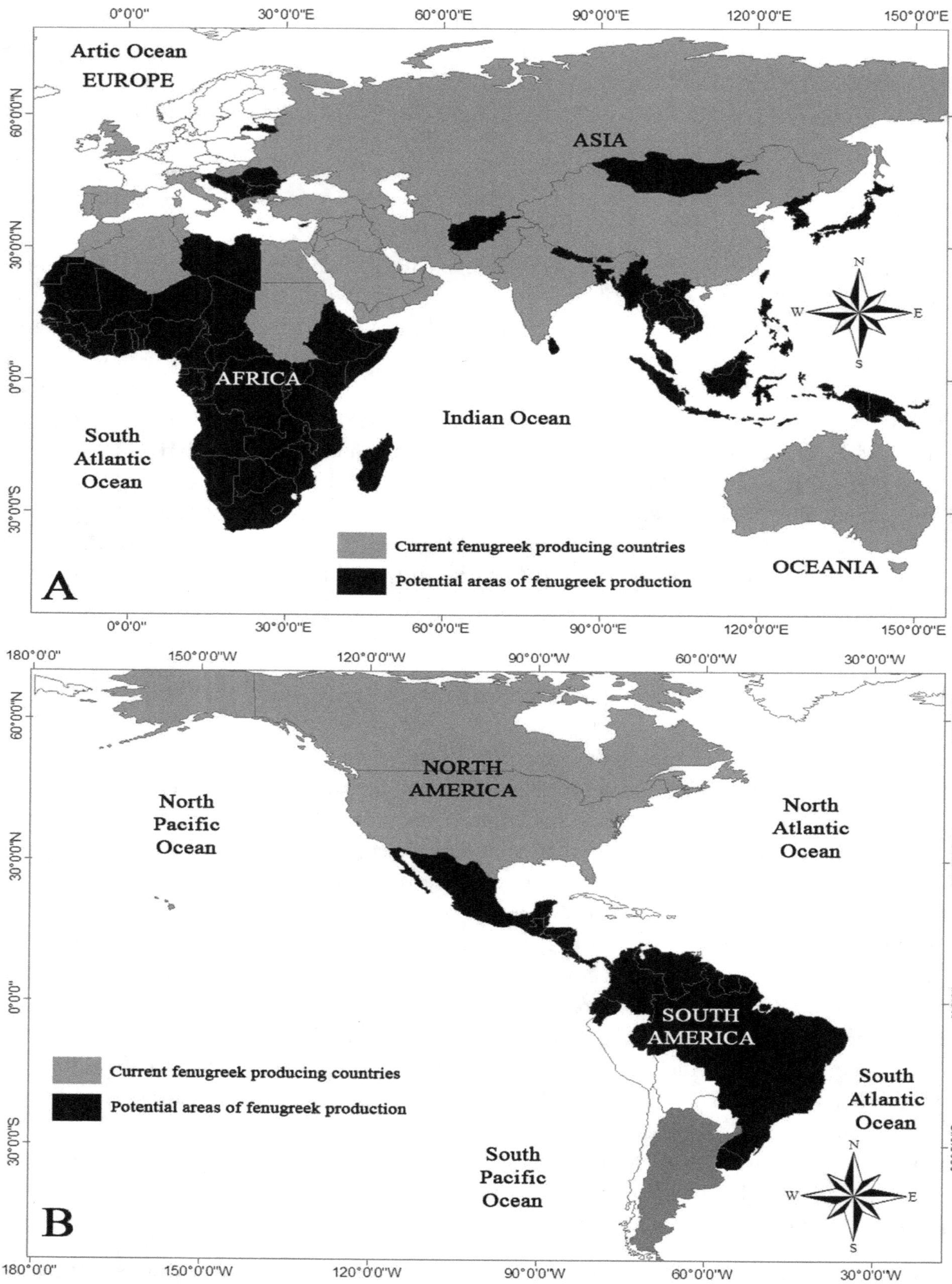

Figure 2. Illustrative map of word (A, B) showing currently grown and potential areas of fenugreek production.

There are widespread uncertainties regarding the probable ancestry of *T. foenum-graecum* which are still unsolved. Though Vavilov [32] introduced the herb as a native species to the Mediterranean region, on a contradictory statement De Candolle [33] and Fazli and Hardman [34] suggested an Asian root for it. They also declared that fenugreek wildly grows in deserts of Mesopotamia, prolific plains of Persia, in Punjab and Kashmir of Pakistan, in middle Asia, and in southern Europe like Greece, Italy and Spain that take advantage of abundant sunshine. As described earlier by De Candolle [33], it is not a reasonable belief to consider southern Europe as the main origin of fenugreek because if this was the case the plant should be far more common not be remaining inconspicuous in this region.

Many experts unanimously agree that the direct wild ancestor of fenugreek is *T. gladiata* Ste. that differs widely from *T. foenum–graecum* in view of the assemblage of attributes like smaller pod size and abnormal seed tuberculation [35]. So it is likely acceptable to believe that the species T. *foenum graecum* was naturally evolved from *T. gladiata* as it had possibly contributed to prevent the extinction of *T. foenum-graecum* [30].

5. Chromosome number

There are many species in the *Trigonella* genus, many of which are diploid. Based on the Darlington and Wylie [36] reports, haploid chromosome numbers of most species in the *Trigonella* genus is 8, 9, 11 or 14 and diploid chromosome number is $2n = 16$. For example, *T. foenum-graecum, T. balansae, T. corniculata, T. sprunerana* Boiss., *T. monspeliaca* L., *T. uncata, T. anguina, T. stellata, T. astroites, T. gladiata, T. cariensis, T. berythea, T. macrorrhyncha, T. cassia, T. foenum-graecum* and *T. homosa* have $2n = 16$ chromosomes [36–41]. However, there are some exceptions. For instance, *T. geminiflora* from Iran and Asia Minor, *T. grandiflora* from Turkey and *T. hamosa* from Egypt have 44 chromosomes; *T. polycerata* from the Mediterranean and Asia have 28, 30 and 32 chromosomes, and *T. ornithopodioides* from Europe was reported to have 18 chromosomes within its genome [30]. While most species in the *Trigonella* genus have $2n = 16$ chromosomes, the results of some studies show that some of species have undergone several rounds of chromosome duplication and have different diploid number of chromosomes. Singh and Singh [42] found some trisomics along with five double trisomics in an auto-tetraploid population which had 18 ($2n + 1 + 1$) chromosomes. They believed that among 13 species of *Trigonella*, only *T. neoana*, have $2n = 30$ chromosomes. Marc and Capraru [43] studied cytogenetic effects of sodium phosphate on meristematic cells of fenugreek root tips and found that it has a negative effect on the mitotic index. Roy and Singh [44] produced tetraploid fenugreek by treating shoot apices with colchicine and Basu [1] also reported that he had produced tetraploid fenugreek ($2n + 2n = 32$) by treating seeds with colchicine.

There are few studies about the variation in chromosome number in fenugreek. For instance, Raghuvanshi and Joshi [45] and Joshi and Raghuvanshi [46] reported that there is an extra B chromosome in some of the fenugreek genotypes. As far as we know, the presence of this type of chromosome can affect plant growth and development [30]. In some researches, it is observed that same species show different behaviors in terms of having B chromosome. For example, some *T. corniculata* species do not contain B chromosome, while the other species have this chromosome. For instance, Singh [47] and Singh and Singh [42] examined *T. corniculata* in some regions of India and did not observe B chromosomes in it, while Lakshmi et al. [48] reported that *T. corniculata* contained two types of pollen mother cells: one with $2n = 16$ and the other with $2n = 16+$ B chromosomes.

6. Molecular genetic diversity

Knowledge of genetic diversity among plants can help to provide beneficial information in the selection of breeding materials for hybridization programs and mapping quantitative trait loci [49]. Review of literatures show that using DNA markers for investigating the genetic diversity of fenugreek does not have a long history in the world. Dangi et al. [50] studied the genetic diversity of two different species of fenugreek (*T. caerulea* and *T. foenum-graecum*) using Random Amplification of Polymorphic DNA' (RAPD) and Inter Simple -Sequence Repeats (ISSR) markers and showed that the genetic diversity in *T. caerulea* was much more than the other species. They also recommended the using of these two methods for grouping the genotypes and determine the genetic relationship among them.

Sundaram and Purwar [51] evaluated genetic diversity and species relation among two taxonomically *Trigonella* species and 61 accession using 18 RAPD primers. These primers made a total of 141 bands of which 74 were polymorphic. Genetic similarity of the genotypes ranged between 0.66 and 0.90, indicating a moderate to high genetic diversity among the populations. The dendrogram obtained from RAPD primers revealed two main clusters. Each cluster had two separate subgroups. This investigation showed that RAPD marker is a useful tool for the evaluation of genetic diversity and relationship among different *Trigonella* species.

Kumar et al. [52] investigated the genetic diversity of five common fenugreek varieties of India using nine RAPD and seven fluorescently labeled amplified fragment length polymorphism (AFLP) primers. These RAPD primers produced a total of 47 bands in the size range of 200–5000 bp with an average polymorphism of 62.4%. AFLP marker produced a total of 669 bands in the size range of 50–538 bp. The results revealed that RAPD markers were more polymorphic than AFLP markers where the reproducibility of AFLP markers was more than RAPD markers.

Ahari et al. [53] assessed the genetic diversity among and within 20 Iranian fenugreek landraces using AFLP markers. Five AFLP primers combinations used in this study produced a total of 147 bands within the molecular weights ranging from 50 to 500 base pairs of which 87% were polymorphic. The results of polymorphism information content (PIC) showed that there was a high polymorphism existed among Kashan (0.79), Broojerd and Kashan (to 0.93) landraces, which shows the moderate and high genetic diversity among these populations. These results demonstrated high efficiency of AFLP markers for investigation the genetic diversity among Iranian fenugreek populations.

Haliem and Al-Huqail [54] investigated the correlation between biochemical characteristics such as acid phosphatase, and glutamate-oxaloacetate transaminase isozymes, and amino acid composition and molecular variations of seven wild *T. foenum-graecum* L.

accessions using RAPD markers. The molecular analysis revealed that RAPD markers were highly polymorphic (94.12%) and can be used in the differentiation of the genotypes effectively.

Al-Maamari et al. [55] investigated the genetic relationship of 20 Omani fenugreek accessions and compare their relationship with four accessions from Iraq and Pakistan using 6 AFLP primer combinations. A total of 1852 polymorphic loci were produced from these combinations. A high level of genetic diversity (H) was found in Omani populations (0.2146) compared to Pakistani (0.0844) and Iraqi (0.1620) populations. They concluded that the average level of genetic variation among fenugreek populations shows their long history of cultivation and frequent exchange of fenugreek genetic material among regions in Oman.

Hora et al. [56] studied the diversity and phylogenetic relationships of different varieties of fenugreek (eight varieties and six populations) collected from northern India using RAPD and ISSR markers. The high similarity coefficient values suggested a diverse genetic diversity in fenugreek populations in India. They concluded that these two molecular markers (RAPD and ISSR) can be used effectively to evaluate genetic diversity and assess genetic relationship.

7. Mutation breeding

Fenugreek becomes more important economically, agronomically and environmentally, day-to-day all over the world. In recent years, revealing the nutritional and medicinal value of fenugreek, its low soil expectations, and a relatively broad adaptation to the different regions, the scope of its cultivation spread from America to India [7, 30, 57]. For example, this plant has been called as a new species in Canada. There are few fenugreek genotypes that are adapted to the climatic conditions of western Canada. In such cases, mutation breeding can be used to generate new genetic variation in an existing gene pool for a certain trait [58]. Such a mutation breeding can be used for a large number of alleles at the same time to correct a particular trait [59]. Colloquially, mutations called every change in the DNA sequence which ultimately leads to a change in the individual's genotype. Gene mutation is a good affair in plant breeding, because it facilitates the selection [60]. Up to now, mutation breeding has created dramatic changes in the species of legume crops [61–63]. For instance, Mahna et al. [64] used mutation breeding to increase the diosgenin content in *T. corniculata* (a close relative of fenugreek). There are a variety of mutagens (chemicals or irradiation) to make mutations in plants.

According to the researches, it can be concluded that most of the mutations are recessive, can be observed to segregate in a 3:1 ratio in diploid crops like fenugreek [35, 42, 65], and for observation of such mutations, we should wait until the second generations [66]. Vice versa, dominant mutations are rare and can be observed in the first generations [65]. Since fenugreek is self-pollinated and the determinate trait is governed by recessive genes [67], mutation breeding can be used to generate mutant plants with a determinate growth habit without losing beneficial adaptations and other agronomic traits in the base population [68].

Application of mutation breeding in fenugreek is expressed in several studies. There are two major types of mutation: spontaneous and induced. Some varieties of fenugreek have been created through spontaneous mutations [35, 42, 69–70]. RH 3129 variety is produced from spontaneous mutation in a Moroccan cultivar and had high level of diosgenin content and twin pods [35, 69, 71]. In creating new varieties of fenugreek, the effect of induced mutations should not be ignored. RH 3112 cultivar with higher diosgenin content and seed yield and RH 3118 cultivar with higher protein content are two main cultivars which are made by induced mutations [35, 42, 69, 70]. Chemical mutation is also important in the production of new varieties of fenugreek. Basu [1] by inducing the seed of Tristar variety using Ethyl Methane Sulfonate (EMS), produced new population with higher height, seed yield, seed number per pod, biomass yield, total number of pods and number of twin pods.

Also, the results show that the impact of chemical mutation is much more than physical one [18, 68–70, 72–74]. Among chemical mutagens, it is observed that EMS can induce mutation successfully in the fenugreek [35, 69, 71]. Basu [1] studied the effect of different levels of EMS on fenugreek (Tristar variety). He found that EMS by alkylating guanine base and mispairing or mismatch pairing in the genome, effectively induced variation in the fenugreek populations and the mutants which were generated by 300 μM EMS had the best characters.

Also the results of various studies show that more than one genotype should be used in mutation breeding program [60, 74]. This is because different genotypes respond differently to a mutagen.

8. Fenugreek tissue culture

One way of producing variation is tissue culture. Several techniques such as somatic embryogenesis, callus regeneration and micropropagation have been reported in fenugreek [75–77]. Malhotra [78] reviewed various studies on in vitro regeneration and callus induction on fenugreek. Aasim et al. [77] performed a successful in vitro shoot regeneration of fenugreek plants on Murashige Skoog medium (MS) medium containing Thidiazuron (TDZ). The reports show that *T. foenum-graecum* L. hypocotyl explants are most responsive to callus induction and proliferation in tissue culture [79]. El-Nour et al. [80] performed a protocol of callus induction in fenugreek (*T. foenum-graecum* L.) on MS and B5 media supplemented with different types and concentrations of growth regulators were tested in order to obtain the best callus formation. The maximum value of callusing index (2.8) was obtained from MS medium containing 1.5 mg/l, 2,4-D using hypocotyls and cotyledons explants. The maximum callus formation observed in the MS media containing 2.0 mg/l naphthalene acetic acid (NAA) was 3.9 ± 0.08 in hypocotyls segment. The callus was compact in cotyledons and variable in hypocotyls segments and the color was creamy.

Shekhawat and Galston [81] examined different culture media and concluded that medium containing 0.1 mg/L of 6-Benzylaminopurine (BAP), zeatin, glutamine and asparagines was suitable for callus induction and differentiation, rapid cell division and growth. Azam and Biswas [75] believed that callus induction and growth were more successful on MS medium supplemented with naphthalene acetic acid (NAA), 2,4-D, kinetin and coconut water. El-Bahr [82] had a different view; he believes that fenugreek callus had its best growth on MS medium containing 3% sucrose and 2 mg 2,4-D.

9. Conclusion

Fenugreek (*T. foenum-graecum* L.) is an annual forage legume and a traditional spice crop that has been grown for centuries across the Indian subcontinent. In addition to South Asia, the crop is also grown in some parts of North Africa, Middle East, Mediterranean Europe, China, SE Asia, Australia and the USA, Canada and Argentina. India is the largest fenugreek producer in the world, but due to high internal consumption, do not have a major share of the global fenugreek trade. The crop has been recommended for the dry and semiarid regions of Asia, Africa and Latin America. The plant has been used traditionally in Indian Ayurvedic medicines as well as in traditional Tibetan and Chinese medication for several centuries. Modern research has also demonstrated that fenugreek seed and leaves are useful in the treatment of a number of diseases including successfully reducing blood sugar and blood cholesterol levels in both animals and human subjects in experimental trials. The reason behind the rich medicinal properties of fenugreek is due to the presence of a wide diversity of important phytochemicals (diosgenin, trigonelline, fenugreekine, galactomannan and 4-hydroxy isoleucine).

Hence, the crop has huge international demand in the associated pharmaceutical, nutraceutical and functional food industries. Our globe represents a wide range of agro-ecosystems on the earth with suitable dry, arid and semiarid climatic regimes suitable for the cultivation of fenugreek. Although the crop is crown to a limited amount in potential regions of fenugreek production, namely Africa, Central and South America and Southeast of Asia, but it has the potential to be grown under larger areas as a chemurgic crop with significant economic and commercial potential for the nation. Furthermore, being a forage legume and a natural nitrogen fixer; it could be easily incorporated in the local crop cycles of different geological regions for replenishing the soil naturally. The crop grows well under rainfed conditions and hence cost of production is lower compared to other commercial crops suitable for Iranian agroclimatic regimes.

Author details

Peiman Zandi[1*], Saikat Kumar Basu[2], William Cetzal-Ix[3], Mojtaba Kordrostami[4], Shahram Khademi Chalaras[5] and Leila Bazrkar Khatibai[6]

*Address all correspondence to: z_rice_b@yahoo.com

1 Institute of Crop Science, Chinese Academy of Agricultural Sciences, Beijing, P. R. China

2 Department of Biological Sciences, University of Lethbridge, Lethbridge, AB, Canada

3 Instituto Tecnológico de Chiná, Colonia Centro Chiná, Campeche, México

4 Department of Biotechnology, Faculty of Agricultural Sciences, University of Guilan, Rasht, Iran

5 Department of Agronomy and Plant Breeding, Rasht branch, Islamic Azad University, Rasht, Iran

6 Department of Plant Breeding, Faculty of Agriculture, Zabol University, Zabol, Iran

References

[1] Basu SK. Seed production technology for fenugreek (*Trigonella foenum-graecum* L.) in the Canadian [Master of Science thesis]. Lethbridge, Alberta, Canada: Department of Biological Sciences University; 2006.

[2] Basu A, Basu SK, Kumar A, Sharma M, Chalghoumi R, Hedi A, Solorio-Sánchez FJ, Ramírez-Avilés L, Balogun MO, Hafez EE, Cetzal-Ix W. Fenugreek (*Trigonella foenum-graecum* L.), a potential new crop for Latin America. American Journal of Social Issues and Humanities. 2014; **4**(3): 148–162.

[3] Basu SK, Agoramoorthy G. Fenugreek (*Trigonella foenum-graecum* L): Production challenges and opportunities for Asia, Africa and Latin America. American Journal of Social Issues and Humanities. 2014; Fenugreek Special Issue (March/April): 1–2.

[4] Zandi P, Basu SK, Bazrkar Khatibani L, Balogun M, Aremu MO, Sharma M, Kumar A, Sengupta R, Li X, Li Y, Tashi S, Hedi A, Cetzal-Ix W. Fenugreek (*Trigonella foenum-graecum* L.) seed: A review of physiological and biochemical properties and their genetic improvement. Acta Physiologia Plantarum. 2015; **37**: 1714. DOI:10.1007/s11738-014-1714-6

[5] Acharya S, Srichamroen A, Basu S, Ooraikul B, Basu T. Improvement in the nutraceutical properties of fenugreek (*Trigonella foenum-graecum* L.). Songklanakarin Journal of Science and Technology. 2006; **28**(1): 1–9.

[6] Mehrafarin A, Qaderi A, Rezazadeh Sh, Naghdi Badi H, Noormohammadi Gh, Zand E. Bioengineering of important secondary metabolites and metabolic pathways in fenugreek (*Trigonella foenum graecum* L.). Journal of Medicinal Plants. 2010; **9**(35): 1–18.

[7] Acharya SN, Thomas JE, Basu SK. Fenugreek: An "old world" crop for the "new world". Biodiversity. 2006; **7**(3&4): 27–30. DOI: 10.1080/14888386.2006.9712808

[8] Acharya SN, Blade S, Mir Z., Moyer JS. Tristar fenugreek. Canadian Journal of Plant Science. 2007; **87**: 901–903. DOI: 10.4141/P06-047

[9] Acharya SN, Thomas JE, Basu SK. Fenugreek (*Trigonella foenum-graecum* L.) an alternative crop for semiarid regions of North America. Crop Science. 2008; **48**: 841–853. DOI: 10.2135/cropsci2007.09.0519

[10] Solorio-Sánchez F, Solorio-Sánchez B, Basu SK, Casanova-Lugo F, Sarabia-Salgado L, Ku-Vera J, Aguilar-Pérez C, Ramírez-Avilés L, Noguera-Savelli E, Cetzal-Ix W, Infante-Cruz Á, Petit-Aldana J, Ayala-Basulto A. Opportunities to grow annual forage legume fenugreek (*Trigonella foenum-graecum L.*) under Mexican silvopastoral system. American Journal of Social Issues and Humanities. 2014; Fenugreek Special Issue (March/April): 86–95.

[11] Zandi P, Shirani Rad AH, Daneshian J, Bazrkar Khatibani L. Agronomic and morphologic analysis of Fenugreek (*Trigonella foenum-graecum* L.) under nitrogen fertilizer and plant density via factor analysis. African Journal of Agricultural Research. 2011; **6**(5): 1134–1140. DOI: 10.5897/AJAR11.004

[12] Basu SK, Thomas JE, Acharya SN. Prospects for growth in global nutraceutical and functional food markets: A Canadian perspective. Australian Journal of Basic and Applied Sciences. 2007; **1**(4): 637–649.

[13] Acharya SN, Acharya K, Paul S, Basu SK. Variation in the antioxidant and anti-leukemic properties among different Western Canada grown fenugreek (*Trigonella foenum-graecum* L.) genotypes. Canadian Journal of Plant Science. 2011; **91**(1): 99–105. DOI: 10.4141/cjps10025

[14] Thomas JE, Basu SK, Acharya SN. Identification of *Trigonella* accessions which lack antimicrobial activity and are suitable for forage development. Canadian Journal of Plant Science. 2006; **86**(3): 727–732. DOI: 10.4141/P05-155

[15] Basu SK, Acharya SN, Thomas JE. Colchicine treatment produces genetic improvement in fenugreek seed size and yield. Graduates studies Association (GSA). Proceedings Multidisciplinary Graduate Research Conference. 2007; **1**(1): 37–43.

[16] Basu SK, Acharya SN, Thomas JE. Foliar spray to improve fenugreek seed yield and reduce maturity duration. Graduates studies Association (GSA). Proceedings Multidisciplinary Graduate Research Conference. 2007; **1**(1): 44–50.

[17] Zandi P, Shirani Rad AH, Daneshian J, Bazrkar Khatibani L. Evaluation of nitrogen fertilizer and plant density effects on yield and yield components of fenugreek in double cropping. Journal of Plant Production (Chamran University, Ahvaz), 2013; **35** (4): 81–91.

[18] Basu SK, Acharya SN, Bandara MS, Friebel D, Thomas JE. Effects of genotype and environment on seed and forage yield in fenugreek (*Trigonella foenum-graecum* L.) grown in western Canada. Australian Journal of Crop Science. 2009; **3**(6): 305–314.

[19] Zandi P, Daneshian J, Shirani Rad AH. Determination of Ideal nitrogen fertilizer rate and plant density in fenugreek under dry farming conditions. In: The regional congress on modern results in agronomy and nanotechnology; 12 October 2010; Quds, Alborz, Iran: Azad University of Quds; 2010.

[20] Basu SK, Acharya SN, Thomas JE. Application of phosphate fertilizer and harvest management for improving fenugreek (*Trigonella foenum-graecum* L.) seed and forage yield in a dark brown soil zone of Canada. KMITL Science and Technology Journal. 2008; **8**(1): 1–7.

[21] Basu SK, Acharya SN, Thomas JE. Genetic improvement of fenugreek (*Trigonella foenum-graecum* L.) through EMS induced mutation breeding for higher seed yield under prairie conditions of western Canada. Euphytica. 2008; **160**: 249–258. DOI: 10.1007/s10681-007-9545-9

[22] Basu SK, Acharya SN, Thomas JE. A report on powdery mildew infestations caused by *Erysiphe polygoni* D.C. in North America grown fenugreek. Journal of Mycopathological Research. 2006; **44**(2): 253–256.

[23] Basu SK, Acharya SN, Cárcamo HA, Thomas JE. Study on the potential insect pests of fenugreek (*Trigonella foenum-graecum* L.) in North America with particular emphasis on

the western flower thrips (*Frankliniella occidentalis* Pergande) in the greenhouse and plant bugs (*Lygus* and *Adelphocoris*, Miridae, Hemiptera) in the field. Journal of Environment and Sociobiology. 2006; **3**(1): 1–7.

[24] Chakraborty N, Chatterjee S, Basu SK, Acharya K. Fungal diseases of fenugreek. American Journal of Social Issues and Humanities. 2014; Fenugreek Special Issue (March/April): 171–185.

[25] Vasilchenko IT. Reports on the species of the genus *Trigonella*. In: Flora and taxonomy of higher plants. Moscow & Leningrad: Publishing house of the Academy of Science of the SSSR (Ser. 1:10); 1953. pp. 331–333. (in Russian)

[26] Hector JN. Introduction to the Botany of Field Crops (Non Cereals), Johannesburg: Central News Agency Ltd.; 1936. 1127p.

[27] Rouk HF, Mangesha H. Fenugreek (*Trigonella foenum-graecum* L.), its relationship, geography and economic importance. Experiment Station Bulletin. No. 20. Dire Dawa, Ethiopia: Imperial Ethiopian College of Agriculture and Mechanical Arts; 1963. pp. 120–127.

[28] Hutchinson J. The Genera of Flowering Plants. Vol. 1. Oxford: Clarendon Press; 1964. pp. 947–952.

[29] Fazli FRY. Studies in steroid-yielding plants of the genus *Trigonella* [PhD dissertation]. England: University of Nottingham; 1967.

[30] Petropoulos GA. Fenugreek, The Genus *Trigonella*. London and New York: Taylor and Francis; 2002. 255 p.

[31] Mehrafarin A, Rezazadeh S, Naghdi Badi H, Noormohammadi Gh, Zand E, Qaderi A. A review on biology, cultivation and biotechnology of fenugreek (*Trigonella foenum-graecum* L.) as a valuable medicinal plant and multipurpose. Journal of Medicinal Plants. 2011; **10**(37): 6–24.

[32] Vavilov NI. Studies in the origin of cultivated plants. Bulletin of Applied Botany and Plant Breeding. Leningrad. 1926; 16(2): 1–248.

[33] De Candolle A. Origin of Cultivated Plants. New York: Hafner; 1964. 468 p.

[34] Fazli FRY, Hardman R. The spice, fenugreek (*Trigonella foenum-graecum* L.): Its commercial varieties of seed as a source of diosgenin. Tropical Science. 1968; **10**: 66–78.

[35] Petropoulos GA. Agronomic, genetic and chemical studies of *Trigonella foenum graecum* L. [PhD dissertation]. England: Bath University; 1973.

[36] Darlington CD, Wylie AP. Chromosome Atlas of Flowering Plants. 2nd ed. London: George Allen & Unwin; 1955. 519 p.

[37] Singh A, Roy RP. Karyological studies in *Trigonella, Indigofera* and *Phaseolus*. The Nucleus (Calcutta). 1970; **13**: 41–54.

[38] Ladizinsky G, Vosa CG. Karyotype and C-banding in *Trigonella* section *foenum-graecum* (Fabaceae). Plant Systematics and Evolutions. 1968; **153**(1–2): 1–5.

[39] Srivastava A, Raghuvanshi SS. Buffering effect of B-chromosome system of *Trigonella foenum graecum* against different soil types. Theoretical and Applied Genetics. 1987; **75**: 807–810. DOI: 10.1007/BF00265609

[40] Reasat M, Karapetyam J, Nasirzadeh A. Karyotypic analysis of *Trigonella* genus of Fars Province. Iranian Journal of Rangelands and Forests Plant Breeding and Genetic Research. 2002; **11**(1): 127–145.

[41] Dundas IS, Nair RM, Verlin DC. First report of meiotic chromosome number and karyotype analysis of an accession of *Trigonella balansae*. New Zealand Journal of Agricultural Research. 2006; **49**: 55–58.

[42] Singh A, Singh D. Karyotype studies in Trigonella. The Nucleus (Calcutta).1976; 19: 13–16.

[43] Marc RC, Capraru G. Influence of sodium phosphate (E 339) on mitotic division in *Trigonella foenum-graecum* L. Scientific Annals of the "Alexandru Ioan Cuza" University of Iasi, Section II a. Genetic and Molecular Biology, 2008; **9**(1): 67–70.

[44] Roy RP, Singh A. Cytomorphological studies of the colchicines-induced tetraploids *Trigonella foenum-graecum* L. Genetica Iberian. 1968; **20**(1–2): 37–54.

[45] Raghuvanshi SS, Joshi S. *Trigonella foenum-graecum* B chromosome. Current Science. 1964; **33**: 654–654.

[46] Joshi S, Raghuvanshi SS. B-chromosome, pollen germination *in situ* and connected grains in *Trigonella foenum-graecum* L. Beitrage zur Biologie der Pflanzen 1968; **44**: 161–166.

[47] Singh A. Studies on the interspecific hybrids of *Trigonella corniculata* and *T. hamosa* and *T. cretica*. Genetica (Dordrecht). 1973; **44**: 264–269.

[48] Lakshmi N, Rao TV, Rao Venkateswara T. Karyological and morphological investigations on some inbred strains of *Trigonella* L. Genetica Iberian. 1984; **36**(3–4): 187–200.

[49] Kordrostami M, Rabiei B, Kumleh HH. Association analysis, genetic diversity and haplotyping of rice plants under salt stress using SSR markers linked to *SalTol* and morpho-physiological characteristics. Plant Systematics and Evolution. 2016; **302**: 871–890. DOI: 10.1007/s00606-016-1304-8

[50] Dangi RS, Lagu MD, Choudhary LB, Ranjekar PK, Gupta VS. Assessment of genetic diversity in *Trigonella foenum-graecum* and *Trigonella caerulea* using ISSR and RAPD markers. BMC Plant Biology. 2004; **4**: 13. DOI: 10.1186/1471-2229-4-13

[51] Sundaram S, Purwar S. Assessment of genetic diversity among fenugreek (*Trigonella foenum-graecum* L.), using RAPD molecular markers. Journal of Medicinal Plants Research. 2011; **5**: 1543–1548.

[52] Kumar V, Srivastava N, Singh A, Vyas MK, Gupta S, Katudia K, Vaidya K, Chaudhary S, Ghosh A, Chikara SK. Genetic diversity and identification of variety-specific AFLP markers in fenugreek (*Trigonella foenum*-graecum). African Journal of Biotechnology. 2012; **11**: 4323–4329.

[53] Ahari DS, Hassandokht MR, Kashi AK, Amri A. Evaluation of genetic diversity in Iranian fenugreek (*Trigonella foenum-graecum* L.) landraces using AFLP markers. Seed and Plant Improvement Journal. 2014; **30**(1): 155–171.

[54] Haliem EA, Al-Huqail AA. Correlation of genetic variation among wild *Trigonella foenum* graecum L. accessions with their antioxidant potential status. Genetics and Molecular Research. 2014; **13**: 10464–10481. DOI: 10.4238/2014.December.12.8.

[55] Al-Maamari IT, Al-Sadi AM, Al-Saady NA. Assessment of genetic diversity in fenugreek (*Trigonella foenum graecum* L.) in Oman. International Journal of Agriculture and Biology. 2014; **16**: 813–818.

[56] Hora A, Malik CP, Kumari B. Assessment of genetic diversity of *Trigonella foenum-graecum* L. in northern India using RAPD and ISSR markers. International Journal of Pharmacy and Pharmaceutical Sciences. 2016; **8**(1): 179–183.

[57] Montgomery JE, King JR, Doepel L. Fenugreek as forage for dairy cattle. In: Proceedings of the 26th Western Canadian Dairy Seminar (WCDS) Advances in Dairy Technology; 4–7 March 2008; Red Deer, Alberta: WCDS; 2006. Vol. 20, Abstract, p. 356.

[58] Fehr WR. Principles of Cultivar Development: Theory and Technique. Vol. II. USA: Macmillan Publishing Company; 1993. 536 p.

[59] Chopra VL. Mutagenesis: Investigating the process and processing the outcome for crop improvement. Current Science. 2005; **89**: 353–359.

[60] Yadav SS, McNeil DL, Stevenson PC (edited). Lentil: An Ancient Crop for Modern Times. Dordrecht: Springer Netherlands; 2007. pp. 1–450. DOI: 10.1007/978-1-4020-6313-8

[61] Sigurbjornsson B, Micke A. Philosophy and accomplishments of mutation breeding. In: Polyploidy and Induced Mutations in Plant Breeding (Proceedings of two Meetings Joint FAO/IAEAO Division and EUCARPIA, Bari, Italy, 1972). Vienna: International Atomic Energy Agency (IAEA); 1974. pp. 303–343.

[62] Sigurbjornsson B. Induced mutations. In: Wood DR, editor. Crop Breeding. Madison, Wisconsin, USA: American Society of Agronomy and Crop Science Society of America; 1983. pp. 153–176.

[63] Toker C, Yadav SS, Solanki IS. Mutation breeding. In: Yadav SS, McNeil D, Stevenson PC, editors. Lentil: An Ancient Crop for Modern Times. Dordrecht, Netherland: Springer; 2007. pp. 209–224. DOI: 10.1007/978-1-4020-6313-8_13

[64] Mahna SK, Raisinghani G, Jain SC. Diosgenin production induced mutants of *Trigonella corniculata*. Fitoterapia. 1994; **65**: 515–516.

[65] Gaul H, Aastveit K. Induced variability of culm length in different genotypes of hexaploid wheat following X-irradiation and EMS treatment. Savrem. Contemporary Agriculture. 1966; **11**: 263–276.

[66] Micke A, Donini B. Induced mutations. In: Hayward MD, Bosemark NO, Romagosa I, editors. Plant Breeding Principles and Prospects. London, UK: Chapman and Hall; 1993. pp. 52–62.

[67] Choudhary AK, Singh VV. An induced determinate mutant in fenugreek (*Trigonella foenum graecum* L.). Journal of Spices and Aromatic Crops. 2001; **10**(1): 51–53.

[68] Basu SK, Acharya SN, Thomas JE. Genetic improvement of fenugreek through EMS-induced mutation breeding for higher seed yield under western Canada prairie condition. Euphytica. 2007; **160**(2): 249–258. DOI: 10.1007/s10681-007-9545-9

[69] Laxmi V, Gupta MN, Dixit BS, Srivastava SN. Effects of chemical and physical mutagens on fenugreek oil. Indian Drugs. 1980; **18**(2): 62–65.

[70] Laxmi V, Datta SK. Chemical and physical mutagenesis in fenugreek. Biological Memoirs. 1987; **13**(1): 64–68.

[71] Petropoulos GA, Kouloumbis P. Botany. In: Petropoulos GA, editor. Fenugreek: The Genus *Trigonella*, Medicinal and Aromatic Plants-Industrial Profiles. London: CRC Press; 2002. pp. 9–17.

[72] IAEA (International Atomic Energy Agency). Manual on Mutation Breeding. 2nd ed. Technical Report Series No. 119, Vienna: IAEA; 1987. 288 p.

[73] Ganapathy S, Nirmalakumari A, Senthil N, Souframanie J, Raveendran TS. Isolation of macro mutations and Mutagenic effectiveness and efficiency in little Millet Varieties. World. Journal of Agricultural Science. 2008; **4**(4): 483–486.

[74] Begum T, Dasgupta T. A comparison of the effects of physical and chemical mutagens in sesame (*Sesamum indicum* L.). Genetics and Molecular Biology. 2010; **33**(4): 761–766. DOI: 10.1590/S1415-47572010005000090

[75] Azam M, Biswas AK. Callus culturing its maintenance and cytological variations in *Trigonella foenum-graecum*. Current Science 1989; **58**: 844–847.

[76] Provorov NA, Tikhonovich IA. Genetic resource for improving nitrogen fixation in legume–shizobia symbiosis. Genetic Resources and Crop Evolution. 2004; **50**(1): 89–99. DOI: 10.1023/A:1022957429160

[77] Aasim M, Khawar MK, Sancak C, Ozcan S. In vitro shoot regeneration of fenugreek. American-Eurasia Journal of Sustainable Agriculture 2009; **3**(2): 135–138.

[78] Malhotra SK. Breading potential of indigenous germplasm of seed spices. In: Singh DK, Chowdhuary H, editors. Vegetable Crops: Genetic Resources and Improvement. New Delhi: New India Publishing House; 2011. pp. 477–497.

[79] Zhang L, Lu YT. Calmodulin-binding protein kinases in plants. Trends in Plant Science. 2003; **8**: 123–127. DOI: 10.1016/S1360-1385(03)00013-X

[80] El-Nour MEM, Lamia S, Mohammed, Bader Eldin AS. In vitro callus induction of fenugreek (*Trigonella foenum-graecum* L.) using differentt media with different Auxins concentrations. Agriculture and Biology Journal of North America. 2014; **4**(3): 243–251. DOI:10.5251/abjna.2013.4.3.243.251

[81] Shekhawat NS, Galston AW. Mesophyll protoplasts of fenugreek (*Trigonella foenum-graecum* L.): Isolation, culture and shoot regeneration. Plant Cell Reports. 1983; **2**(3): 119–121. DOI: 10.1007/BF00269333.

[82] El-Bahr MK. Influence of sucrose and 2, 4-D on *Trigonella foenum-graecum* tissue culture. African Journal of Agricultural Science. 1989; **16**(1–2): 87–96.

4

Olea europaea subsp. *africana* (Oleaceae)

Nontokozo Z. Msomi and Mthokozisi. B. C Simelane

Abstract

Background: Medicinal plants have been used as a key source for medication and they remain to provide new therapeutic remedies to date. Extracts of *Olea europaea* subsp. africana *Oleaceae* (leaf, bark and root) are used extensively in Africa to treat various diseases traditionally. Phytochemistry has identified phenols, terpenoids and coumarins in different parts of the plant. However, little pharmacological studies have been done on *Olea europaea* subsp. *africana*. The present review aims to compile available information on the ethnobotany, phytochemistry, pharmacology and toxicology of *Olea africana*.

Materials and methods: Information available pertaining *Olea europaea* subsp. *africana* was collected through electronic search using (Google Scholar, PubMed and Science Direct).

Results: *Olea africana* has been used throughout Africa traditionally for various ailments. Phytochemical studies have led to the isolation of compounds, namely oleuropein, esculin, ursolic acid, scopolin and oleanolic acid. Studies have shown that the leaf extract contains antihypertensive, diuretic, anti-atherosclerotic, antioxidant, antidiarrhoeal and hypoglycaemic activities. Conclusion: *Olea africana* has been used expansively for treating ailments traditionally, but pharmacological studies are seldom published. Further research is required to extend existing therapeutic potential of the African olive.

Keywords: *Olea europaea* subsp. *africana*, ethnobotany, phytochemistry, pharmacology, toxicology

1. Introduction

Medicinal plants are defined as any plant containing substances which can be used for curative purposes in one or more parts of its organ, which are precursors for the production of useful drugs [1, 2]. A vast number of these plant species have been used in treating numerous ailments for decades [3, 4]. In Africa, the use of traditional medicine dates back 4000 years ago before the use of orthodox medicine [5]. According to the World Health Organization, traditional medicine still remains the primary healthcare system for an estimated 80% of the population in Africa, because of its affordability and accessibility [2, 6]. South Africa has a profound native knowledge on plants used as traditional remedies [5]. An estimated 30,000 species of higher plants are found in South Africa and 3000 of these species have been used in phytomedicine across the country [7]. It is approximated that 3 million of the South African population uses phytomedicine for primary health purposes [5, 7].

Plant fragments such as leaves, bark, roots, flowers and seeds can be used to derive traditional remedies [8]. These can be prepared not only from a single plant but a combination of plant concoctions [9], aiding in ailments such as influenza, arthritis, heart burn, kidney infections, high blood pressure, etc. [8]. Traditional medicine has also contributed to the management of epidemic diseases such as HIV/AIDS [10], malaria [11] and diabetes [2]. The therapeutic potential of medicinal plants is due to the existence of phytochemicals which comprise of tannins, alkaloids, flavonoids, essential oils and chemical compounds established as subordinate metabolites in plants [4]. It has been reported that at least 25% of commercial drugs are derivatives from plants [2], such as picrotoxin and aspirin [4], and various others are analogues made by chemical synthesis fabricated from isolated compounds from plants [12]. However, biomedical literature data are miniature regarding the safety, quality and efficacy of the plants used in traditional medicine [3]. Therefore, there has been a sudden growth in the interest of studying and using medicinal plants which have led to the isolation of active chemical compounds for therapeutic significance [13]. The plant species from the family *Oleaceae* have been used extensively in traditional medicine in Asia, Southern Africa, European Mediterranean islands, Spain, Italy, etc. [14, 15]; the family *Oleaceae* is a family of dicotyledons [16], containing 600 species in 25 genera, and some genera are wide and arise in several continents [17]. Species of the family are trees, shrubs or woody climbers including the olive tree [16, 17].

2. Olea

The genus *Olea* descends from the Greek "elaia" and the Latin "oleum," [16, 18], but it is known in other languages as Olivo (Spanish), Olive (English, French and German), Oliva (Russian, Latin and Italian), Zaitun (Arabic-Persian, Hindi, Urdu and numerous Indian languages) and Zayit (Hebrew) [19]. The genera *Olea* are classified into the subfamily *Oleideae* [20], containing 35 species [21] which extant throughout the Mediterranean, Europe, Africa, Iran and Asia [16]. The olive is thought to have a cultivation history of several 1000 years [19]. It holds historic importance in the context of religion, and it is quoted in the Christian and Hebrew Bibles and the Koran [16, 18].

The olive shrub is rarely consumed as a natural fruit due to its bitter taste but used as oil or table olive [16, 22], and its wild and cultivated forms are considered as a significant botanical research subject [22]. The traditional use of leaves includes treatment for fever, malaria, bacterial infections, diabetes, inflammatory disorders and hypertension [23]. The decoction of leaves is also used as a mouthwash to treat aphthous, gingivitis and glossitis [23]. The preparation of the bark concoction is taken to treat tapeworm infestation [16]. Olive oil is used externally in the treatment of insect stings and burns [19]. Previous studies established that olive leaves have antioxidant, anti-inflammatory [23], anticancer, antihypertensive and antidiabetic properties [16]. These activities have been shown to be displayed by compounds isolated from the olive tree including iridoids, secoiridoids, lignans, biophenols, flavonoids, flavone glycosides, isochromans and terpenoids [16, 19]. Six species of the olive tree are currently recognized: subsp. *europaea*, subsp. *maroccana*, subsp. *cerasiformis*, subsp. *guanchica*, subsp. *laperrinei* and subsp. *africana* [18].

2.1. *Olea europaea* subsp. *africana*

The African species of *Olea europaea*, previously acknowledged as *Olea africana* subsp. *cuspidata*, was defined as *Olea europaea* subsp. *africana* (Mill) in the early 1980s [4, 14]. In Africa, it is commonly known as the wild olive and vernacular names are motholoari (Sotho), olienhout (Afrikaans) and umquma (Xhosa and Zulu) [14, 24].

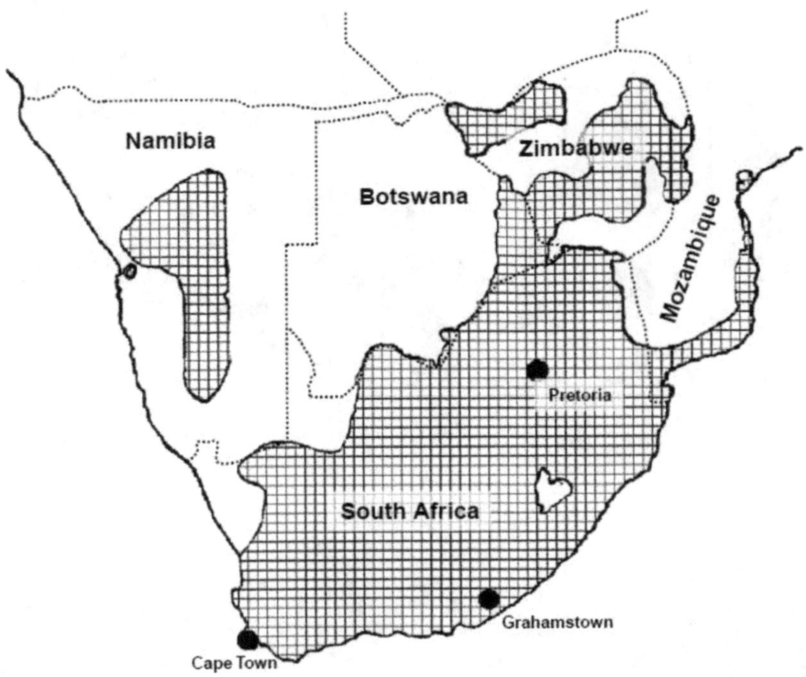

Figure 1. Distribution of wild olives in Southern Africa (Mkize et al.) [25].

2.1.1. *Geographical distribution*

Olea africana is widely distributed in Africa from the southern tip to the north through east Tropical African into Eritrea [14, 15]. The plant is documented in the following countries: South Africa, Tanzania, Sudan, Namibia, Kenya and Ethiopia [15]. In the Asian continent, *O. africana* is significant in Afghanistan, northern India, Kashmir and Pakistan [15]. The African olive cultivates in a varied range of natural surroundings, from rocky mountain slopes, riverbanks, forest, bush and grassfields [4] (**Figure 1**).

2.1.2. Botanical description

The wild olive tree is a shrub which grows to 5–10 m in height, irregularly reaching 18 m [26]. The trees mature into a wild, rounded pattern with a solid upper layer and twisted trunk when exposed to dry conditions [15]. The bark is grey to brownish and flaky once it matures [15]. Flowers are greenish white in colour, 6–10 mm long, with a sweet aroma and held insecurely in axillary or occasionally terminal heads [15, 26]. The ovoid fruit are thinly fleshy, about 7–10 mm in dimension, and upon maturation it turns black or dark brown [15] (**Figures 2–6**; **Table 1**).

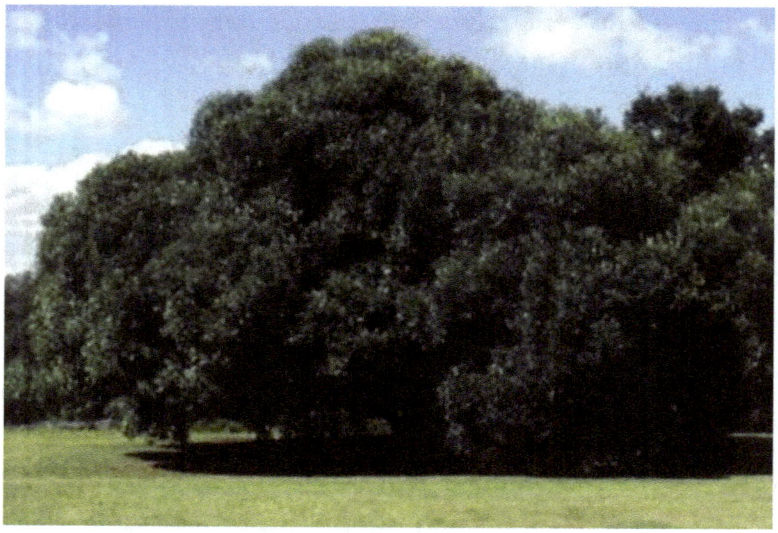

Figure 2. *Olea africana* shrub (plantzafrica.com).

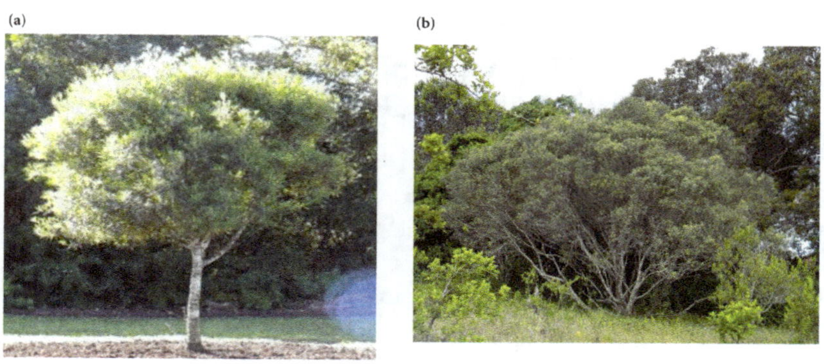

Figure 3. *Olea africana*: Young specimen (a) and mature specimen with twisted trunk (b) (www.KumbulaNursery.co.za).

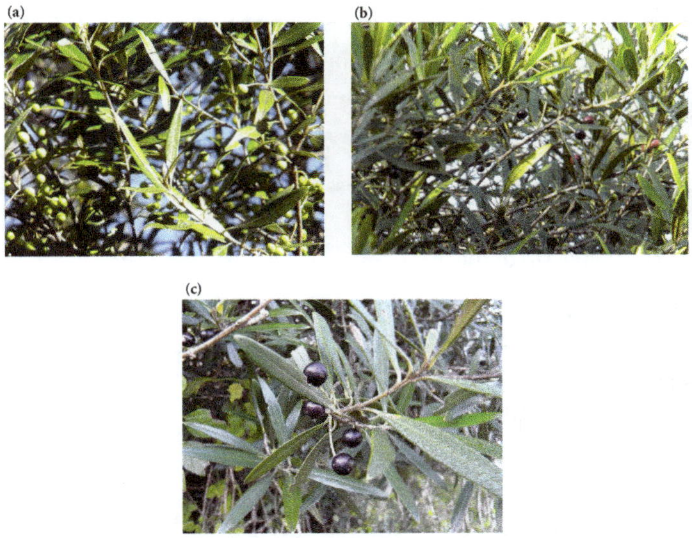

Figure 4. Ovoid fruit of *Olea africana*: Unripe fruit (a), fruits turn red before ripening (b) and ripe fruits (c) (www.KhumbulaNursery.co.za).

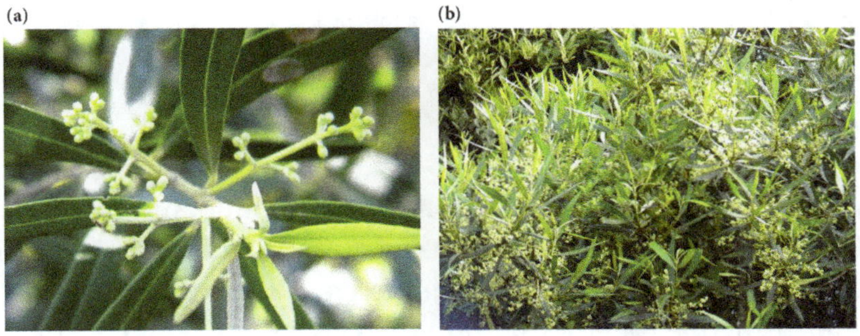

Figure 5. Tiny flower buds (a) and blossomed flowers hidden in the foliage (b) (www.KhumbulaNursery.co.za).

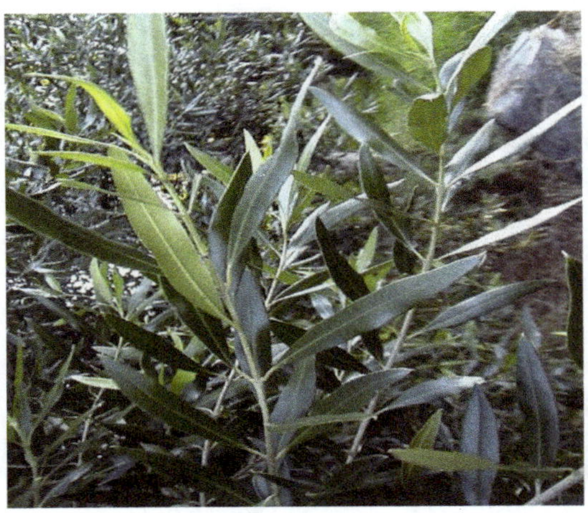

Figure 6. Wild olive foliage (esc.nsw.gov.au).

Taxon	Leaf characteristics	Field characteristics/comments
African wild olive *Olea europaea* subsp. *Africana*	• 6–10 cm in length • 10–25 mm wide • Light green to yellowish brown in the lower part of the leaf • Hooked apex on the tip of the leaf • Yellowish green mid veins	• Fruit are purple black, thinly fleshed drupe about 6–7 mm in diameter • The tree is dense with a twisted trunk, which has dark green glossy leaves. It is weedy in coastal areas

Table 1. Leaf characteristics of the African olive (Cuneo and Leishman, 2006).

2.1.3. Photochemistry

Phytochemicals are various biologically active compounds that occur naturally in plants, which provide potential medicinal benefits for humans [27]. These chemicals assemble in several parts of the plant including the flower, stems, seed, roots and leaves [27]. Phytochemical screening of the African wild olive has led to the separation of phenolic compounds, known as oleuropein, tyrosol and hydroxytyrosol [28] flavonoids [24], triterpenoids (oleanolic acid, ursolic acid) [14] (erythrodiol and uvaol) [29] and coumarin glucosides (esculin and scopolin) [30].

2.1.3.1. Phenols

Plant phenols are aromatic secondary metabolites, containing antioxidant and antimicrobial properties [31]. The compound oleuropein is a coumarin-like compound, which is profuse in the family *Oleaceae* [32], considered as the main active compound in the olive leaf [27, 33]. It gives olives its bitter principle together with hydroxytyrosol [34], a constituent of oleuropein derived from it through enzymatic hydrolysis [4, 34]. Tyrosol is another structurally related compound that co-occurs with oleuropein [28]. As secoiridoid compounds, they are bound glycosidically, produced from the secondary metabolism of terpenes [32]. In the *Oleaceae* family, it results from the oleoside form of glucoside, which is characterized by an exocyclic 8,9-olefinic functionality [32]. In a previous study, these secoiridoids have been isolated from methanolic and ethyl acetate leaf extracts of the wild olive [28] (**Figure 7**).

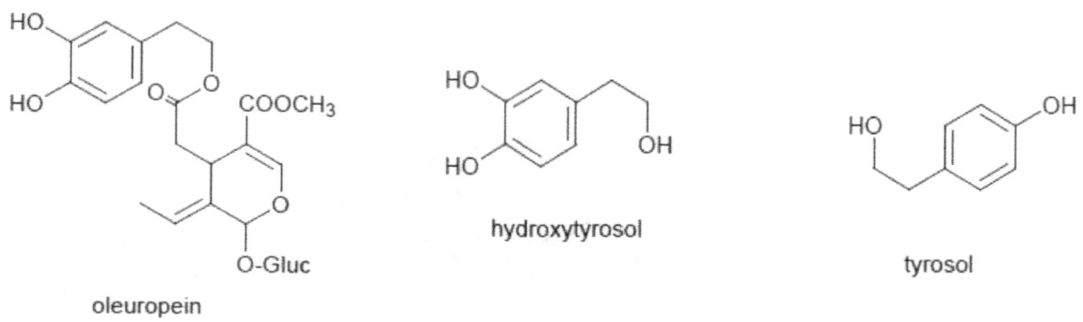

Figure 7. Biochemical structures of phenolic compounds found in olives (Ryan and Robards [31]).

2.1.3.2. Triterpenoids

Triterpenoids are a vastly varied group of natural products, including steroids, extensively dispersed in plants [35]. These compounds are accumulated by plants in their glycosylated form (saponin) [35]. Oleanolic acid (**Figure 8**) is a biologically active pentacyclic triterpenoid with pharmacologic activities, such as anticancer, hepatoprotective effects, antioxidant and anti-inflammatory [36]. Oleanolic acid is often in existent with its isomer ursolic acid (**Figure 9**) [36]. Ursolic acid is biologically used as an antioxidant, anticancer and anti-inflammatory chemical [37]. Erythrodiol and uvaol are triterpenoids belonging to the oleanane and ursane classes [29]. These compounds have been stated to possess antimalarial, antifungal, antileishmanial, antibacterial and anti-inflammatory activities [29]. Triterpenoids isolated from *O. africana* in previous studies were of dichloromethane [29], ethyl acetate and methanol leaf extracts [14, 28] (**Figure 10**).

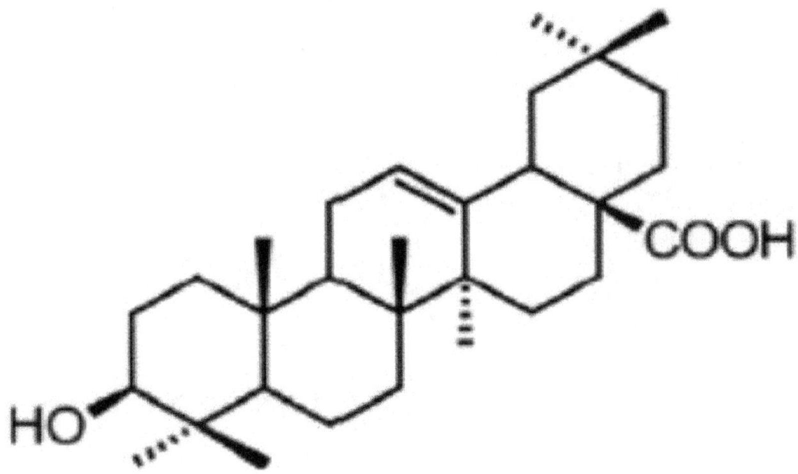

Figure 8. Biochemical structure of oleanolic acid (Pollier and Goossens [36]).

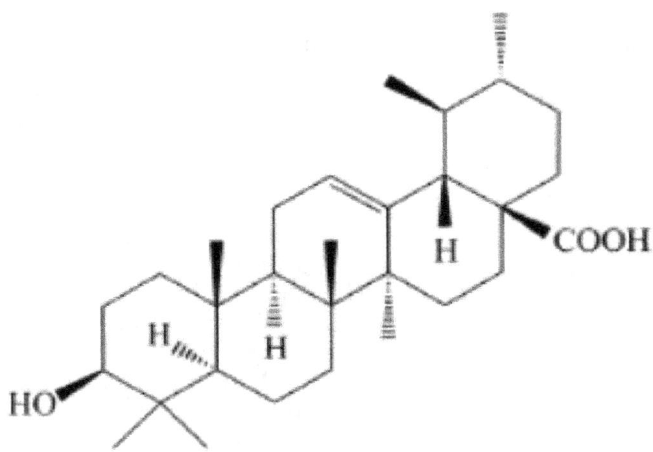

Figure 9. Biochemical structure of ursolic acid (Ikeda et al. [37]).

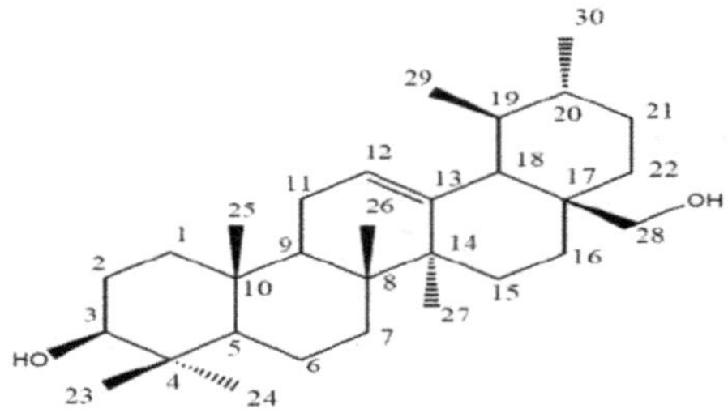

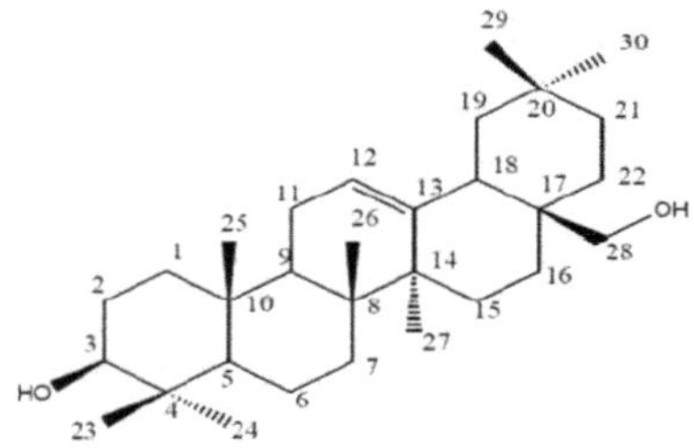

Figure 10. Biochemical structures of uvaol and erythrodiol (Douglas et al. [29]).

2.1.3.3. Coumarins

Coumarins are derived from 1,2-benzopyrones, containing of a large class of phenolic elements originating in plants [38, 39] and distributed in the following families: *Guttiferae, Caprifoliaceae, Rutaceae, Umbelliferae, Clusiaceae, Nyctaginaceae, Oleaceae* and *Apiaceae* [39]. Coumarins have received attention in the following therapeutic fields: chemotherapy, multiple sclerosis and organ transplants [38]. The bark of *O. africana* has been reported to contain coumarin glucosides, esculin and scopolin [30] (**Figures 11** and **12**).

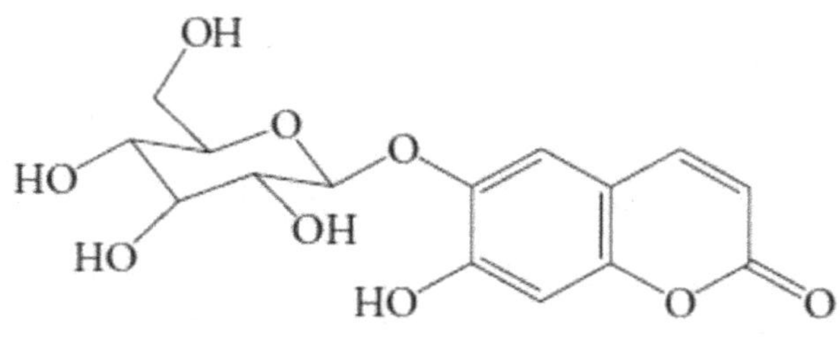

Esculin

Figure 11. Chemical structure of esculin (Venugopala et al. [39]).

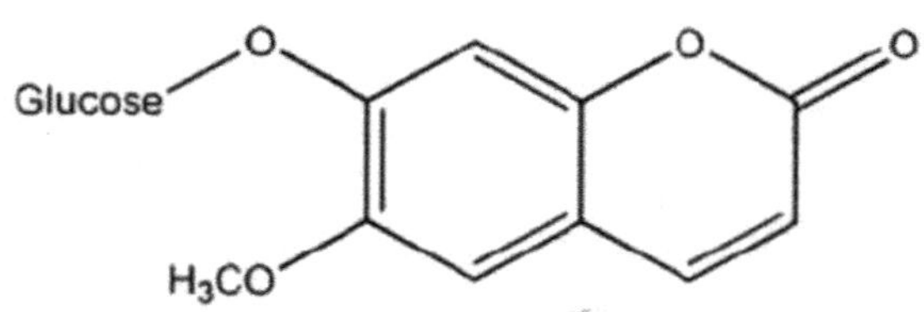

Scopolin

Figure 12. Chemical structure of scopolin (Malik et al.) [40].

2.1.4. Medicinal uses

The wild olive tree has been stated to be "the most important plant" from 120 plants being used in traditional medicine [14]. *O. africana* has a number of traditional uses medically that are summarized in **Table 2**. The bark, leaves, roots and fruits are used in different forms, alone or sometimes in combination [28].

Traditional use	References
• Dried and powdered leaf is applied on fresh wounds as a styptic	[28]
• Sap from the bark is used for bone-setting (fracture)	[41]
• Leaves are used as a treatment for malaria, urinary tract infections, backaches and kidney problems	[4]
• Leaf infusions are used as lotion for the treatment of eye infections or to relieve sore throats	[15, 42]
• The scraped bark is used to treat headaches and bladder infections. Smoke from a fire made with kindling is believed to clear the head and blood after excessive drinking	[43]
• The plant is used traditionally as a hypotensive, febrifuge, diuretic, tonic and emollient, for headaches and bladder and urinary infections	[14]
• Powered leaf stops nosebleeds by using it as a snuff. Leaves are used as tea. Sugar and boiled ripe fruits are administered for coughs	[28]
• The leaf and stem bark decoctions are treatment for anaplasmosis and also retained afterbirth	[12]
• Bark, which is dried, pound and powdered, is applied for eye illnesses. Boiled bark is administered for itchy rashes	[44]
• Boiled bark is administered to treat tapeworms	[45]
• Decoction of stem bark is used to treat helminthiasis, asthma, rheumatism and lumbago in Samburu district, Kenya	[46]
• Bark, root and leaf infusions are taken to relieve colic, leaf infusion taken to treat sore throats and diphtheria	[47]
• Fruit infusion treats bloody stool and diarrhoea	[48]
• Decoction of the fruits and leaves is used in treating blood pressure in the Transkei region	[49]

Table 2. Traditional uses of *Olea europaea* subsp. *africana* in Africa.

2.1.5. Pharmacology

2.1.5.1. Antidiarrhoeal activity

A study by Amabeoku and Bamuamba [24] investigated the methanolic leaf extract of *O. africana* for antidiarrhoeal activity in mice. The use of the plant in the Western Cape rural areas in treating diarrhoea is extensive. Albino mice were administered with the methanol leaf extract at doses ranging from 25 to 75 mg/kg, 15 min before the administration of castor oil at a dosage of 0.7 ml (orally (p.o)). It was observed that the methanol leaf extract doses from 50 to 75 mg/kg expressively reduced the occurrence of diarrhoea by notably decreasing the number of mice affected with diarrhoea. The plant extract dose of 25 mg/kg was able to protect 50% of the animals affected with diarrhoea; therefore, signifying it did not have a significant effect on the occurrence of diarrhoea. This study showed that *O. africana* methanolic leaf extract was able to significantly antagonize diarrhoea, by possibly exerting its activity through reducing intestinal motility [24].

2.1.5.2. Antihypertensive, antiatherosclerotic, hypoglycaemic and antioxidant activity

Somova et al. [14] stated that the African wild olive leaf can prevent atherosclerosis and hypertension and improve insulin resistance. The experimental animals were treated at a dosage of 60 mg/kg b.w with ethyl acetate leaf extract, as this fraction is known to contain the active compound oleuafricein. Hemodynamic screening was evaluated for 42 days monitoring the administration of the drug, heart rate, systolic and diastolic blood pressure. The Lipschitz test was conducted to record the excreted urine after 5 h and after 24 h. On completion of the study, the animals were starved overnight and killed. Following killing, blood glucose was estimated, and glutathione peroxidase and superoxide dismutase were assayed. These biochemical parameters showed that treatment with *O. africana* leaf extract after 6 weeks exhibited effective hypoglycaemic, antiatherosclerotic, antihypertensive and antioxidant activity. It was obtained that *O. africana* contains 0.27% combination of ursolic and oleanolic acid accountable for the bioactivities [14].

A study by Abdel-Sattar et al. [50] reported antihypertensive, hypoglycaemic and antioxidant properties of *O. africana* methanol leaf extract. The antioxidant activity was studied by exploring scavenging activity of 1,1-diphenyl-2-picrylhydrazyl free radical. The Olive leaf extract reduced the radical to a yellow-coloured diphenylpicrylhydrazine, confirming its antioxidant property. Experimental animals were treated with the extract for 42 days at a dosage of 200 mg/kg to evaluate hypertension and three dosage levels (100, 300 and 500 mg/kg) for antihyperglycaemic activity. The results obtained were partial reduction of L-N-nitroarginine methyl ester (L-NAME) which triggered hypertension compared to the control group. The Olive leaf revealed blood glucose lowering activity against streptozotocin (STZ) which elicited hyperglycaemia in rats. The highest dose of the extract (500 mg/kg) exhibited a significant decrease in blood glucose level by 69.6% on the fourth week of treatment relative to the control group. *O. africana* was exhibited to have protective activity against diabetes induced by STZ and hypertension induced by L-NAME. The antihyperglycaemic activity was accredited to be caused by an increase in glucose uptake in skeletal muscle, antioxidant activity, inhibition of liver gluconeogenesis and insulinomimetic effect [33].

2.1.5.3. Antibacterial activity

A study by Douglas et al. [29] evaluated the antibacterial activity of the leaves of *O. africana*. The bacterial strains *Staphylococcus aureus* ATCC 25923, *Escherichia coli* ATCC 25922, *Pseudomonas aeruginosa* ATCC 87853 and *Bacillus subtilis* BCCM 1735 were used for this study. The crude extracts displayed comparatively elevated action against bacteria in Gram-positive strains with the methanol extract exhibiting the highest antibacterial activity. The triterpenoids (uvaol and erythrodiol) isolated from the plant exhibited adequate antibacterial activity. However, in the *E. coli* strain, the compounds showed no significant activity, as this strain has been stated to have multi-resistance against antibiotics. Erythrodiol presented higher bioactivity compared to uvaol against *S. aureus* [29].

A study by Douglas and Jeruto [51] investigated antibacterial activity of *O. africana* leaf extracts (methanol, ethyl acetate and dichloromethane) against *Pseudomonas aeruginosa, Bacillus subtilis, Escherichia coli* and *Staphylococcus aureus*, by means of micro-broth diffusion method. The bacterium strain *S. aureus* was the most susceptible to dichloromethane extract (15 mg/mL) displaying a zone of inhibition of 19.40 mm. The strains *P. aeruginosa, E. coli* and *B. subtilis* were inhibited effectively with the methanol extract (25 mg/mL) with zones of inhibition 17.40, 17.20 and 19.20 mm, respectively [51]. These studies therefore assume that *O. africana* could be used traditionally in treating symptoms of infection and inflammation by bacteria [29, 51].

2.1.5.4. Toxicology

Amabeoku and Bamuamba [24] examined *O. africana* methanolic leaf extract in groups of eight per dose (400, 800, 1200, 1600, 2000, 2400, 2800, 3200, 3600 and 4000 mg/kg). It was observed that the mortality rate increased as the dosage increased from 2800 to 4000 mg/kg. The doses from 2000 to 4000 mg/kg indicated the animals to be hypoactive. The dose at 3475 mg/kg was determined to be the LD50 value for the plant [24]. Somova et al. [14] investigated the effect of the African wild olive leaves on Sprague-Dawley rats using the doses 20, 40, 60 and 80 mg. It was observed using the brine shrimp test that the leaf extract had a toxicity with LC50 of 1.25 at a dosage of 60 mg/kg which was relatively low. The reference substances, ursolic and oleanolic acid, showed low toxicity with LC50 of 0.95 and 0.10 mg/mL, respectively [14]. These studies therefore conclude that the African wild olive is non-toxic and can be used as medical drug.

3. Conclusion

Olea africana has a varied range of documented medicinal uses such as treatment for eye infections, urinary tract infections, headaches, sore throat, diuretics and hypertension. However, little is known pharmacologically regarding the African olive. The mentioned pharmacological studies found the plant to have hypoglycaemic, antihypertensive, antibacterial, antidiarrhoeal, anti-atherosclerotic and antioxidant activities. These bioactivities are elicited by compounds isolated from the plant including oleuropein, ursolic and oleanolic acid. Further scientific research is required to attain the traditional therapeutic potential, identification of potential mechanism of action and toxicity of the African olive.

Author details

Nontokozo Z. Msomi and Mthokozisi. B. C Simelane*

*Address all correspondence to: simelanem2@ukzn.ac.za

Department of Biochemistry, School of Life Science, University of KwaZulu-Natal, Pietermaritzburg, South Africa

References

[1] Okigbo RN, Anuagasi CL, Amadi JE. Advances in selected medicinal and aromatic plants indigenous to Africa. Journal of Medicinal Plants Research. 2009;3(2):86–95. ISSN: 1996–0875

[2] Borokini TI, Omotayo FO. Phytochemical and ethnobotanical study of some selected medicinal plants from Nigeria. Journal of Medicinal Plants Research. 2010;6(7):1106–1118. doi:10.5897/JMPR09.430

[3] Ojewole JAO. Anticonvulsant effect of *Rhus chirindensis* (Baker F.) (Anacardiaceae) stem bark aqueous extract in mice. Journal of Ethnopharmacology. 2008;117:130–135. doi: 10.1016/j.jep.2008.01.026

[4] Masoko P, Makgapeetja DM. Antibacterial, antifungal and antioxidant activity of *Olea africana* against pathogenic yeast and nosocomial pathogens. BMC Complementary and Alternative Medicine. 2015;15(409):1–9. doi:10.1186/s12906-015-0941-8

[5] Dyubeni L, Buwa LV. An ethnobotanical study of plants used for the treatment of ear, nose and throat (ENT) infections in Nkonkobe Municipality, South Africa. Journal of Medicinal Plants Research. 2012;6(4):2721–2726. doi:10.5897/JMPR10.869

[6] World Health Organisation. Progress report on decade of traditional medicine in the African region. WHO Regional Office for Africa [Internet]. 2011. Available from: http://www.afro.who.int/index.php?option=com_docman&task=doc_download&gid=6665. [Accessed: 2016-08-18]

[7] Xego S, Kambizi L, Nchu F. Threatened medicinal plants of South Africa: case of the family Hyacinthaceae. African Journal of Traditional, Complementary and Alternative Medicines. 2016;13(3):169–180. doi:10.4314/ajtcam.v3i3.20

[8] Ndhlala AR, Stafford GI, Finnie JF, Van Staden J. Commercial herbal preparations in KwaZulu-Natal, South Africa: the urban face of traditional medicine. South African Journal of Botany. 2011;77:830–843. doi:10.1016/j.sajb.2011.09.002

[9] Deutschländer MS, van de Venter M, Roux S, Louw J, Lall N. Hypoglycaemic activity of four plant extracts traditionally used in South Africa for diabetes. Journal of Ethnopharmacology. 2009;129:619–624. doi:10.1016/j.jep.2009.04.052

[10] Kisangau DP, Lyaruu HVM, Hosea KM, Joseph CC. Use of traditional medicines in the management of HIV/AIDS opportunistic infections in Tanzania: a case in the Bukoba rural district. Journal of Ethnobiology and Ethnomedicine. 2007;3(9):1–8. doi: 10.1186/1746-4269-3-29

[11] Simelane MBC, Shonhai A, Shode FO, Smith P, Singh M, Opoku AR. Anti-plasmodial activity of some Zulu medicinal plants and of some triterpenes isolated from them. Molecules. 2013:18:12313–12323. doi: 10.3390/molecules181012313

[12] Muthee JK, Gakuya DW, Mbaria JM, Kareru PG, Mulei CM, Njonge FK. Ethnobotanical study of anthelmintic and other medicinal plants traditionally used in Loitoktok district of Kenya. Journal of Ethnopharmacology. 2011;135:15–21. doi:10.1016/j.jep.2011.02.005

[13] Ojewole JAO. Analgesic, anti-inflammatory and hypoglycaemic effects of Rhus chirindensis (Baker F.) [Anacardiaceae] stem-bark aqueous extract in mice and rats. Journal of Ethnopharmacology. 2007;113:338–345. doi:10.1016/j.jep.2007.06.025

[14] Somova LI, Shode FO, Ramnanan P, Nadar A. Antihypertensive, antiatherosclerotic and antioxidant activity of triterpenoids isolated from *Olea europaea,* subspecies africana leaves. Journal of Ethnopharmacology. 2003;84:299–305. pii:S0378–8741(02) 00332-X

[15] Cuneo P, Leishman MR. African Olive (Olea europaea subsp. Cuspidata) as an environmental weed in eastern Australia: a review. Cunninghamia. 2006;9(4):545–577. ISSN: 545–577

[16] Hashmi MA, Khan A, Hanif M, Farooq U, Perveen S. Traditional uses, phytochemistry, and pharmacology of Olea europaea (Olive). Evidence-Based Complementary and Alternative Medicine. Hindawi Publishing Corporation. 2015;2015:1–29. doi: 10.1155/2015/541591

[17] Wallander E, Albert VA. Phylogeny and classification of Oleaceae based on RPS16 and TRNL-F sequence data. American Journal of Botany. 2000;87(12):1827–1841.

[18] Kaniewski D, Van Campo E, Boiy T, Terral JF, Khadari B, Besnard G. Primary domestication and early uses of the emblematic olive tree: palaeobotanical, historical and molecular evidence from the Middle East. Biological Reviews. 2012;87:885–899. doi: 10.1111/j.1469-185X.2012.00229.x

[19] Khan H, Khan SA. Blessed tree of olive. Asian Journal of Pharmaceutical and Clinical Research. 2016;9(3):32–34.

[20] Besnard G, Greene PS, Serville A. The genus Olea: molecular approaches of its structure and relationships to other Oleaceae. Acta Botanica Gallica. 2002;149(1):49–66. doi: 10.1080/12538078.2002.10515928

[21] Hegazi ESS, Hegazi AA, Naguib MM, El-Attar HA. Anatomical study on the junction and location of abscission zone of olive fruit pedicels as affected by chemical loosening agents. Journal of Horticultural Science and Ornamental Plants. 2016;8(1):19–25. doi: 10.5829/idosi.jhsop.2016.8.1.1168

[22] Sheidaia M, Noormohammadi Z, Dehghani A, Parvini F, Hoshiar-Parsian H, Hosseini-Mazinani M. Intra-specific morphological and molecular diversity in brown olive (Olea Cuspidata) of Iran. Science Asia. 2010;36:187–193. doi:10.2306/scienceasia1513-1874.2010.36.18

[23] Haloui E, Marzouk Z, Marzouk B, Bouftira I, Bouraoui A, Fenina N. Pharmacological activities and chemical composition of the *Olea europaea* L. leaf essential oils from 14

Aromatic and Medicinal Plants Tunisia. Journal of Food, Agriculture and Environment. 2010;8(2):204–208. ISSN: 1459–0263

[24] Amabeoku GJ, Bamuamba K. Evaluation of the effects of Olea europaea L. subsp. africana (Mill.) P.S. Green (Oleaceae) leaf methanol extract against castor oil-induced diarrhoea in mice. Journal of Pharmacy and Pharmacology. 2010;62:368–373. doi:10.1211/jpp/62.03.0012

[25] Mkize N, Hoelmer KA, Villet MH. A survey of fruit-feeding insects and their parasitoids occurring on wild olives, *Olea europaea* ssp. *cuspidata,* in the Eastern Cape of South Africa. Biocontrol Science and Technology. 2008;18: 991-1004. doi: 10.1080/09583150802450154

[26] Orwa C, Mutua A, Kindt R, Jamnadass R, Simons A. Agroforestree Database: a tree reference and selection guide version 4.0. World Agroforestry Centre, Kenya [Internet]. 2009. Available from: http://www.worldagroforestry.org/af/treedb/. [Accessed: 2016-4-28]

[27] Saxena M, Saxena J, Nema R, Singh D, Gupta A. Phytochemistry of medicinal plants. Journal of Pharmacognosy and Phytochemistry. 2013;1(6):168–182. ISSN:2278–4136

[28] Long HS, Tilney PM, Wyk BEV. The ethnobotany and pharmacognosy of *Olea europaea* subsp. africana (Oleaceae). South African Journal of Botany. 2010;79:324–331. doi: 10.1016/j.sajb.2009.12.005

[29] Douglas K, Kiplimo JJ, Chirchir D. Phytochemistry and antibacterial activity of extracts from medicinal plant Olea africana. African Journal of Pharmacy and Pharmacology, Biochemistry and Behavior. 2016;10(15):330–336. doi:10.5897/AJPP2016.4543

[30] Tsukamoto H, Hisada S, Nishibe S. Coumarin and secoiridoid glucosides from bark *Olea africana* and *Olea capensis*. Chemical and Pharmaceutical Bulletin. 1985;33(1):396–399.

[31] Ryan D, Robards K. Phenolic compounds in olives. Analyst. 1998;123:31–44. doi: 10.1039/A708920A

[32] Soler-Rivas C, Espin JC, Wichers HJ. Oleuropein and related compounds. Journal of the Science of Food and Agriculture. 2000;80:1013–1023.

[33] Elberry AA, Harraz FM, Gharei SA, Gabr SA, Nagy AA, Abdel-Sattar E. Methanolic extract of Marrubium vulgare ameliorates hyperglycemia and dyslipidemia in strepto28 zotocin-induced diabetic rats. International Journal of Diabetes Mellitus. 2015;3:37–44. ISSN: 0975–8585

[34] Visiolil F, Bellosta S, Galli C. Oleuropein, the bitter principle of olives, enhances nitric oxide production by mouse macrophages. Life Sciences. 1998;62(6):541–546. pii:S0024-3205(97)01150-8

[35] Sawai S, Saito K. Triterpenoid biosynthesis and engineering in plants. Frontiers in Plant Science. 2011;2(25):1–8. doi:10.3389/fpls.2011.00025

[36] Pollier J, Goossens A. Oleanolic acid. Phytochemistry. Elsevier. 2012;77:10–15. doi: 10.1016/j.phytochem.2011.12.022

[37] Ikeda Y, Murakami A, Ohigashi H. Ursolic acid: an anti- and pro-inflammatory triterpenoid. Molecular Nutrition and Food Research. 2008;52:26–42. doi:10.1002/mnfr.200700389

[38] Bourgaud F, Hehn A, Larbat R, Doerper S, Gontier E, Kellner S, Matern U. Biosynthesis of coumarins in plants: a major pathway still to be unravelled for cytochrome P450 enzymes. Phytochemistry Reviews. 2006;5:293–308. doi:10.1007/s11101-006-9040-2

[39] Venugopala KN, Rashmi V, Odhav B. Review on natural coumarin lead compounds for their pharmacological activity. BioMed Research International. Hindawi Publishing Corporation. 2013;2013:1–14. doi:10.1155/2013/963248

[40] Malik J, Karan M, Vasisht K. Attenuating effect of bioactive coumarins from Convolvulus pluricaulis on scopolamine-induced amnesia in mice. Natural Product Research. 2016;30(5):578-582. doi: 10.1080/14786419.2015.1025398

[41] Kareru PG, Gachanja AN, Keriko JM, Kenji GM. Antimicrobial activity of some medicinal plants used by herbalists in Eastern Province, Kenya. African Journal of Traditional, Complementary and Alternative Medicines. 2008;5(1):51–55. ISSN: 0189–6016

[42] Agrawal M, Nandini D, Sharma V, Chauhan NS. Herbal remedies for treatment of Hypertension. International Journal of Phamaceutical Sciences and Research. 2010;1(5): 1–21. ISSN: 0975–8232

[43] Grace OM, Prendergast HDV, Jäger AK, Van Staden J. Bark medicines used in traditional healthcare in KwaZulu-Natal, South Africa: an inventory. South African Journal of Botany. 2003;69(3):301–363. ISSN: 0254–6299

[44] Kipkore W, Wanjohi B, Rono H, Kigen G. A study of the medicinal plants used by the Marakwet Community in Kenya. Journal of Ethnobiology and Ethnomedicine. 2014; 10(24):1–22. doi:10.1186/1746-4269-10-24

[45] Fratkin E. Traditional medicine and concepts of healing among Samburu Pastoralists of Kenya. Journal of Ethnobiology. 1996;16(1):63–97.

[46] Nanyingi MO, Mbaria JM, Lanyasunya AL, Wagate CG, Koros KB, Kaburia HF, Munenge RW, Ogara WO. Ethnopharmacological survey of Samburu district, Kenya. Journal of Ethnobiology and Ethnomedicine. 2008;4(14):1–12. doi:10.1186/1746-4269-4-14

[47] Reida KA, Maesa A, Van Staden J, De Kimpe N, Mulholl DA, Verschaeve L et al. Evaluation of the mutagenic and antimutagenic effects of South African plants. Journal of Ethnopharmacology. 2006;106(1):44–50. doi:10.1016/j.jep.2005.11.030

[48] Bisi-Johnson MA, Obi CL, Kambizi L, Nkomo M. A survey of indigenous herbal diarrhoeal remedies of O.R. Tambo district, Eastern Cape Province, South Africa. African Journal of Biotechnology. 2010;9(8):1245–1254. ISSN: 1684–5315

[49] Bhat RB. Medicinal plants and traditional practices of Xhosa people in the Transkei region of Eastern Cape South Africa. Indian Journal of Traditional Knowledge. 2014;13(2):292–298.

[50] Abdel-Sattar EA, Abdallah HM, Khedr A, Abdel-Naim AB. Chemical and biological assessment of African Olive leaf extract. Research Journal of Pharmaceutical, Biological and Chemical Sciences. 2012;3(4):155-172. ISSN: 0975-8585

[51] Douglas K, Jeruto J. Phytochemistry and antimicrobial activity of extracts from medicinal plants *Tithonia diversifolia* and *Olea africana*. British Journal of Pharmaceutical Research. 2016;12(3):1–7. doi:10.9734/BJPR/2016/26566

5

Aromatherapeutic Textiles

Angela Cerempei

Abstract

Only innovative products will be sustainable to open up new markets and new horizons for textile industry. As a response to consumer demand, in recent years textile manufacturers are demonstrating increasing interest in added value products by getting the insect repellents, cosmetics, antimicrobials, phase-change materials, fire retardants, counterfeiting, polychromic and thermochromic effects. Aromatherapy application in textile industry led to a series of value-added products that give besides comfort a number of other properties (anti-acne, antimicrobial, fragrance, anti-inflammatory sedation, or soothing properties). In recent years, aromatherapeutic textiles were applied in many fields such as food, cosmetics, medicine, tobacco, textiles, leather, papermaking and pharmaceutical industries. The purpose of this chapter was to present the essential oils used in textile finishing, textile supports used for aroma finishing, embedding methods and the controlled release of essential oils.

Keywords: aromatherapy, essential oils, textile materials

1. Introduction

Although medicinal plants have been used for centuries as remedies for human diseases, in recent years, they have reached a great interest due to their low toxicity, pharmacological activities and economic viability. It shows a more pronounced shift from chemical and nonsustainable products to natural products that are not harmful, biodegradable and with health and wellness benefits [1]. After Mahboob et al., a good part of the population prefer traditional medicine because of the scarcity and cost-effectiveness of this sector.

Natural additives from plants can be compounds, groups of compounds, or essential oils [2]. Among natural additives, essential oils present a particular interest due to multiple benefits it shows such as antiviral, antifungal, antibacterial, antioxidant, antiparasitic, insecticidal, radical-scavenging properties, anti-inflammatory, antiseptic, germicide, healing and emollient effects.

Essential oils are made up of complex mixtures of several hydrocarbons (alcohols, terpenes, aldehydes, esters, phenols, oxides and ketones) and are obtained by conventional or advanced methods (**Figure 1**) [3, 4].

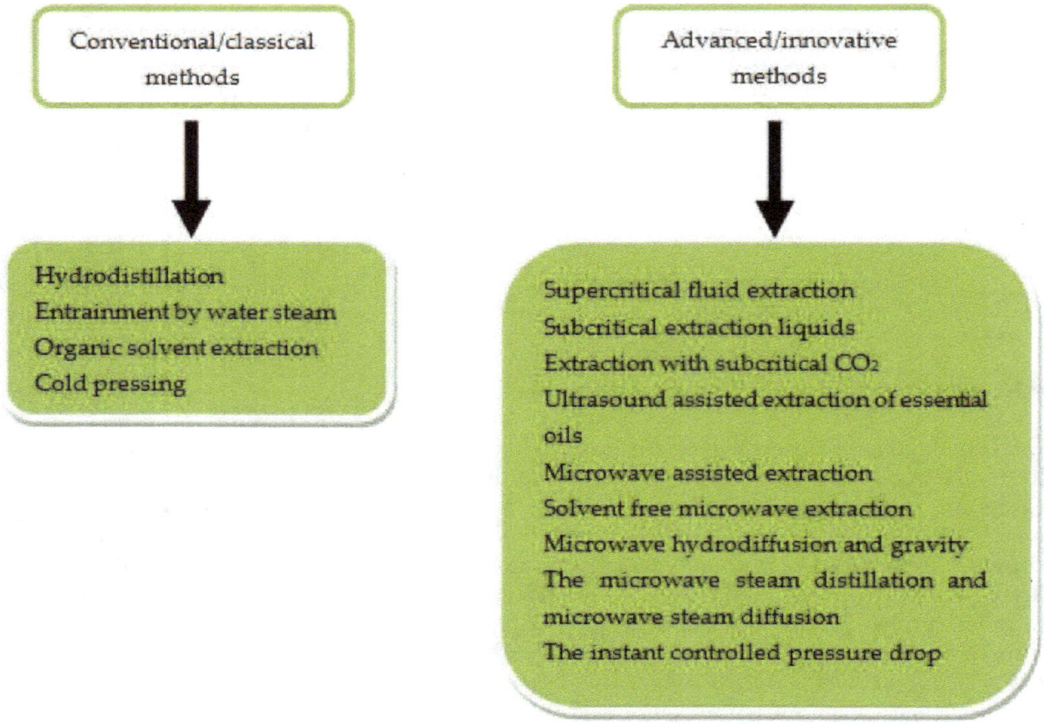

Figure 1. Extraction methods of essential oils.

Essential oils are fat soluble and thus they have the ability to permeate the skin membranes and drained into the systemic circulation, which reaches all targets organs as described by Radulovic et al. [5] and Kandori [6]. Essential oils are considered "vital force" of the plants. The role of these oils in plants is similar to that of the blood in the body. Fat-soluble structure of essential oils is similar to that of cells and tissues in the human body. This makes them compatible with human proteins and allows them to be easily identified and accepted by the body. Due to the fat-soluble structure and very small-size molecules, essential oils serve as transport agents that easily penetrates the cell membrane. Only one application of essential oils is sufficient to stimulate and revitalize the entire body. Recent research has shown that essential oils are able to penetrate the barrier blood/brain due to their small size (≤500 amu) [7].

2. Chemical composition of essential oils

Essential oils represent less than 5% from vegetal dry matter and are complex mixtures of volatile compounds extracted from plants [8].

Chemical composition of the main essential oils used in textile industry, identified by gas chromatography (GC) and GC-mass spectrometry (GC-MS), is presented in **Table 1**:

Essential oil	Chemical type	Main compounds	Composition (%)	References
Peppermint	Oxygenated compounds	Menthol	36	[11]
		Menthone	21.24	
		Menthyl acetate	6.92	
		Eucalyptol	6.58	
		Isomenthone	4.71	
		Neomenthol	4.06	
	Bicyclic sesquiterpene	β-Caryophyllene	2.07	
	Monoterpenes	Pulegone	1.72	
		D-Limonene	2.09	
		β-Pinene	1.02	
		Menthofuran	3.00	
Citronella	Oxygenated compounds	Citronellal	55.24	[12]
		Citronellol	13.41	
		Geraniol	26.29	
Thyme	Oxygenated compounds	Carvacrol	14.1–77.6	[13]
		Thymol	0.5–27.8	
		Borneol	0.2–16.3	
	Monoterpenes	γ-Terpinene	3.8–6.6	
		p-Cymene	3.5–7.9	
		α-pinene	1.2–7.8	
Ocimum sanctum L.	Oxygenated compounds	Carvacrol	2.04	[14]
		Eugenol	61.30%	
	Bicyclic sesquiterpene	β-Caryophyllene	11.89%	
	Monocyclic sesquiterpenes	Germacrene-D	9.14%	
	Tricyclic sesquiterpene	α-Cubebene	2.54%	
	Byclic sesquiterpenes	β-Selinene	1.34%	
Lavender	Monoterpenes	α-Pinene	3.4%	[15]
	Oxygenated monoterpenes	1,8-cineole	33.0%	
		Camphor	23.1%	
		α-Bisabolool	14.1%	
	Monoterpene	β-Pinene	4.1%	
Sage	Oxygenated monoterpenes	1,8-cineole	13.7%	
		Camphor	23.8%	
	Bicyclic monoterpene	cis-thujone	5.9%	
		Camphene	5.2%	
Rosemary	Bicyclic Monoterpenes	α-Pinene	28.2%	

Essential oil	Chemical type	Main compounds	Composition (%)	References
	Oxygenated monoterpenes	1,8-cineole	7.4%	
		Camphor	7.9%	
	Oxygenated compounds	Borneol	6.5%	
Chamomile	Monoterpenes	Sabinene	27.9%	
		β-Pinene	16.0%	[16]
		Limonene	2.0%	
	Oxygenated compounds	4-terpineol	1.4%	
	Monoterpenes	α-Pinene	43.9%	
Lemongrass	Oxygenated compounds	α-Citral (geranial)	43.356	[17]
		β-Citral (neral)	36.548	
		Geranyl N-butyrate	2.661	
	Sesquiterpenes	β-Caryophyllene	1.998	
	Monoterpene	cis-Verbenol	1.495	
		Camphene	1.005	
Citrus	Monoterpenes	Limonene	84.73–98	[18, 19]
		β-Pinene	1.37–3.36	
		Sabinene	0.28	
		α-Pinene	0.27–1.06	
		Myrcene	1.2–2.16	
	Oxygenated compounds	Octanol	0.34–0.54%	
		L-α-Terpineol	2.80	
		Terpinen-4-ol	1.18	
Geranium	Oxygenated compounds	Citronellol	26.7	[20]
		Geraniol	13.4	
		Nerol	8.7	
		Citronellyl formate	7.1	
		Geranyl formate	2.5	
	Sesquiterpenes	β-Caryophyllene	1.5	
		10-epi-g-Eudesmol	4.4	
	Oxygenated compounds	Geranyl propionate	1.00	
		Geranyl tiglate	1.0	
		Geranyl butyrate	1.4	
Turmeric	Sesquiterpenes	α-Phellandrene	33.9	[21]
	Oxygenated monoterpenes	Eucalyptol (1,8-cineole)	10.6	
	Monoterpenes	Terpinolene	21.1	

Essential oil	Chemical type	Main compounds	Composition (%)	References
		α-Pinene	1.7	
		Myrcene	3.3	
		p-Cymene	5.6	
		γ-Terpinene	2.9	
	Oxygenated compounds	Carvacrol	2.2	
		Curlone	1.3	
Eucalyptus	Monoterpenes	α-Pinene	3.8	[22]
	Sesquiterpenes	α-Phellandrene	1.9	
		Aromadendrene	19.7	
		Allo-aromadendrene	2.5	
		Ledene	3.1	
	Oxygenated monoterpenes	Eucalyptol (1,8-cineole)	19.8	
		Isovaleraldehyde	2.4	
	Oxygenated Sesquiterpenes	Epiglobulol	6.4	
		Globulol	23.6	
		Eudesmol	2.1	

Table 1. Chemical composition of essential oils.

2.1. Terpene hydrocarbons

Terpenes are found in a wide variety of essential oils and many of them are of industrial importance [4]:

- *Monoterpene hydrocarbons*: Monoterpene consists of two isoprene units and can be classified into three categories: acyclic, monocyclic and bicyclic. The chief sources of the monoterpenes and their derivatives are the essential oils obtained by distillation or extraction under pressure of various plant parts [9].
- *Sesquiterpenes*: Sesquiterpenes are made of isoprene units and have empirical formula of $C_{15}H_{24}$. Some plant-derived sesquiterpenoids have been identified as anti-inflammatory and anti-carcinogenic species [10].

2.2. Oxygenated compounds

- *Phenols* (thymol, eugenol, carvacrol and chavicol);
- *Alcohols* (linalol, menthol, borneol, santalol, nerol, citronellol and geraniol);
- *Aldehydes* (citral, myrtenal, cuminaldehyde, citronellal, cinnamaldehyde and benzaldehyde);

- *Ketones* (carvone, menthone, pulegone, fenchone, camphor, thujone and verbenone);
- *Esters* (linalyl acetate, geraniol acetate, eugenol acetate and bornyl acetate);
- *Lactones* (nepetalactone, bergaptene, costuslactone, dihydronepetalactone and alantrolactone);
- *Coumarins* (warfarin, acenocumarol and phenprocoumon);
- *Ethers* (linalyl acetate, geraniol acetate, eugenol acetate and bornyl acetate);
- *Oxides* (bisabolone oxide, linalool oxide, sclareol oxide and ascaridole).

3. Application of essential oils in textile field

Due to essential oils that can act both at local level and through odor, they have great important applications in many fields such as food, cosmetics, medicine, tobacco, textile, leather, papermaking, pharmaceutical and perfume industries [23].

Essential oils add much value to the textile materials. The most commonly used essential oil in aroma finishing is lavender essential oil due to its properties: anti-acne, antibacterial, calming, anti-inflammatory, treatment of eczema and dermatitis. The most used essential oils in the textile industry are presented in **Table 2**.

Introducing the concept of aromatherapy, textile materials came with increasing consumer demands in terms of quality, comfort and functionality of textiles. There was a shift in their

Essential oil	Final product destination/effect	References
Peppermint	Sedative, stimulatory, antiviral, and antibacterial properties	[24]
Citronella	Mosquito repellent	[25]
Thyme *Ocimum sanctum* L.	Antimicrobial natural textiles	[26, 27]
Lavender	Garment's packaging and storage system Health and well-being Medical applications in treatments at skin level Antibacterial textiles	[28–30]
Chamomile	Garment's packaging and storage system Health and well-being	[31]
Moluccella spinosa L.	Antibacterial activity for historical textiles	[32]
Lemongrass	Antibacterial and antifungal properties	[33]
Citrus species	Medical textiles Fragrant textiles Cosmetic textiles	[34–37]
Geranium	Health-care textiles	[38]
Turmeric	Food-packaging materials	[39]
Eucalyptus	Antibacterial wound dressing	[40]
Rosemary Sage Lavender	Health-care textiles Antimicrobial skin-care textiles Nonwoven textile shoe insoles	[41–43]

Table 2. Major essential oils used in textile finishing.

values. Instead of wanting the finest natural materials, people look at beauty through engineering, innovative design, smart appearance and added value of products [44].

Aroma finish is a process by which the textile materials are treated with bioactive systems (e.g., chitosan/essential oil, alginate/essential oil systems) and finally get the multifunctional properties such as therapeutic effects and a feeling of well-being and freshness in the wearer.

Aromatherapy textiles are used in medicine and alternative healing, home textiles, body-care textiles, household cleaning and cosmetic products.

Aromatherapeutic textiles first appeared on the market were scented women's tights. Hosiery and intimate apparel have been the more widely explored product categories to apply aroma finishing. In recent years, a number of companies around the world turned their attention to aromatherapy textiles. Woolmark™ is applying aroma technology to hosiery, lingerie, socks, outdoor clothing, underwear, carpeting and other interior textiles. The Invista Company, owner of fiber brands such as LYCRA®, TACTEL® and SUPPLEX®, launched the LYCRA® Body Care Collection that includes moisturizing and fragrance features in the yarns to enhance the wearer's sense of well-being in the intimate apparel category. The Nike clothing brand has also explored encapsulation methods to a limited extent [45, 46].

Cooperation of specialists from medical and textile fields leads to rapid development in various fields, such as medical, barrier, hygiene and controlled-release textiles. Textiles used for obtaining aroma products are presented in **Table 3**.

Textiles	Destination	References
Linen/cotton blended fabric 100% eco-friendly cotton knitted fabrics Cotton/ regenerated bamboo (50/50) knitted fabrics Flax knitted fabrics	Antimicrobial protection	[47–57]
knitted fabrics (plain stitch) of polyamide	Cosmeto-textiles	[48]
Pure cotton Polyester/coton (40:60) blend fabrics Silk Synthetic fibres (polyamide or polyester)	Flavors and fragrances in textile applications	[49–52, 55, 56]
100% Viscose Hydroentangled nonwoven	Medical textiles	[53]
Nylon net fabrics Cotton fabrics	Mosquito repellent efficiency	[54]

Table 3. Textiles used in aromatherapy.

4. Embedding techniques of essential oils

Losses by evaporation and difficulties in their controlled release make essential oils commercial application limited. In this case, nanocarrier systems (lipid-based particles, nanoemulsions and biocompatible polymer-based particles) can provide an ideal solution for realizing a controlled and targeted delivery of the essential oil. In the last few years, the application of a biocompatible and biodegradable polymer-based formulations as a controlled-release form has generated immense interest [58]. Because polymers (e.g., chitosan, alginates, starch, poly (DL-lactide-co-glycolide), poly-ε-caprolactone, polyethylene glycol, gum Arabic, maltodextrin, modified starches, mesquite gum) are friendly for the environment and safe for human health, they are commonly used in medicine, pharmacy, textiles, food and other fields [59]. As known, essential oils are adsorbed by the skin from the textile fabric through a mechanism of controlled release [60].

Bioactive systems are applied to the textile materials by a variety of techniques such as follows.

4.1. Microencapsulation techniques

Microcapsules are spherical or irregular shape (1–100 μm) containing one or more active ingredients (core) coated by synthetic or natural polymer (shell) material which gives controlled release of core materials. The core may contain a solid or liquid substances, solutions or suspensions and mixture of solids or liquids.

The shell material is generally formed of a polymer that must meet some conditions:

- Physicochemical compatibility with the core material
- Flexibility
- Impermeability
- Stability

Compatibility from core and wall material is an important criterion for efficacy microcapsules. Core size plays an important role in the diffusion, permeability, or controlled release of the active compound. The wall material protects temporarily or permanently the core from external factors and may be:

- Permeable
- Semipermeable (wall material is impermeable to the active compound and permeable to liquids with low molecular weight)
- Waterproof (membrane protects the active compound from external factors. Active compound is released by breakage or degradation of the wall) [61]

The main used methods of microencapsulation are shown in **Table 4** [62].

Microcapsules (core-shell system) in terms of morphology can be classified into mononuclear and polynuclear matrix (**Figure 2**).

Microencapsulation techniques			
Chemical methods	Simple coacervation Complex coacervation Coacervation phase separation Solvent extraction Solvent evaporation In situ polymerization Interfacial polymerization Nanoencapsulation Matrix polymerization Liposome polymerization	Physical methods	Spray drying Spray chilling Pan coating Rotary disk atomization Air-suspension coating Stationary nozzle coextrusion Multiorifice-centrifugal process Centrifugal extrusion

Table 4. Encapsulation process.

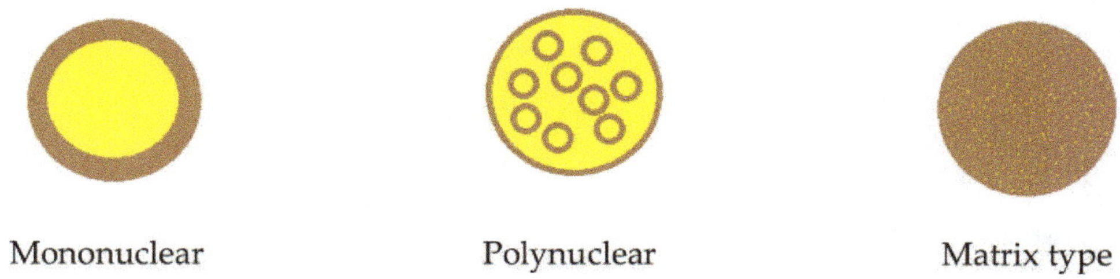

Figure 2. Morphology of microcapsules.

The microcapsules have many advantages, among which the most important are:

- protection of biologically active compound against environment;
- extends the life of biologically active compound by avoiding degradation reactions (oxidation and dehydration);
- controlled release of biologically active compound;
- microorganisms and enzyme immobilization.

The main useful shell materials used for obtaining microcapsules are presented in **Figure 3**.

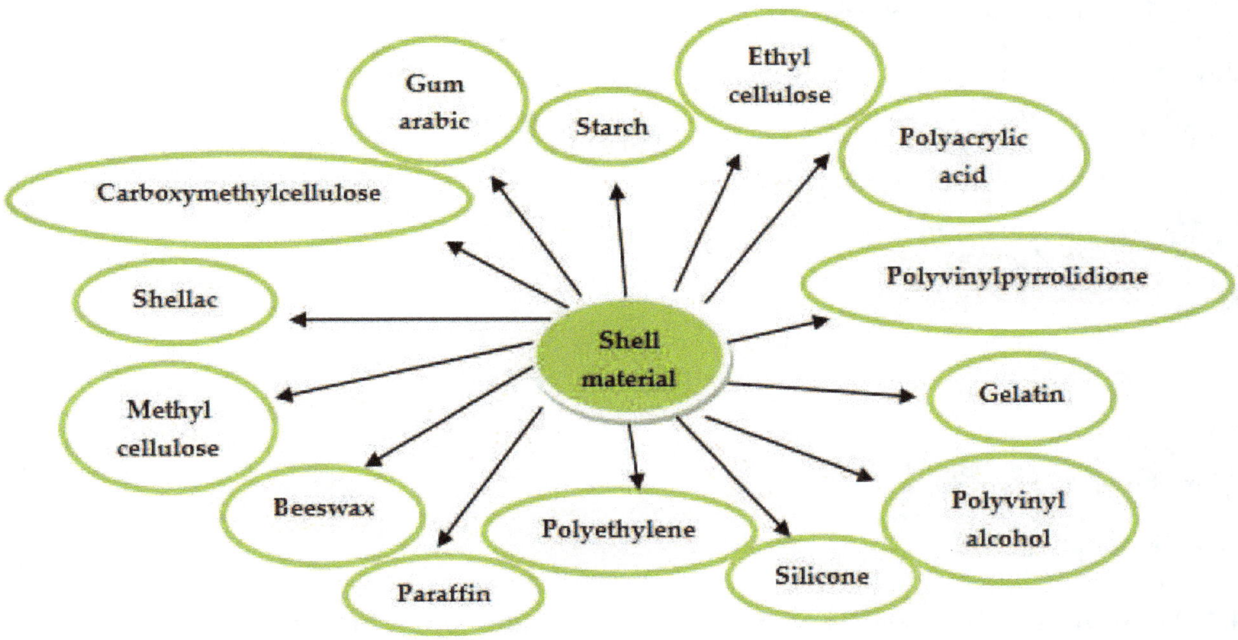
Shell material
Gum arabic
Starch
Ethyl cellulose
Polyacrylic acid
Carboxymethylcellulose
Polyvinylpyrrolidione
Shellac
Gelatin
Methyl cellulose
Polyvinyl alcohol
Beeswax
Polyethylene
Silicone
Paraffin

Figure 3. The main useful shell materials.

4.2. Application of biologically active compounds in the form of hydrogels

Hydrogel is a water-swollen and cross-linked polymeric network produced by the reaction of one or more monomers. The hydrogels can be classified on different bases as detailed below [63]:

Hydrogel source:

- Natural

- Synthetic hydrogels

Polymeric composition:

- Homopolymeric hydrogels

- Copolymeric hydrogels

- Multipolymer interpenetrating polymeric hydrogel

Hydrogels configuration:

- Amorphous hydrogels

- Semicrystalline

- Crystalline

Type of cross-linking:

- Chemically cross-linked networks

- Physical cross-linked networks

Physical appearance of hydrogels:

- Matrix

- Film

- Microsphere

Network electrical charge:

- Nonionic

- Ionic

- Amphoteric

- Zwitterionic

4.3. Application of biologically active compounds in the form of polymer matrices

There are various materials that can be used to attach the biologically active compounds, such as synthetic polyelectrolytes, natural polyelectrolytes, inorganic nanoparticles, fats, dyes, or polyvalent ions.

Generally, for polymer matrices, two classes of materials were used:

Natural materials [64] include

- Carbohydrates: agarose, carrageenan, alginate, chitosan, gellan gum and hyaluronic acid

- Proteins: collagen, gelatin, fibrin, elastin, silk fibroin

Synthetic polymers [65]: aliphatic polyesters, polyacrylates, polyamides, polyepoxides, polyphosphazenes and poly(ethylene glycol).

4.4. Functional coatings

Functional coatings are applied to textile surfaces for decorative, protective, or functional purposes. The term "functional coatings" describes systems that presents besides basic functions (protective and decorative) and additional functions [66].

Functional coatings can be classified according to their characteristics [67] as follows:

- Functional coatings with optical properties (fluorescent, phosphorescent, or photochromic coatings)
- Functional coatings with physicochemical properties (hydrophilic or hydrophobic coatings)
- Functional coatings with thermal properties (heat-resistant coatings)
- Functional coatings with mechanical properties (anti-abrasive coatings)
- Functional coatings with electric/magnetic properties (antistatic, conductive, dielectric, or piezoelectric coatings)
- Functional coatings with hygienic properties (antimicrobial coatings)

4.5. Application of biologically active compounds by activating the textile support

Plasma treatment of textile materials is an alternative to chemical treatments in order to obtain new characteristics of the final product.

Usually, it is used in low-pressure plasma treatments and atmospheric pressure plasma treatments of textiles (ex. for hydro- and oleo-repellence). For the enhancement of the wettability of different fabrics, the plasma treatment with a dielectric barrier discharge [68] is most often used.

The main plasma treatment effects are increasing the hydrophilic character, enhancing adhesion (composite materials, coated and laminated textiles), improving dyeing and printing properties, hydrophobicity and oleophobicity, deposition of fiber coatings (metallic coatings and polymer coatings), surface cleaning, inactivation of microorganisms, influencing physical properties of fibers (optical, mechanical and electrical properties), shrink-proofing of wool, improving the efficiency of wet-finishing processes and formation of radicals [69].

4.6. Controlled release of essential oil

Micro-encapsulation ensures the storage life of essential oils and can effectively control the release rate of the biologically active compounds.

Controlled release of biologically active compounds from shell material can be classified as [70] follows:

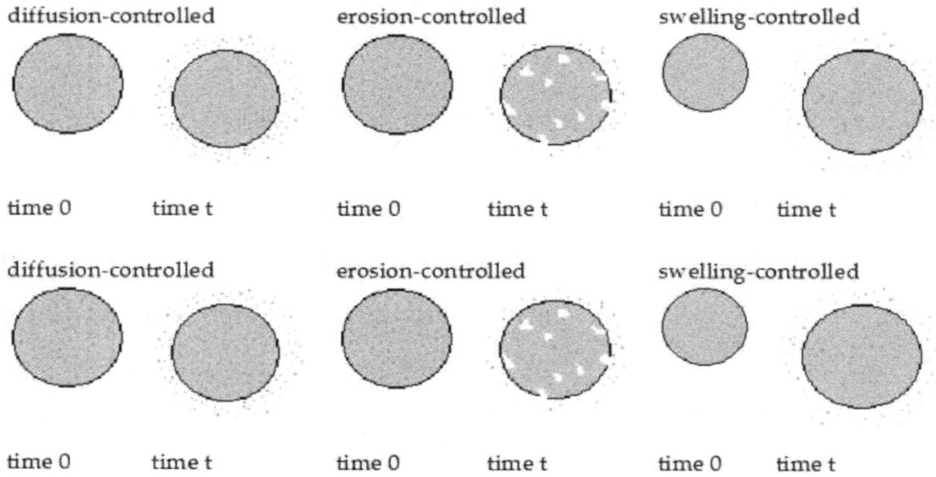

The methods for investigating the kinetics of biologically active compound release from controlled-release formulation can be classified into three categories [71]:

- Statistical methods
- Model-dependent methods: zero-order, first-order, Higuchi, Korsmeyer-Peppas model, Baker-Lonsdale model, Weibull model and so on
- Model-independent methods: difference factor (f_1), similarity factor (f_2)

The most used methods to investigate the release profile of essential oils are model-dependent methods. For empirical/semi-empirical mathematical modeling of biologically active compounds from polymeric layer, the Korsmeyer-Peppas model is generally favorable and is based on the Fickian diffusive release from a thin polymeric film [72]:

$$M_t/M_\infty = k \cdot t^n \quad (1)$$

where

K—Peppas release rate constant;

t—time (s);

Mt/M_∞—fraction of active compound released at time t;

n—the release exponent.

Transport mechanisms of active principle function are shown in **Table 5**.

The release mechanism for the biologically active compound from the textile supports is primarily based on the diffusion process of the oil molecules. The main mechanism of essential oils release from shell materials is presented in **Table 6**.

Release exponent (n)	Active compound transport mechanism	dM_t/dt as a function of time
$n = 0.5$	Fickian diffusion	$t^{-0.5}$
$0.5 < n < 1$	Non-Fickian transport	t^{n-2}
$n = 1$	Case II transport	Zero-order release
$n > 1$	Super case II transport	t^{n-1}

Table 5. Transport mechanism of biologically active compound.

Essential oil	Shell material	Release mechanism	References
Rosemary	Chitosan film	Non-Fickian mechanismZero-order mechanism	[73]
Geranium	Chitosan matrix	Fickian mechanism	[74]
Citronella	GelatinGum Arabic	Fickian mechanismNon-Fickian mechanism	[75]
CloveThyme	Orabase	Mixed mechanism	[76]
Tea tree	Sodium alginate/quaternary ammonium salt of chitosan	Ritger-Peppas mode	[77]
Calendula officinalis L.	Chitosan grafted with sodium acrylate-co-acrylamide	Non-Fickian (coupling of Fickian diffusion and relaxation of entangled chains of the encapsulating polymer)	[78]
Coriandrum sativum L.	Chitosan/alginate/inulin microcapsules	Non-Fickian transport mechanism (diffusion or diffusion-swelling-controlled process)	[79]
Peppermint Eucalyptus	Polyvinyl pyrolidine (PVP)Ethyl cellulose (EC)	Zero-order release kinetic	[80]
Cardamom	Alginate-whey protein	Fickian diffusion	[81]

Table 6. Controlled release kinetics.

5. Conclusions

Aromatherapeutic textiles are a good choice for people who want to maintain harmony between their physical and psychological comfort. Applying of essential oils on textile materials shows great potential for the value-added textiles. Aromatherapy textiles application in various fields (cosmeto-textiles, home textiles, sport wears, medical textiles, etc.) made them indispensable in day-to-day life.

Author details

Angela Cerempei

Address all correspondence to: angela.cerempei@yahoo.com

Faculty of Textiles, Leather and Industrial Management, Department of Chemical Engineering in Textile and Leather, "Gheorghe Asachi" Technical University, Iasi, Romania

References

[1] West AJ, Annett-Hitchcock KE. A critical review of aroma therapeutic application for textiles. Journal of Textile and Apparel, Technology and Management. 2014;**9**(1):1–13.

[2] Boulekbache-Makhlouf L, Rigoub P, Remini H, Adjaouda A, Khoudjaa NK, Madani K. Essential oils composition, antibacterial and antioxidant activities of hydrodistillated extract of Eucalyptus globulus fruits Z. Bey - Ould Si Saida, H. Haddadi - Guemghar, L. Boulekbache - Makhlouf, P. Rigoub, H. Remini, A. Adjaouda, N.K. Khoudjaa, K. Madani. Industrial Crops and Products. 2016;**89**:167–175.

[3] Ghosha S, Chipot N. Embedding aromatherapy essential oils into textile fabric using β-cyclodextrin inclusion compound. Indian Journal of Fibre & Textile Research. 2015; **40**:140–143.

[4] El Asbahani A, Miladi K, Badri W, Sala M, Aït Addi EH, Casabianca H, El Mousadik A, Hartmann D, Jilale A, Renaud FNR, Elaissari A. Essential oils: from extraction to encapsulation. International Journal of Pharmaceutics. 2015;**483**:220–243.

[5] Radulovic N, Dekic M, Radi ZS, Palic R. Chemical composition and antimicrobial activity of the essential oils of *Geranium columbinum* L. and *G. lucidum* L. (Geraniaceae). Turkish Journal of Chemistry. 2011;**35**:499–512.

[6] Kandori I. Diverse visitors with various pollinator importance and temporal change in important pollinators of *Geranium thunbergii* (Geraniaceae). Ecological Research. 2002; **17**:283–294.

[7] Balabai, I.V. Rasteniea, coterie nas leceat/ I.V. Balabai, A.C. Nistrean, Chisinau, 1988, 351 pages.

[8] Abraham MH, Gola JRM, Gil-Lostes J, Acree Jr. WE, Cometto-Muñizc JE. Determination of solvation descriptors for terpene hydrocarbons from chromatographic measurements. Journal of Chromatography A. 2013;**1293**:133–141.

[9] Rachwalik R, Hunger M, Sulikowskic B. Transformations of monoterpene hydrocarbons on ferrierite type zeolites. Applied Catalysis A: General. 2012;**427–428**:98–105.

[10] Duhamela N, Martin D, Larcher R, Fedrizzia B, Barker D. Convenient synthesis of deuterium labelled sesquiterpenes. Tetrahedron Letters. 2016;**57**(40):4496–4499.

[11] Skalicka-Woz′niak K, Walasek M. Preparative separation of menthol and pulegone from peppermint oil (*Mentha piperita* L.) by high-performance counter-current chromatography. Phytochemistry Letters. 2014;**10**:xciv–xcviii.

[12] Timung R, Barik CR, Purohit S, Goud VV. Composition and anti-bacterial activity analysis of citronella oil obtained by hydrodistillation: process optimization study. Industrial Crops and Products. 2016;**94**:178–188.

[13] Jamali CA, Kasrati A, Bekkouche K, Hassani L, Wohlmuth H, Leach D, Abbad A. Phenological changes to the chemical composition and biological activity of the essential oil from Moroccan endemic thyme (Thymus maroccanus Ball). Industrial Crops and Products. 2013;**49**:366–372.

[14] Kumar A, Shukla R, Singh P, Dubey NK. Chemical composition, antifungal and antiaflatoxigenic activities of *Ocimum sanctum* L. essential oil and its safety assessment as plant based antimicrobial. Food and Chemical Toxicology. 2010;**48**(2):539–543.

[15] J. González-Rivera, C. Duce, D. Falconieri, C. Ferrari, L. Ghezzi, A. Piras, M.R. Tine. Coaxial microwave assisted hydrodistillation of essential oils from five different herbs (lavender, rosemary, sage, fennel seeds and clove buds): chemical composition and thermal analysis. Innovative Food Science & Emerging Technologies. 2016;**33**:308–318.

[16] Bouchekrit M, Laouer H, Hajji M, Nasri M, Haroutounian SA, Akkal S. Essential oils from *Elaeoselinum asclepium*: chemical composition, antimicrobial and antioxidant properties. Asian Pacific Journal of Tropical Biomedicine. 2016; http://dx.doi.org/10.1016/j.apjtb.2016.07.014

[17] Leimann FV, Gonçalves OH, Machado RAF, Bolzan A. Antimicrobial activity of microencapsulated lemongrass essential oil and the effect of experimental parameters on microcapsules size and morphology. Materials Science and Engineering: C. 2009;**29**(2):430–436.

[18] Zarrad K, Hamouda AB, Chaieb I, Laarif A, Mediouni-Ben Jemâa J. Chemical composition, fumigant and anti-acetylcholinesterase activity of the Tunisian *Citrus aurantium* L. essential oils. Industrial Crops and Products. 2015;**76**:121–127.

[19] AL-Jabri NN, Hossain MA. Chemical composition and antimicrobial potency of locally grown lemon essential oil against selected bacterial strains. Journal of King Saud University – Science. 2016; http://dx.doi.org/10.1016/j.jksus.2016.08.008

[20] Sienkiewicz M, Poznańska-Kurowska K, Kaszuba A, Kowalczyk E. The antibacterial activity of geranium oil against Gram-negative bacteria isolated from difficult-to-heal wounds. Burns. 2014;**40**(5):1046–1051.

[21] Zaibunnisa AH, Norashikin S, Mamot S, Osman H. An experimental design approach for the extraction of volatile compounds from turmeric leaves (*Curcuma domestica*) using pressurised liquid extraction (PLE). LWT—Food Science and Technology. 2009;**42**(1):233–238.

[22] Bey-Ould Si Saida Z, Haddadi-Guemghara H, Boulekbache-Makhloufa L, Rigoub P, Reminia H, Adjaouda A, Khaled Khoudjaa N, Madania K. Essential oils composition,

antibacterial and antioxidant activities of hydrodistillated extract of Eucalyptus globulus fruits. Industrial Crops and Products. 2016;**89**:167–175.

[23] Hu J, Xiao Z, Zhou R, Ma S, Wang M and Li Z. Properties of aroma sustained-release cotton fabric with rose fragrance nanocapsule. Chinese Journal of Chemical Engineering. 2001;**19**(3):523–528.

[24] Ciobanu A, Mallard AI, Landy D, Brabie D, Nistor D, Fourmentin S. Retention of aroma compounds from Mentha piperita essential oil by cyclodextrins and crosslinked cyclodextrin polymers. Food Chemistry. 2013;**138**:291–297.

[25] Specos MM, García JJ, Tornesello J, Marino P, Vecchia MD, Tesoriero MV, Hermida LG. Microencapsulated citronella oil for mosquito repellent finishing of cotton textiles. Transactions of the Royal Society of Tropical Medicine and Hygiene. 2010;**104**(10):653–658.

[26] Walentowska J, Foksowicz-Flaczyk J. Thyme essential oil for antimicrobial protection of natural textiles. International Biodeterioration & Biodegradation. 2013;**84**:407–411.

[27] Ravindra KB, Murugesh Babu K. Study of antimicrobial properties of fabrics treated with *Ocimum sanctum* L. (tulsi) extract as a natural active agent. Journal of Natural Fibers. 2016;**13**(5):619–627.

[28] West A, Annett-Hitchcock K. The development of an herb-infused bag that regenerates aromatherapy textiles. International Journal of Designed Objects. 2016;**10**(2):17–30.

[29] Cerempei A, Ciobanu L, Muresan E, Măluţan C, Butnaru R. Textile materials functionalised with natural biologically active compounds. Romanian Biotechnological Letters. 2010;**15** (5):5537–5544.

[30] Balasubramanian K, Kodam KM. Encapsulation of therapeutic lavender oil in an electrolyte assisted polyacrylonitrile nanofibres for antibacterial applications. RSC Advances. 2014;**4**(97):54892–54901.

[31] West A, Annett-Hitchcock K. The development of an herb-infused bag that regenerates aromatherapy textiles. International Journal of Designed Objects. 2016;10(2):7–30.

[32] Casiglia S, Ben Jemia M, Riccobono L, Bruno M, Scandolera E, Senatore F. Chemical composition of the essential oil of *Moluccella spinosa* L. (Lamiaceae) collected wild in Sicily and its activity on microorganisms affecting historical textiles. Natural Product Research. 2015;**29**(13):1201–1206.

[33] Dutra JAP, Carvalho SG, Villanova JCO, Ayres E. Preparation of β-cyclodextrin/latex dispersion for coating of cellulose fabric. M. Cotrim. Journal of Renewable Materials. 2016;**4**(1):9–17.

[34] Wolffenbüttel AN, Zamboni A, dos Santos MK, Borille BT, Augustin OA, Mariotti KC, Leal MB, Limberger RP. Chemical components of Citrus essential oils from Brazil. Natural Products Journal. 2015;**5**(1):14–27.

[35] Kumari P, Rose NM, Jeet Singh SS. Microencapsulation of lime essential oil for fragrant textiles. Annals of Agri Bio Research. 2015;**20**(1):152–157.

[36] Chelaru C, Ignat M, Albu M, Meghea A. Polymeric microcapsules for cosmetic applications, based on Lemon essential oil (*Citrus limon*). UPB Scientific Bulletin, Series B: Chemistry and Materials Science. 2015;**77**(4):101–112.

[37] Lee AR, Han CH, Yi E. Preparation and characterization of melamine-formaldehyde microcapsules containing Citrus unshiu essential oil. Fibers and Polymers. 2014;**15** (1):35–40.

[38] Cerempei A, Muresan EI, Cimpoesu N. Biomaterials with controlled release of geranium essential oil. Journal of Essential Oil Research. 2014;26(4):267–273.

[39] Navarro S, Finkelman S. Protecting food packaging materials by natural nontoxic insect repellents. Acta Horticulturae. 2014;**1015**:137–144.

[40] Khajavi R, Abbasipour M, Barzi MG, Rashidi A, Rahimi MK, Mirzababa HH. Eucalyptus essential oil-doped alginate fibers as a potent antibacterial wound dressing. Advances in Polymer Technology. 2014;**33**(2):n/a.

[41] Cerempei A, Muresan EI, Sandu I, Chirila L, Sandu IG. Textile materials with controlled release of rosemary essential oil. Revista de Chimie. 2014;**65**(10):1154–1157.

[42] Cerempei A, Abramiuc D, Popescu C, Muresan R, Muresan A. Textile materials treated with antimicrobial skin care emulsion optimized by mathematical modelling. Industria Textila. 2014;**65**(4):213–218.

[43] Boh B, Knez E. Microencapsulation of essential oils and phase change materials for applications in textile products. Indian Journal of Fibre and Textile Research. 2006;**31** (1):72–82.

[44] Monllor P, Angeles Bonet M, Cases F. Characterization of the behaviour of flavour microcapsules in cotton fabrics. European Polymer Journal. 2007;**43**:2481–2490.

[45] Wang CX, Chen ShL. Aromachology and its applications in the textile field. Fibres & Textiles in Eastern Europe. 2005;**13**(6):41–44.

[46] "Hand-book of Technical Textiles" Edited by A.R. Horrocks and S.C. Anand. Published by Woodhead Publishing Limited in association with The Textile Institute. 2010.

[47] Walentowska J, Foksowicz-Flaczyk J. Thyme essential oil for antimicrobial protection of natural textiles. International Biodeterioration & Biodegradation. 2013;**84**:407–411.

[48] Alonso C, Martí M, Barba C, Lis M, Rubio L, Coderch L. Skin penetration and antioxidant effect of cosmeto-textiles with gallic acid. Journal of Photochemistry & Photobiology, B: Biology. 2016;**156**:50–55.

[49] Sharaf S, Higazy A, Hebeish A. Propolis induced antibacterial activity and other technical properties of cotton textiles. International Journal of Biological Macromolecules. 2013; **59**:408–416.

[50] Hu J, Xiao Z, Zhou R, Ma S, Wang M, Li Z. Properties of aroma sustained-release cotton fabric with rose fragrance nanocapsule. Chinese Journal of Chemical Engineering. 2011;**19** (3):523–528.

[51] Badulescu R, Vivod V, Jausoved D, Voncina B. Grafting of ethylcellulose microcapsules onto cotton fibers. Carbohydrate Polymers. 2008;**71**(1):85–91.

[52] Ghosh S, Chipot N. Embedding aromatherapy essential oil into textile fabric using β-cyclodextrin inclusion compound. Indian Journal of Fibre and Textile Research. 2015; **40**:140–143.

[53] Chinta SK, Landage Abhishek SM, Sonawane KD and Jalkate CB. Medical textiles – application of essential oil as antimicrobial agent on nonwoven. G.J.B.B. 2012;**1**(1):75–80.

[54] Raja ASM, Kawlekar S, Saxena S, Arputharaj A, Patil PG. Mosquito protective textiles—a review. International Journal of Mosquito Research. 2015;**2**(4):49–53.

[55] Alonso D, Gimeno M, Sepúlveda-Sánchez JD, Shirai K. Chitosan-based microcapsules containing grapefruit seed extract grafted onto cellulose fibers by a non-toxic procedure. Carbohydrate Research. 2010;**345**(6):854–859.

[56] Rodrigues SN, Martins IN, Fernandes IP, Gomes PB, Mata VG, Barreiro MF, Rodrigues AE. Scentfashion®: Microencapsulated perfumes for textile application. Chemical Engineering Journal. 2009;**149**(1–3):463–472.

[57] Rîmbu C, Cerempei A, Muresan R, Guguianu E, Ursache M, Borhan O, Muresan A. Eco-friendly antibacterial finish for natural knitted fabrics. TEKSTİL ve KONFEKSİYON. 2015;**25**(4):359–364.

[58] Cerempei A, Muresan EI, Cimpoesu N. Biomaterials with controlled release of geranium essential oil. Journal of Essential Oil Research. 2014;**26**(4):267–273.

[59] González JW, Yeguerman C, Marcovecchio D, Delrieux C, Ferrero A, Fernández Band B. Evaluation of sublethal effects of polymer-based essential oils nanoformulation on the german cockroach. Ecotoxicology and Environmental Safety. 2016;**130**:11–18.

[60] Mureşan A, Cerempei A, Dunca S, Muresan R, Butnaru R. Aromatherapeutic characteristics of cotton fabrics treated with rosemary essential oil. Cellulose Chemistry and Technology. 2009;**43**(9–10):435–442.

[61] Patil DK, Agrawal DS, Mahire RR, More DH. Synthesis, characterization and controlled release studies of ethyl cellulose microcapsules incorporating essential oil using an emulsion solvent evaporation method. American Journal of Essential Oils and Natural Products. 2016;**4**(1):23–31.

[62] Dubey R, Shami TC, Bhasker Rao KU. Microencapsulation technology and applications. Defence Science Journal. 2009;**59**(1):82–95.

[63] Ahmed EM. Hydrogel: Preparation, characterization and applications: a review. Journal of Advanced Research. 2015;**6**:105–121.

[64] Gasperini L, Mano JF and Reis RL. Natural polymers for the microencapsulation of cells. Journal of the Royal Society Interface. 2014;11(100):20140817. http://dx.doi.org/10.1098/rsif.2014.0817

[65] Olabisi RM. Cell microencapsulation with synthetic polymers. Journal of Biomedical Materials Research A. 2015;**103**(2):846–859.

[66] Edge M, Allen NS, Turner D, Robinson J, Seal K. The enhanced performance of biocidal additives in paints and coatings. Progress in Organic Coatings. 2001;**43**:10–17.

[67] Functional Coatings. Edited by Ghosh SK, 2006 WILEY-VCH Verlag GmbH & Co. KGaA, Weinheim.

[68] Zanini S, Freti S, Citterio A, Riccardi C. Characterization of hydro- and oleo-repellent pure cashmere and wool/nylon textiles obtained by atmospheric pressure plasma pre-treatment and coating with a fluorocarbon resin. Surface & Coatings Technology. 2016;**292**:155–160.

[69] Morent R, De Geyter N, Verschuren J, De Clerck K, Kiekens P, Leys C. Non-thermal plasma treatment of textiles. Surface & Coatings Technology. 2008;**202**:3427–3449.

[70] Tramón C. Modeling the controlled release of essential oils from a polymer matrix—a special case. Industrial Crops and Products. 2014;**61**:23–30.

[71] Dash S, Narasimha Murthy P, Nath L, Chowdhury P. Kinetic modeling on drug release from controlled drug delivery systems. Acta Poloniae Pharmaceutica—Drug Research. 2010;**67**(3):217–223.

[72] Maleki M, Amani-Tehrana M, Latifia M, Mathur S. Drug release profile in core–shell nanofibrous structures: a study on Peppas equation and artificial neural network modeling. Computer Methods and Programs in Biomedicine. 2014;**113**:92–100.

[73] Muresan A, Cerempei A, Dunca S, Muresan R and Butnaru R. Aromatherapeutic characteristics of cotton fabrics treated with Rosemary essential oil. Cellulose Chemistry and Technology. 2009;**43**(9–10):435–442.

[74] Cerempei A, Muresan EI and Cimpoesu N. Biomaterials with controlled release of geranium essential oil. Journal of Essential Oil Research. 2014;**26**(4):267–273.

[75] Bezerra FM, Carmona OG, Carmona CG, Lis MJ, de Moraes FF. Cellulose. Controlled release of microencapsulated citronella essential oil on cotton and polyester matrices. 2016;**23**:1459–1470.

[76] Labib GS, Aldawsari H. Innovation of natural essential oil-loaded Orabase for local treatment of oral candidiasis. Drug Design, Development and Therapy. 2015;**9**:3349–3359.

[77] Chen M, Hu Y, Zhou J, Xie Y, Wu H, Yuana T, Yang Z. Facile fabrication of tea tree oil-loaded antibacterial microcapsules by complex coacervation of sodium alginate/quaternary ammonium salt of chitosan. RSC Advances. 2016;**6**:13032–13039.

[78] Shruthi SB, Roy P, Sailaja RRN, Sengupta C. Encapsulation and release characteristics of Marigold oleoresin in chitosan grafted sodium acrylate-co-acrylamide. Advanced Materials Letters. 2016;**7**(10);795–801.

[79] Dima C, Pătraşcu L, Cantaragiu A, Alexe P, Dima Ș. The kinetics of the swelling process and the release mechanisms of *Coriandrum sativum* L. essential oil from chitosan/alginate/inulin microcapsules. Food Chemistry. 2016;**195**:39–48.

[80] Kumar A, Aggarwal G, Singh K, Harikumar SL. Comparison of vegetable and volatile oils as skin permeation enhancers for transdermal delivery of losartan potassium. Der Pharmacia Lettre. 2014;**6**(1):199–213.

[81] Zandi M, Dardmeh N, Pirsa S, Almasi H. Identification of cardamom encapsulated alginate–whey protein concentrates microcapsule release kinetics and mechanism during storage, stew process and oral consumption. Journal of Food Process Engineering. DOI: 10.1111/jfpe.12314, 2015.

6

Evaluation of Genetic Diversity in *Chlorophytum borivilianum* (Santp. and Fernan.) Using Molecular Markers: An Endangered Medicinal Plant

Sanghamitra Samantaray and
Umakanta Ngangkham

Abstract

Chlorophytum borivilianum is a traditional medicinal plant distributed throughout the tropics and subtropics. In the present investigation, RAPD and ISSR analyses were used to assess the genetic diversity among 21 accessions collected from different geographical regions of India using 20 RAPD primers and 6 ISSR primers. RAPD and ISSR primers revealed 92.26% and 82.76% polymorphism, respectively. Similarity in coefficient values ranged from 0.321 to 0.707 for RAPD and 0.363 to 0.846 for ISSR markers. The dendrogram developed by RAPD and ISSR marker-based analysis grouped the 21 accessions into different clusters. Mantel test employed for detection of goodness of fit established the cophenetic correlation value for both the primer systems and it was observed to be significant. Clustering of accessions within groups was also similar based on RAPD- and ISSR-derived dendrograms. In our study, both marker systems were similar except for the percentage polymorphism which was found to be greater using RAPD, thus indicating the greater effectiveness of RAPD primers for estimating genetic variation of *C. borivilianum*.

Keywords: *Chlorophytum borivilianum*, ISSR, RAPD, Diversity, medicinal plant

1. Introduction

All the plants considerably possess some medicinal or perfumery or mixed properties. In the course of time, the human beings were able to distinguish between the harmful and useful plants. The world Health Organization (WHO) has listed over 21,000 plant species that have been reported for medicinal uses around the world. Among these, over 100 botanicals are reported to have consistent large demand and are traded in major drug markets in the world.

In the developing countries, about 80% of the people depend upon the traditional system of the medicine, as it shows no or less side effects [1]. India is considered as a veritable emporium of medicinal and aromatic plants. In India, about 2500 plant species belonging to more than 1000 genera are used by traditional healers and about 500 plant species are utilized by 159 different pharmaceutical companies [2].

Many of the medicinal plant species are facing threats of extinction due to over and improper exploitation, habitat loss, degradation of land, urbanization, etc. On the other hand, the increasing global demand for the medicinal plants necessitates an accelerated cultivation and conservation of them. However, before the widespread domestication of such plant species is implemented, it would be important to determine their genetic diversity so that the useful genotypes could be effectively used as cultivars by farmers or breeders and it would, in turn, facilitate the efficient conservation, management and utilization of the species. For the purpose of conservation and to carry out successful breeding programmes, proper identification of the plant is of prime importance, for which an accurate, reliable and more authentic system of classification is required. Conventionally, identification and classification of plant groups are solely based on similarities and dissimilarities in morphological features, particularly, the floral character which are considered to be consistent. As already established, expression of morphological characters is the outcome of interaction between the environment and the genotype and is highly influenced by climatic and edaphic factors. Certain biochemical markers such as isozymes and storage proteins are used for identification of cultivars as well as characterization of somaclonal variation. However, the number of genetic loci generated with chemical/ biochemical (isozymes) were quite lower than detected with DNA markers [3]. Molecular techniques are very much useful not only to identify the genotypes for authentication but also to assess and exploit the genetic variability [4]. DNA fingerprinting of all the genetic resources of the medicinal plants is necessary to generate a molecular database as well as to utilize the information in a systematic manner.

During last 20 years, the advent of the PCR and the DNA sequencing techniques has allowed a very significant development of this approach, which leads to great change in the traditional vision of the classification of the organisms. The DNA marker systems are considered to be the best tools for determining the genetic diversity, as they are unlimited in number, show high polymorphism and are independent of environmental interaction, i.e. they are highly heritable. The application of the DNA marker systems in agricultural research has progressed rapidly over the past few years, especially, in the area of cultivar identification and characterization [5] as well as determination of population diversity in many plant species [6]. Among these, random amplified polymorphic DNA (RAPD) and inter-simple sequence repeats (ISSR) markers provide a larger number of potential markers that are useful for the analysis of genetic diversity, often using fast, simple and reliable protocols that minimize the amount and quality of DNA required. Genetic diversity in a population is considered to represent its evolutionary potential. Genetic variation has implications for conservation at the species level. Evidently, molecular markers could be used to derive genetic relationship with an increased level of accuracy and also can provide valuable data on diversity through their ability to detect variation at the DNA level.

Chlorophytum borivilianum Santapau and Fernandes belong to the family Liliaceae and are popularly known as safed musli. It is an important medicinal plant. Its peeled and dried fasciculated roots are considered to be a wonder drug in traditional Indian systems of medicine due to its aphrodisiac and natural tonic properties [7]. About 100 Ayurvedic preparations are available in the Indian market using *C. borivilianum* as a major ingredient [8]. Its roots are widely used for various therapeutic applications in the Ayurvedic and Unani [9] systems of medicine. Though many tribal communities of India use the fresh leaves of safed musli as Pot herb [10], however, the roots are the useful part of the plant for medicinal purposes. Dried roots of Chlorophytum contain 42% carbohydrate, 8–9% protein, 3–4% fibre and 2–17% saponin [11]. It is known to cure many physical illness and weaknesses. In recent years, its effectiveness in increasing male potency has become very popular and is now considered as an alternative to 'Viagra'. Excessive collections from its natural stands and destructive harvesting techniques coupled with poor seed germination and low vegetative multiplication ratio have made this species endangered and simultaneously provided the justification for its conservation. The cost of genetic conservation should be reduced ensuring representation of maximum genetic variation for which a set of accessions should be selected to represent the genetic diversity of a base collection with minimum redundancy [12]. Thus, the present study aimed at characterizing the genetic diversity in 21 accessions of *C. borivilianum* collected from different regions of India using RAPD and ISSR.

2. Materials and methods

2.1. Plant materials

A total of 21 accessions of *C. borivilianum* were collected from different parts of India (Gujarat, Rajasthan, Madhya Pradesh and Maharashtra) and maintained under uniform growth conditions at DMAPR, Anand, Gujarat (**Figure 1**). The name and place of collection of the material used in the study are given in **Table 1**. *C. borivilianum* is reported in Bastar Forests (Chhattisgarh), Dangs forest (Gujarat), Mount Abu, Mahi and Aravalli hills (Rajasthan) of India. It is also reported to occur in some parts of Pakistan. It is now widely cultivated in different parts of India like Andhra Pradesh, Rajasthan, Gujarat and Maharashtra on commercial basis. The CAMP workshop at IIFM, June 1999 reported the natural habitat of this plant as endangered.

2.2. Molecular characterization

2.2.1. Isolation, purification and quantification of genomic DNA

Since isolation of DNA from *C. borivilianum* was encountered with lots of problems, because of the high polysaccharides and saponin contents, a method was standardized for isolation of genomic DNA of this species. Total genomic DNA was extracted from young leaves derived from field-grown plants following the CTAB method [13] with major modifications. At the time of homogenization of the leaves, 20 mg PVP and 6.5 mM dithiothreitol (DTT) were added. The extraction buffer consisted of 4% (w/v) CTAB (cetyl trimethyl ammonium

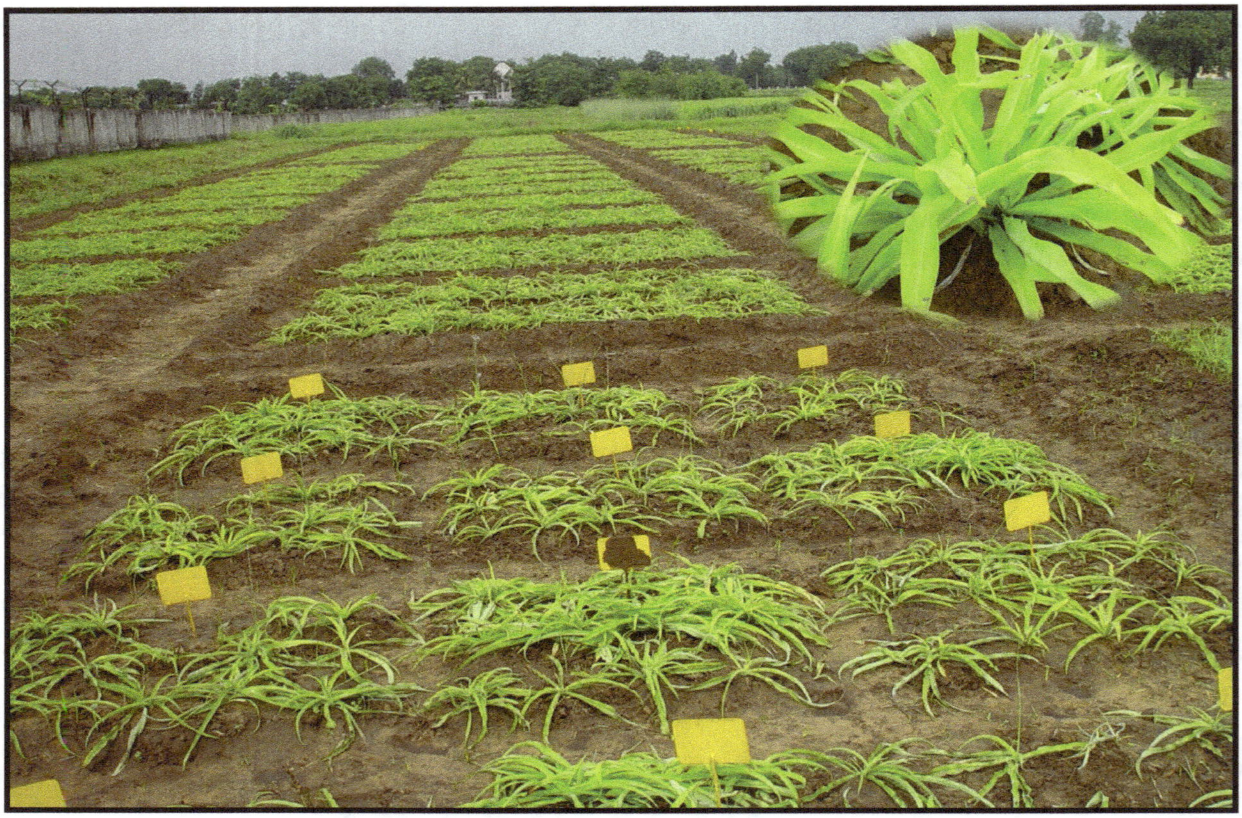

Figure 1. An overview of 21 accessions of *C. borivilianum* collected from different regions of India and grown in the field.

bromide), 3 M NaCl, 20 mM EDTA (pH, 8.0), 100 mM Tris-Cl (pH, 8.0), 50 mM ascorbic acid, 40 mM diethyl dithiocarbamic acid and 2% (v/v) ß-mercaptoethanol. The quality and quantity of the DNA were checked by 0.8% agarose gel followed by spectrophotometric measurement.

2.2.2. RAPD and ISSR analysis

RAPD analysis was performed using randomly and arbitrarily 10-base primers (Operon Technologies Inc., Alameda, California). A preliminary screening was carried out using 100 RAPD primers following the protocol of Williams et al. [14] with minor modifications. ISSR analysis was carried out using ISSR primers (Banglore Genei, India) based on the protocol of Zietkiewicz et al. [15] with some modifications. The amplified products were separated in 1.5% agarose gel for both the markers used. After electrophoresis, the gel was visualized under the UV light and photographed in a gel documentation system (Syngene, United Kingdom). The sizes of the amplicons were determined by comparing them with that of the ladder.

2.2.3. Scoring of the data for RAPD and ISSR

The data were scored as 1 for the presence and 0 for the absence of the band for each primer-accession combination for RAPD and ISSR analysis.

Sr. no.	Germplasm (name)	Place of collection
1	Ch1	Madhya Pradesh
2	Ch2	Madhya Pradesh
3	Ch3	Madhya Pradesh
4	Ch4	Madhya Pradesh
5	Ch5	Madhya Pradesh
6	Ch6	Madhya Pradesh
7	Ch7	Madhya Pradesh
8	Ch8	Madhya Pradesh
9	Ch9	Madhya Pradesh
10	Ch10	Rajasthan
11	Ch11	Rajasthan
12	Ch12	Rajasthan
13	Ch13	Rajasthan
14	Ch14	Rajasthan
15	Ch15	Maharashtra
16	Ch16	Maharashtra
17	Ch17	Maharashtra
18	Ch18	Gujarat
19	Ch19	Gujarat
20	Ch20	Gujarat
21	Ch21	Gujarat

Table 1. Detailed information of 21 accessions of *C. borivilianum*.

2.2.4. Data analysis

2.2.4.1. Resolving power (Rp)

Resolving power of the primer/primer combination was calculated as per Prevost and Wilkinson [16] as: $Rp = \Sigma IB$ [IB (band informativeness) = $1- [2 \times (0.5 - P)]$, P is the proportion of the 21 accessions containing the loci.

2.2.4.2. PIC and primer index

The primer index (PI) was calculated from the polymorphic index (PIC). The polymorphic index was calculated as $PIC = \Sigma P_{2i}$, P_i is the band frequency of the *i*th allele [17] Here, the PIC was considered to be 1-p2-q2, where p is the band frequency and q is no band frequency [18]. The PIC value was then used to calculate the RAPD and ISSR primer index. PI is the sum of the PIC of all the markers amplified by the same primer.

2.2.4.3. Jaccard's similarity

Jaccard's coefficient of similarity [19] was measured and a dendrogram based on similarity coefficients generated by the unweighted pair group method using arithmetic averages (UPGMA) [20], and the sequential agglomerative hierarchial and nested (SHAN) clustering was obtained. The entire analysis was performed using the statistical package NTSYS-pc 2.02e [21].

2.2.4.4. Cophenetic correlation

The correlation among different dendrograms generated from the data obtained from RAPD and ISSR was calculated separately and the cophenetic correlation for both the markers was also calculated from the total data.

2.2.4.5. Principal co-ordinate analysis

To visualize the genetic variation among 21 accessions of *C. borivilianum* in detail, PCA was performed with 20 RAPD markers and 06 ISSR markers. This technique helps in converting a set of variables into a few dimensions using which the genotypes under study can be depicted in a two- or three-dimensional space [22] so that the variations of several individuals will be condensed into a set of limited axes. Such a graphical analysis helps in identifying the individuals that tend to cluster together. Principal co-ordinate analysis was also performed using the NTSYS-pc 2.02C software.

To study the efficiency of each marker technique, the Mantel 'Z' test was performed for the comparison of each marker system with the combined data and between the marker systems [23].

3. Results

The present work pertains to the study of genetic diversity among 21 accessions of *C. borivilianum* collected from different regions of India (Gujarat, Madhya Pradesh, Maharashtra and Rajasthan) using molecular markers.

3.1. RAPD analysis

A total of 100 random decamer oligonucleotide primers from 20 numbers from each series (OPA, OPC, OPD, OPP and OPT) were screened using an accession (Ch12; Raj 4) of *C. borivilianum* for primer optimization out of them 20 primers showed the distinct and reproducible amplicons. Twenty primers produced 168 loci out of which 155 were polymorphic and 13 were monomorphic in nature. Among the polymorphic loci, five loci were found unique in nature (**Figure 2**). The amplicons were observed in the range of 250 to >3000 base pair. The resolving power and primer index of the primers varied from 12.762 to 3.810 and 0.499 to 0.245, respectively. Best resolving power was observed in the primer OPA16 and the minimum (3.810) with primer OPT18. The maximum RAPD primer index (RPI) (0.499) was observed with the

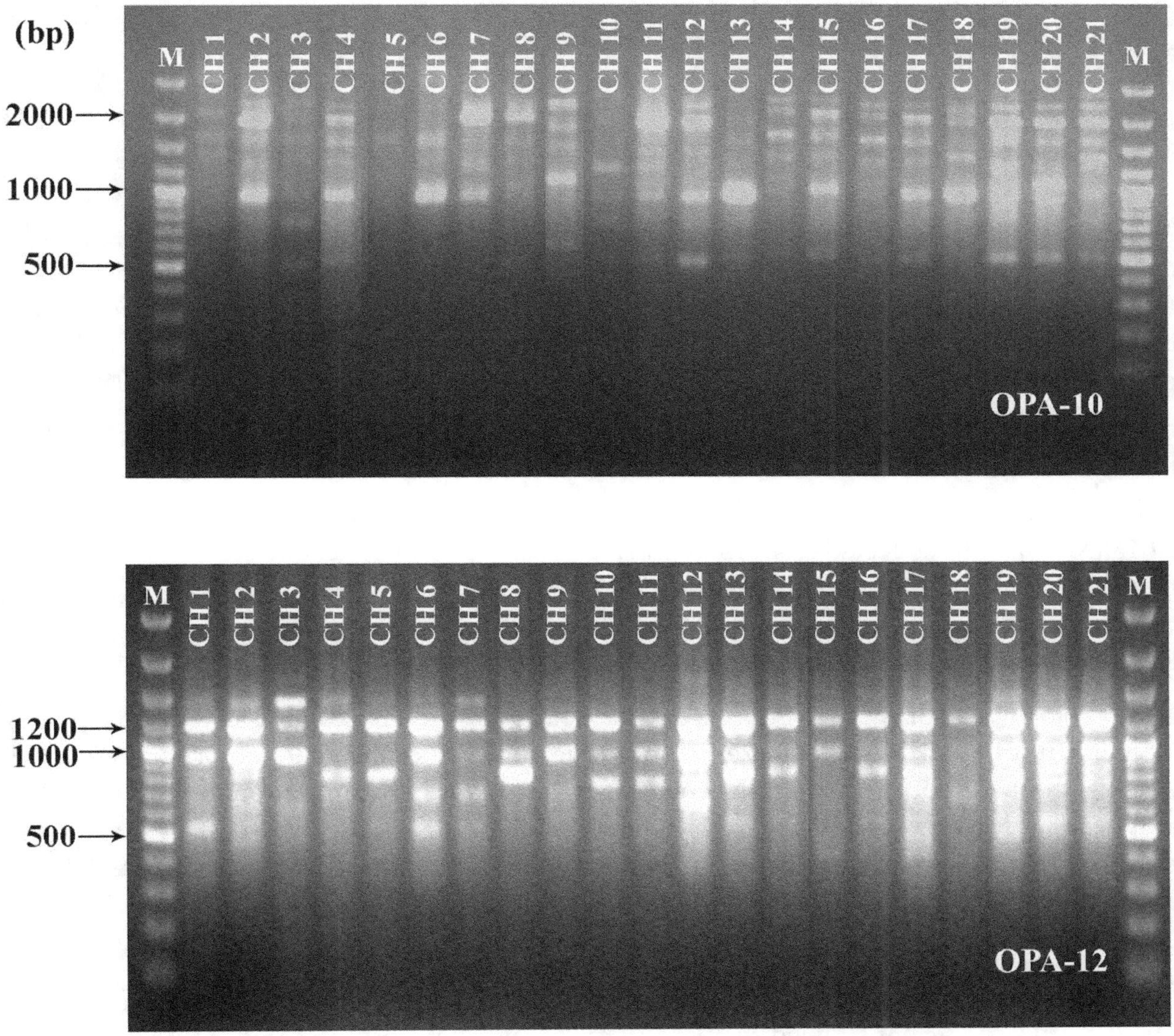

Figure 2. RAPD banding pattern in 21 accessions of *C. borivilianum* with OPA10 and OPA12 primer [M: 100 bp DNA ladder, Lane 2-22: Ch1–Ch21].

primer OPA07, OPA08, OPA10, OPC20 and OPP12 and the minimum (0.245) with primer OPT16.

The Jaccard's coefficient showed that MH2 and MH3 were most closely related with a similarity value of 0.707 followed by MH3 and Akola with similarity value of 0.697. The matrix value ranged from 0.321 to 0.707. It was observed that MP5 and Guj2 were most remotely placed with the similarity coefficient of 0.321. The average similarity coefficient was 0.639 between any two accessions taken into account.

The dendrogram constructed by the UPGMA method of pooled RAPD data led to the segregation of the 21 accessions into two distinct groups. All accessions were distributed between 39 units. Surprisingly, the first contained only one accession, Ch8 collected from Madhya Pradesh and second contained remaining 20 accessions collected from different diversified regions (Madhya Pradesh, Rajasthan, Maharashtra and Gujarat) though they belong to same species. The second major cluster divided into two sub-major clusters out of which one sub-major cluster IIA contained four accessions (Ch1, Ch4, Ch5 and Ch7) collected from Madhya Pradesh with ~47% similarity and the another one (Group IIB) clutched Ch2 and Ch3 collected from Madhya Pradesh depicting 47% genetic variability. The third sub-major cluster (Group IIC) comprised four accessions Ch6 (Madhya Pradesh collection), Ch15, Ch16 and Ch17 collected from Maharashtra showing genetic similarity at the level of 68%. Another group, IID, consisted of two accessions (Ch12 and Ch13) collected from Rajasthan and other two Ch19 and Ch21 of Gujarat collections. Another group (IIE) holds two accessions (Ch18 and Ch20) collected from Gujarat showed 51% (approx.) genetic diversity. Accession no. Ch10 and Ch11 of Rajasthan collections fall in group IIF depicting 52% genetic similarity whereas cluster (IIG) containing two accessions (Ch9 and Ch14) showed genetic variability of about 51% collected from Madhya Pradesh and Rajasthan, respectively.

The cophenetic correlation showed maximum (0.7065) correlation between Ch15 (MH2) and Ch16 (MH3); both collected from Maharashtra. The average cophenetic correlation between two accessions was found to be 0.584.

3.2. ISSR analysis

A total of 10 ISSR primers were used out of which 06 primers resulted in amplification of 29 loci. Out of 29 loci, 24 loci were polymorphic and 05 loci were monomorphic in nature. Among the polymorphic loci, only one (01) locus was found to be unique in nature. The amplicons were observed in the range of 180 to >3000 base pair (**Figure 3**). The resolving power of the primers varied from 1.905 to 8.667 while the primer index varied from 0.091 to 0.499. Best resolving power (8.667) was observed in the primer (CA)8AT and the minimum (1.905) with primer (CA)6GG. The maximum ISSR primer index (0.499) was observed with the primer (CT)9G and the minimum (0.091) with primer (CA)6GG.

The Jaccard's coefficient showed that Ch13 (Raj 5 was most closely related) to Ch 14 (Raj 11) with a similarity value of 0.846 followed by Ch7 (MP7) and Ch10 (Raj1) with a similarity value of 0.833. The matrix value ranged from 0.363 to 0.846. The Rajasthan collected accession (Ch11) and Ch18 (Dangs) of Gujarat collections were most remotely placed with the similarity coefficient of 0.363. Between any two accessions, the average similarity coefficient was observed as 0.627.

Six (06) ISSR primers were used to construct a dendrogram by using the UPGMA method which led to the segregation of the accessions into two distinct groups. All accessions were distributed between 36 units. The resultant dendrogram formed a cluster with the 18 accessions in one group and the other 3 accessions into a separate group. Again 18 accessions discriminated into several groups. Group I consisted of only three accessions, Ch9, Ch11 and Ch19 collected from Madhya Pradesh, Rajasthan and Gujarat, respectively that showed about 35% genetic variability. Group II comprises five groups such as IIA, IIB, IIC, IID and IIE. Group IIC is the largest, which comprises six accessions, Ch3, Ch6 and Ch7 collected from Madhya Pradesh, Ch 10 and Ch12 from Rajasthan and Ch18 collected from Gujarat showed 61% genetic similarity.

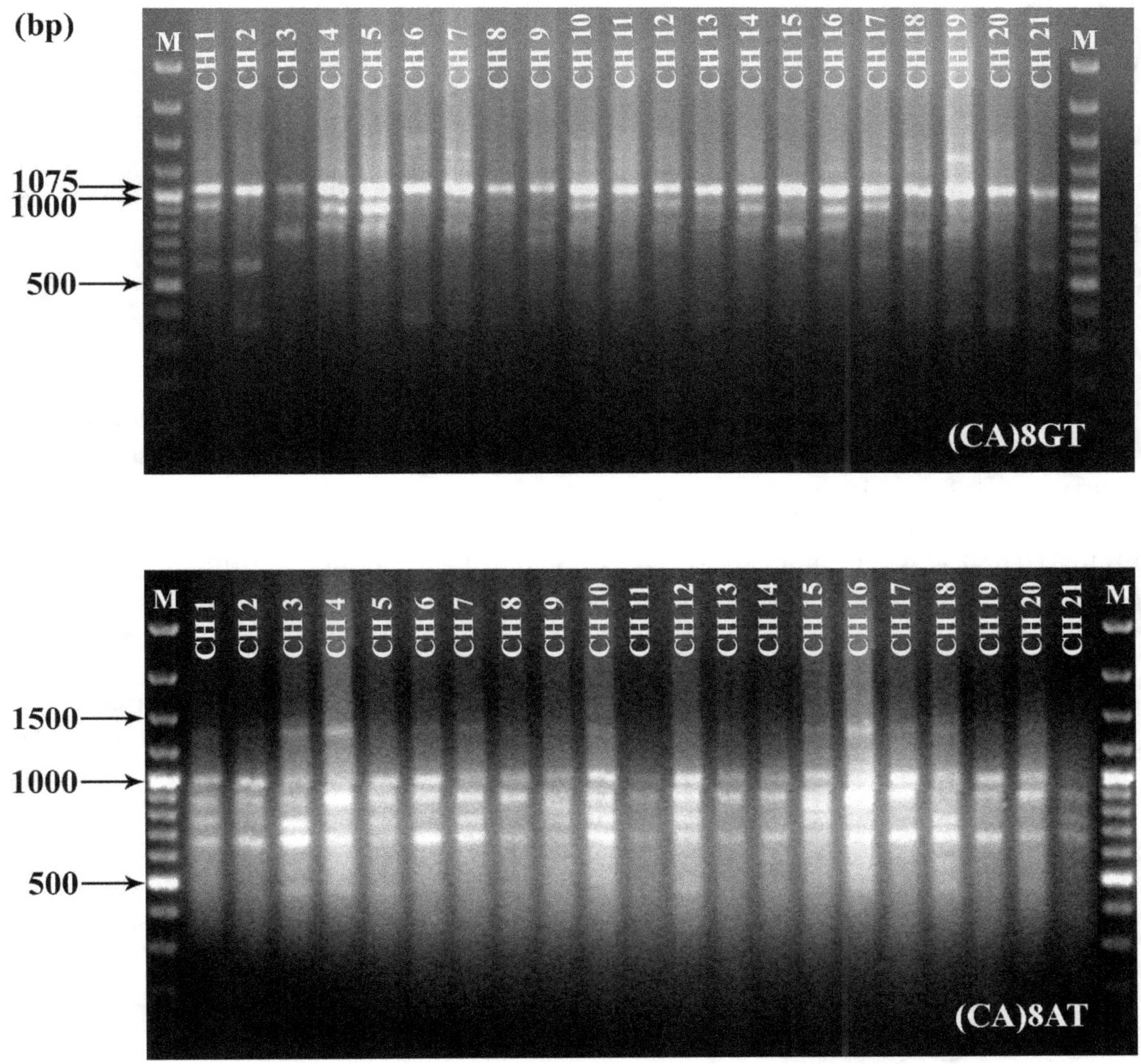

Figure 3. ISSR banding pattern in 21 accessions of *C. borivilianum* (CA)8GT and (CA)8AT primer [M: 100 bp DNA ladder, Lane 2-22: Ch1–Ch21].

The second largest Group IIB holds five accessions from which Ch2 and Ch8 collected from Madhya Pradesh, Ch13 and Ch14 from Rajasthan and Ch20 collected from Gujarat showed about genetic variation of about 40%. IID formed a group with three accessions, Ch 15, Ch16 and Ch17 of Maharashtra collections showing about 70% genetic similarity among them. The smallest Group IIE consisted accessions Ch4 and Ch5 of Madhya Pradesh showed 30% genetic variability between them.

The cophenetic correlation showed the maximum cophenetic correlation value (0.846) between Ch13 (Raj5) and Ch16 (Raj11); both are collected from Rajasthan. The average cophenetic correlation between two accessions was found to be 0.605.

3.3. Combined RAPD and ISSR data analysis

Both RAPD and ISSR produced a total of 197 loci of which 179 loci were polymorphic and 18 loci were monomorphic. A dendrogram was constructed by pooled RAPD and ISSR data using Jaccard's similarity coefficient and SHAN clustering.

The Jaccard's similarity coefficient showed a wide range of correlation among all the accessions. The average similarity coefficient between any two accessions was approximately 0.565. Maximum similarity (0.709) was observed between Ch15 and Ch16. However, Ch 8 and Ch17 were found distantly related with a similarity coefficient value of 0.423.

3.4. RAPD- and ISSR-derived dendrogram analysis from Jaccard's coefficient

The dendrogram constructed from combined RAPD and ISSR data segregates a single accession (Ch 8) of Madhya Pradesh Collection from the rest of the accessions sharing a node at 48% level of genetic variation (**Figure 4**). The subsequent sub-cluster contained five groups (IIA, IIB, IIC, IID and IIE). The accessions (Ch1, Ch4 and Ch5) formed a group (IIA) which were collected from Madhya Pradesh. Then group IIB consisted of Ch2 and Ch3 collected from Madhya Pradesh showed 47% genetic variability. The IID holds five accessions out of which Ch12 and Ch13 of Rajasthan collections and Ch19, Ch20 and Ch21 of Gujarat collections showed 52% genetic similarity. Thereafter Group IIC consisted of four accessions among which Ch6 collected from Madhya Pradesh and three accessions such as Ch15,

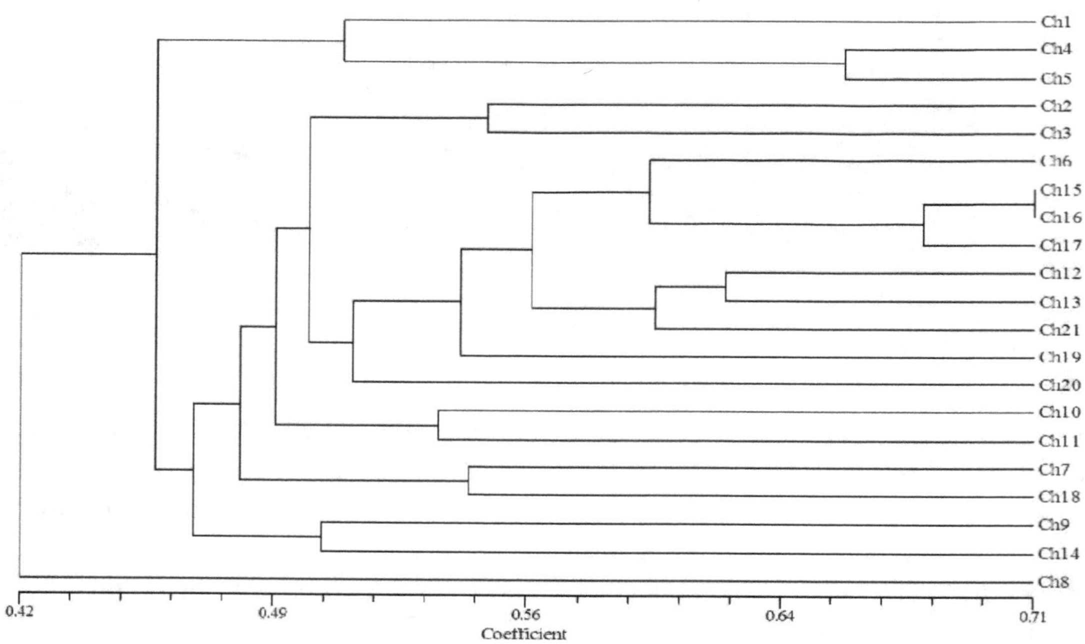

Figure 4. Clustering pattern of 21 accessions of *C. borivilianum* based on combined RAPD and ISSR markers.

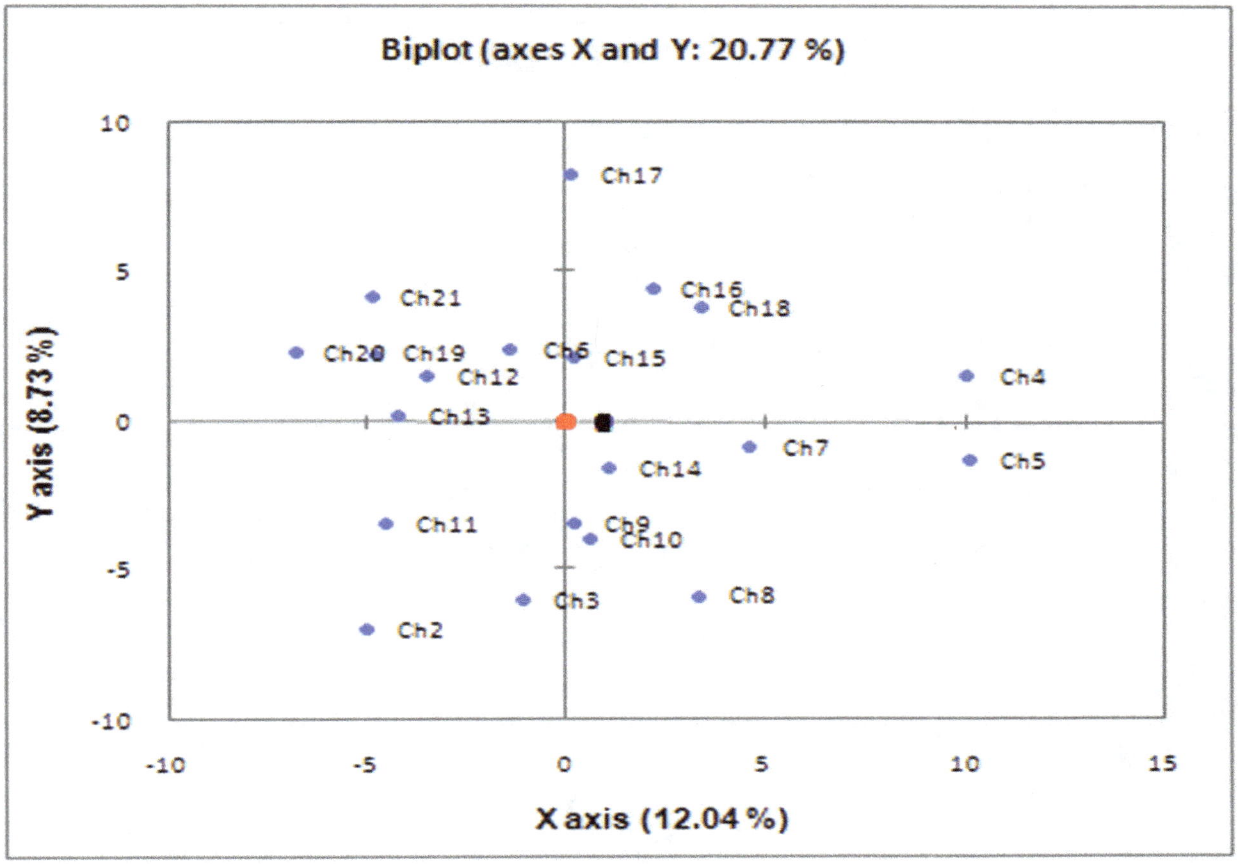

Figure 5. Principal co-ordinate analysis (PCA) in 21 accessions of *C. borivilianum* based on RAPD and ISSR markers.

Ch16 and Ch17 collected from Maharashtra shared 68% genetic similarity among them. About 47% variability was observed between Ch10 and Ch11 of Rajasthan collections which fall in Group IIE. In this study, it was observed that genetic relation/ variability among the accessions were found more or less similar to RAPD analysis. The maximum cophenetic correlation value (0.707) existed between Ch15 (MH2) and Ch16 (MH3); both were collected from Maharashtra. The average cophenetic correlation between two accessions was found to be 0.590.

As can be seen in **Figure 5**, the accessions of *C. borivilianum* were more dispersed on the PCA, which is a reflection of broad genetic base of this species. In general, the result of PCA is in agreement with the dendrogram and is a further confirmation of the genetic relationships delineated by cluster analysis.

Matrix comparison showed the *r* value for RAPD, ISSR and combined RAPD and ISSR to be 0.720, 0.696 and 0.707, respectively, which indicates significant fitness among all the markers studied.

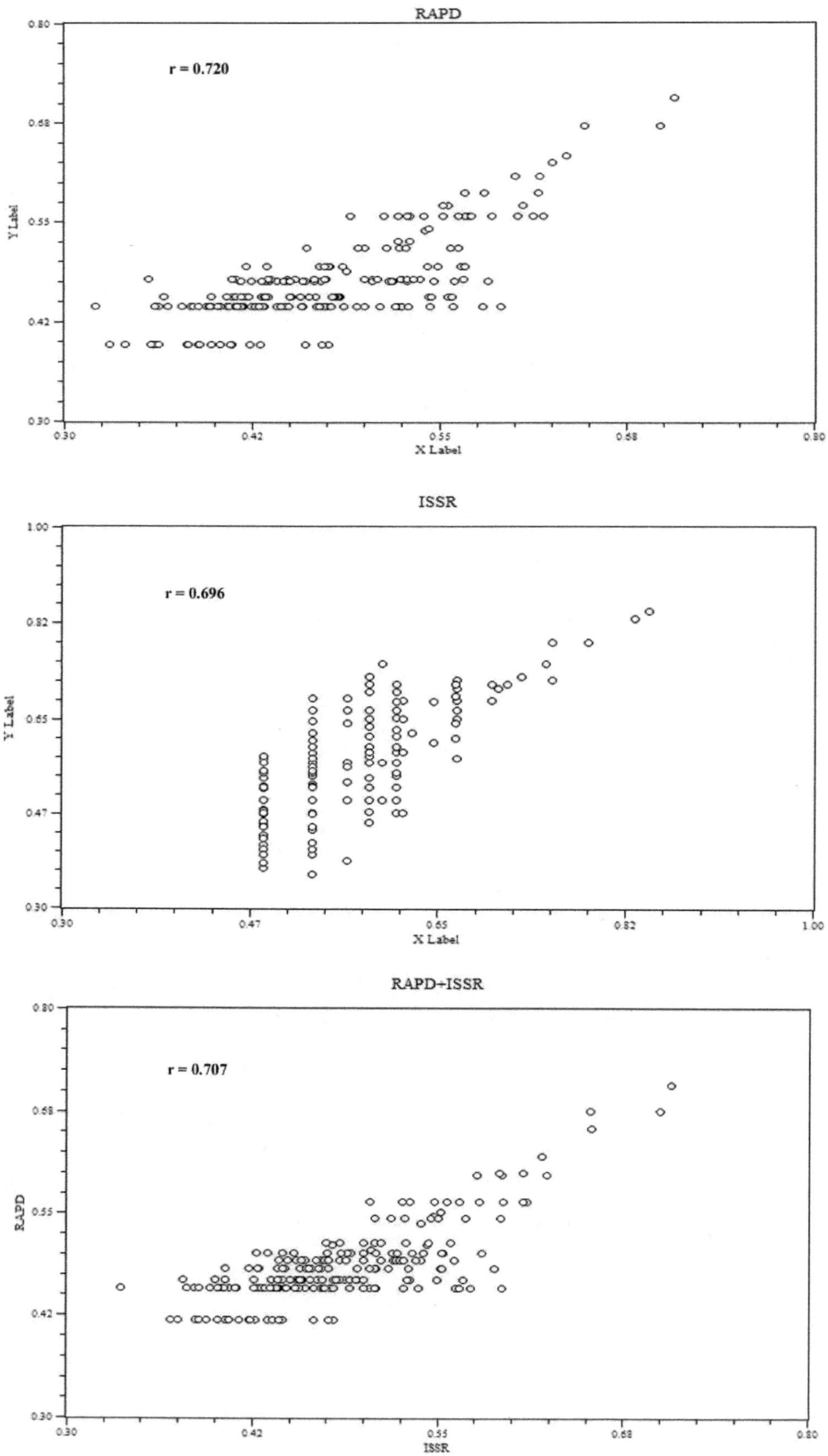

Figure 6. Matrix comparison of combined RAPD and ISSR markers in 21 accessions of *C. borivilianum*.

The programme takes two symmetric similarity or dissimilarity matrices and plots, one matrix against the other element by element (but with the diagonal values ignored). It also computes the product-moment correlation, *r*, and the Mantel test statistic, *Z*, to measure the degree of relationship between the two matrices (**Figure 6**).

4. Discussion

C. borivilianum is an important traditional and ancient crop of India. Due to its high-therapeutic value, this species is being over-exploited for which it was listed in the endangered category. Therefore, their cultivation area has expanded rapidly during last few decades to cope up with the current internal demand and export. However, it would be important to determine their genetic variation so that the useful genotypes could be effectively used as cultivars by farmers or breeders and it would, in turn, facilitate the efficient conservation, management and utilization of the species. Nevertheless, genetic support to the cultivar development programme still remains limited relative to the scenario in many traditional crops where enormous genetic resource knowledge and saturated linkage maps have become available. Molecular markers can demonstrate genetic similarities and differences between accessions even when a classical morphological description is severely limited. To resolve the nomenclature problem, identification of duplicates and also to develop new cultivars, 21 different accessions of *C. borivilianum* were characterized using RAPD and ISSR markers to assess the variability within and among them. DNA markers are considered to be the most suitable means for estimating genetic diversity because of their abundance polymorphism and the fact that they are independent of the environment [24]. Quite considerable genetic variability does exist among different accessions.

Characterization of genetic resource collection has been greatly facilitated by the availability of a number of molecular marker systems. Different types of molecular markers have been used to assess the genetic diversity in crop species, but no single technique is universally ideal. Therefore, the choice of the technique depends on the objective of the study, sensitivity level of the marker system, financial constraints, skill and facilities available [25].

The molecular markers best studied for detecting genetic diversity should be relatively easy and inexpensive to use and should rapidly evolve enough variable within populations [26]. There are numerous DNA-based molecular marker systems suitable for genetic diversity assessment. Random amplified polymorphic DNA (RAPD) and inter-simple sequence repeat (ISSR) marker, in addition to its suitability of genetic diversity study, are highly polymorphic, reproducible, cost effective and require no prior information of sequence [27]. These facts suggest RAPD and ISSR could be unbiased tools to evaluate the changes of diversity in agronomically important crops [28].

RAPD generated a total of 168 bands ranging from 300 to >3000 bp of which 7.73% were monomorphic common to all accessions, 2.97% were unique present in four accessions and 92.26% were polymorphic in many of the accessions. This high degree of polymorphism detected with 20 RAPD primers indicates a high marker index. This is consistent with the results obtained by Shin et al. [29] in watermelon and Galderisi et al. [30] in fig. Some RAPD primers (OPA16, OPA18) produced more markers probably because genomic DNA sequences possess high frequency of annealing sites [31]. ISSR markers have been used to evaluate the genetic diversity in several medicinal plants [32–35]. The larger number of polymorphic markers (as compared to number of primers used) generated by ISSR-PCR can be attributed to the fact that the centromeric region contains a large amount of repeated sequences [36]. A higher level of polymorphism was detected by both RAPD and ISSR in our study corroborated to other reports [37, 38].

The present results showed that molecular markers, ISSR and RAPD, efficiently identify *C. borivilianum* accessions allowing the characterization of all the different accessions. Moreover, both ISSR and RAPD markers exhibited their efficiency for genotype identification in other medicinal and aromatic plants earlier [39–41].

Though RAPD and ISSR markers demarcated 21 accessions into several groups, clustering of accessions within groups was not similar. A possible explanation for the difference in resolution of RAPD and ISSR is that the two marker techniques targeted different portions of the genome. The inter-simple sequence repeats target regions lying within the micro-satellite, and the amplification loci of RAPD are mainly in the gene expression region [14, 15]. These differences may also be attributed to marker sampling errors and/or the level of polymorphism detected reinforcing the importance of the number of loci and their coverage of the overall genome in obtaining reliable estimates of genetic relationships among cultivars [42, 43]. The putatively similar bands originating for RAPDs in different individuals are not necessarily homologous, although they may share the same size in base pairs. This result sometimes may lead to wrong results when calculating genetic relationships [44].

The dendrogram did not indicate any clear pattern of clustering according to the locations from where germplasm were collected, indicating little and no location specificity among *C. borivilianum* germplasm except in Maharashtra collections. A similar result was observed earlier in 22 accessions of Shisham (*Dalbergia sissoo*) collected from different regions of India using RAPD and ISSR markers [45]. Since different dendrograms were obtained; no conclusive common grouping could be drawn from ISSR and combined RAPD-ISSR analyses. These results suggest that the manner of polymorphism differs because of marker specificity. In addition, the relation is assumed to depend on the genome coverage and sequence type recognized by each marker system [42, 46]. On comparing the diversity from different places of Madhya Pradesh, it was evident that *Chlorophytum* accessions from Madhya Pradesh were more diverse (52%) compared to Maharashtra (31%). Since *C. borivilianum* has been vegetatively propagated for a considerable time, it is reasonable to assume that part of the diversity detected in this study, is of ancient inheritance or accumulation of somatic point mutation in the course of vegetative reproduction events.

Matching the clustering result with their collection sites revealed that the geographical distribution of most accessions was not found to be defined. The majority of accessions in subgroup IIC were from different places of Madhya Pradesh and Rajasthan. Similarly, three of five accessions in the sub-group IID were collected from Maharashtra whereas two were from Madhya Pradesh. Similar conclusions were made by Padmesh et al. [47] in *Andrographis paniculata* where one accession collected from Thailand was shown to cluster with genotypes of different parts of Tamil Nadu. All the genotypes in sub-group IIA were from different places of Madhya Pradesh exhibiting 37% diversity. Without exception, two accessions in group IA from Madhya Pradesh showed 79% similarity; it was evident from the dendrogram that most of the accessions assessed, were clustered according to their geographical region.

On the basis of percent of polymorphism (RAPD = 92.26 and ISSR = 82.76), RAPD markers were marginally more informative than ISSR in the assessment of genetic diversity in *C. borivilianum*. This is corroborated with the findings in *Caldesia grandis, Dalbergia sissoo* and *Prunus armeniaca* [45, 48, 49]. This may be because of the fact that two marker techniques targeted different portions of the genome. Some researchers have considered RAPD markers to represent segments of DNA with non-coding regions and to be selectively neutral [50, 51]. Some studies have shown that RAPD markers are distributed throughout the genome and may be associated with functionally important loci [52]. Nevertheless, RAPD have been sometimes been associated with a lack of reproducibility [53]. However, if the PCR conditions are well controlled, a high level of reproducibility is attainable [54]. In this study, a considerable effort has been made to optimize the components of PCR, including the concentrations of $MgCl_2$, dNTP, primer, *Taq* DNA polymerase and the quality and concentration of template DNA.

The Mantel test on the similarity matrices produced by RAPD and ISSR markers showed significant correlation ($r = 0.7638$; $p < 0.001$) between RAPD and ISSR markers in their ability to detect genetic relationships between *Chlorophytum* accessions. The coefficient correlation value, $r = 0.7591$, 0.7263 and 0.7638 for RAPD, ISSR and combined RAPD and ISSR analyses, respectively. This result is corroborated with the earlier report of Dai et al. [55].

In this study, superiority of RAPD markers over ISSR were observed with regards to polymorphism detection, as RAPD detected 92.26% as compared to 82.76% for ISSR markers. This is in contrast to the results as obtained for other several plant species where ISSR was proved to be superior as compared to RAPD [44, 56–58]. More polymorphism, in the case of RAPD than ISSR markers might be due to the fact that out of 10 primers used in the study, only 6 primers amplified 609 numbers of fragments for ISSR. While in the case of RAPD, all the 20 primers which were used in the investigation amplified 3528 number of fragments. The same polymorphism pattern was observed in jatropha, podophyllum and apricot [59–61]. RAPD also provides marker even for cultivars identification [62] determining hybridity among the sexual cross made intentionally to exploit the genetic variability [63, 64] and germplasm evaluation [31].

To conserve the diversity of genetic resources, a large number of accessions are to be conserved for which problems are encountered in documentation, conservation, multiplication and evaluation. Therefore, to minimize the cost of genetic conservation ensuring representation of maximum genetic variation, a set of accessions (core collection) should be selected to represent the genetic diversity of a base collection with minimum redundancy [12]. From the PCA of the 38 accessions, it was evident that some of the accessions were found overlapping each other depicting redundancy which should be eliminated. Since there are different strategies for developing a core collection using morphological or marker data, however molecular markers are more stable and efficient in estimating the genetic relatedness among the individuals [65, 66].

The molecular analyses of RAPD and ISSR markers were extremely useful for studying the genetic relationship/variability between and among *C. borivilianum* accessions. Also, the phylogenetic analysis on the basis of RAPD- and ISSR-derived dendrograms supports the fact that region-specific variation are there, which is because of the multiple generations of the selection carried out after their introduction.

5. Conclusion

The present findings demonstrate the use of RAPD and ISSR markers in estimating genetic diversity and identifying a core collection in *C. borivilianum* for which genotypes representing maximum genetic diversity need to be conserved followed by accessions which complement the previous one. Moreover, sample duplication could be detected in the germplasm collection followed by selection of a core collection to enhance the efficiency of germplasm management for use in crop improvement and conservation. Based on polymorphic features among the accessions of *C. borivilianum* based on RAPD and ISSR study, it may be recommended that any future conservation plans for this species should be specifically designed to include representative accessions with the highest genetic variation for both *in situ* conservation and germplasm collection expeditions. The unique bands that could be identified are likely to provide tags for future genetic improvement as well as in authenticating the genotypes. Further investigation using more sophisticated markers may be helpful for the accuracy and resolution of genetic diversity. ISSR and RAPD markers along with chemical fingerprinting and morphological characters could now be used as coherent tools for the development of core collection of *C. borivilianum*. The RAPD markers along with ISSR markers should complement one another during genetic identification, by coding different regions of *C. borivilianum* genome. Conversion of specific RAPD/ISSR segments into sequenced characterized amplified region (SCAR) markers could enhance the value of these markers for the identification of any variety/ cultivars developed.

Acknowledgements

The authors wish to acknowledge the support from the Directorate of Medicinal and Aromatic Plants Research (DMAPR) Boriavi, Anand for providing necessary facilities. The authors are also thankful to K.A. Geetha, Principal Scientist (Plant Breeding) for providing the material for the study.

Author details

Sanghamitra Samantaray* and Umakanta Ngangkham

*Address all correspondence to: smitraray@gmail.com

ICAR-National Rice Research Institute, Cuttack, Odisha, India

References

[1] Sharma R. (2003). Medicinal Plants of India—An Encyclopedia. Daya Publishing House; New Delhi: 333 p.

[2] Chopra AK, Khanna DR, Prasad G, Malik DS, Bhutiani R. (eds.). Medicinal Plants: Conservation, Cultivation and Utilization. 2007. Daya Publishing House; New Delhi.

[3] Kongkiatngam P, Waterway MJ, Fortin MG, Coulman BE. Genetic variation within and among cultivars of red clover (*Trifolium pratense*): comparison of morphological, isozyme and RAPD markers. Euphytica. 1995;**84**: 237–246.

[4] Whitkus R, Doebley J, Wendel JF. Nuclear DNA markers in systematics and evolution. In: Phillips L. and Vasil I. K. (eds), DNA–Based Markers in Plants. Kulwer Academic Publishers; Dordrecht, The Netherlands: 1994. pp. 116–141.

[5] Nybom H. DNA fingerprinting-A useful tool in fruit breeding. *Euphytica*. 1994;77: 59–64.

[6] Ipek M, Simon P. Genetic Diversity in Garlic (*Allium sativum* L.) as Assessed by AFLPs and Isozymes. *American Society for Horticultural Science 98th Annual Conference & Exhibition*. July 2001; 22 – 25.

[7] Singh A, Chauhan HS. Safed musli (Chlorophytum borivilianum): distribution, biodiversity and cultivation. Journal of Medicinal and Aromatic Plant Science. 2003;**25**: 712–719, 2003.

[8] Oudhia P.: My experiences with wonder crop Safed Moosli. In: Souvenir. International Seminar on Medicinal Plants and Quality Standardization, VHERDS, Chennai, India, 9–10 June, 2001a.

[9] Oudhia P, Tripathi RS. Scope of cultivation of important medicinal plants in Chhattisgarh plains. In: Proc. National conference on Health care and Development of Herbal Medicines, IGAU, Raipur (India), 29–30 Aug. 1997, 1999: pp.71–78.

[10] Oudhia P, Joshi BS. The decreasing availability of natural medicinal plants in Chhattisgarh: A study. In: Abstr. VI National Science Conference, Mahatma Gandhi Gramoday Chitrakut Vishwavidyalaya, Chitrakut, India: 2000;18.

[11] Bordia PC, Joshi A, Simlot MM. Safed Musli. In: K.L. Chadha and Rajendra Gupta (eds.), Advances in Horticulture Vol. II. Medicinal and Aromatic Plants. Malhotra Publishing House, New Delhi. 1995; pp. 429–451.

[12] Franklin OH, Brown AHD. Plant Genetic Resources Today- A Critical Appraisal. In: Crop Genetic Resources: Conservation and Evaluation. Holden, JHW and Williams JT (eds) Allen and Unwin; Winchester, Massachusetts, USA: 1984; pp. 187–196.

[13] Doyle JJ, Doyle JL. Isolation of plant DNA from fresh tissue. Focus. 1990;**12**: 13–15.

[14] Williams JGK, Kubelic AR, Livak KJ, Rafalsky JA, Tingey SV. DNA polymorphisms amplified by arbitrary primer are useful as genetic markers. Nucleic Acid Research. 1990;**18**: 6531–6535.

[15] Zietkiewicz E, Rafalski A, Labuda D. Genome fingerprinting by simple sequence repeats (SSR)-anchored PCR amplification. Genomics. 1994;**20**: 176–183.

[16] Prevost A, Wilkinson MJ. A new system of comparing PCR primers applied to ISSR fingerprinting of potato cultivars. Theoretical andApplied Genetics. 1999;98: 107–112.

[17] Smith JSC, Chin ECL, Shu H, Smith OS, Wall SJ, Senior ML, Mitchell SE, Kresovich S, Ziegle J. An evaluation of the utility of SSR loci as molecular markers in maize (Zea mays L.): comparison of data from RFLPs and pedigree. Theoretical and Applied Genetics. 1997;**95**: 163–173.

[18] Ghilslain M, Zhang D, Fazardo D, Huamann Z, Hismans RH. Marker-assisted sampling of the cultivated Andean Potato Solanum fureja collection using RAPD markers. Genetic Resources and Crop Evolution. 1999;**46**: 547–555.

[19] Jaccard P. Nouvelles researches sur la distribution florale. Bull. Soc. Vaud. Sci. Nat. 1908;**44**: 223–270.

[20] Sneath PHA, and Sokal R. Numerical Taxonomy. Freeman, San Francisco, CA, USA. 1973.

[21] Rohlf, FJ. NTSYS-PC: Numerical taxonomy and Multivariate Analysis System. Exeter Software, New York, USA. 1997.

[22] Ludwig AJ, Reynolds FJ. Statistical Ecology—A Primer on Methods and Computing. John Wiley and Sons, New York, USA. 1988.

[23] Mantel NA. The detection of disease clustering and a generalized regression approach. Cancer Research. 1967;**27**: 209–220.

[24] Gepts P. The Use of Molecular and Biochemical Markers in Crop Evolution Studies. In: Hecht MK (eds) Evolutionary Biology, 27. Plenum Press, New York, 1993; pp. 51–94.

[25] Yoseph B, Boltha AM, Myburg AA. A comparative study of molecular and morphological methods of describing genetic relationship in traditional Ethiopian highland maize. African Biotechnology. 2005;**4**(7): 586–595.

[26] Esselman EJ, Jiangqiang J, Croford DJ, Windus JL, Wolf AD. Clonal diversity in the rare *Calamagrostis porteri* ssp. Insperata (Poaceae): Comparative results for allozymes and Random amplified polymorphic DNA (RAPD) and Inter simple sequence repeat (ISSR) markers. Molecular Ecology. 1999;**8**(3): 443–451.

[27] Bornet BC, Muller FP, Branched M. Highly informative nature of inter simple sequence repeats (ISSR) sequences amplified using tri and tetra nucleotide primers from DNAs of cauliflower (Brassica oleracea var. Botrytus L). Genome. 2002;**45**: 890–896.

[28] Brantestam AK, Bothmer RV, Dayteg C, Rashal I, Tuvesson S, Weibull J. Inter simple sequence repeat analysis of genetic diversity and relationships in cultivated barley of Nordic and Baltic origin. Hereditas. 2004;**141**(2): 186–187.

[29] Shin JS, Lee SJ, Park KW. Genetic diversity in *Citrullus vulgaris* L. germplasm through RAPD analysis. Korean Journal of Breeding. 1995;**27**(1): 94–107.

[30] Galderisi U, Cipollaro M, Di Bernardo G, De Masi L. Identification of the edible fig 'Bianco del Cilento' by random amplified polymorphic DNA analysis. Horticultural Science. 1999;34: 1263–1265.

[31] Virk PS, Ford-Lloyd BV, Jackson MT, Newbury HJ. Use of RAPD for the study of diversity within plant germplasm collections. Heredity. 1995;**74**: 170–179.

[32] Zhou Y, Zhou C, Yao H, Liu Y, Tu R. Application of ISSR markers in detection of genetic variation among Chinese yam (*Dioscorea opposita* Thunb) cultivars. Life Science Journal. 2008;**5(4)**: 6–12.

[33] Wang Z, Feng SG, Lu JJ, Shi NN, Liu JJ. Phylogenetic study and molecular identification of 31 *Dendrobium* species using inter-simple sequence repeat (ISSR) markers. Scientia Horticulturae. 2009;**122**:440–447.

[34] Tamhankar S, Ghate V, Raut A, Rajput B. Molecular profiling of "Chirayat" complex using inter simple sequence repeat (ISSR) markers. Planta Medica. 2009;**75**(11): 1266–1270.

[35] Ding G, Li X, Ding X, Qian L. Genetic diversity across natural populations of *Dendrobium officinale*, the endangered medicinal herb endemic to China, revealed by ISSR and RAPD markers. Russian Journal of Genetics. 2009;**45(3)**: 327–334.

[36] Bhuyan N, Basanta KB, Sharma RN. Genetic diversity analysis in traditional lowland rice (Oryza sitiva) of Assam using RAPD and ISSR markers. Current Science. 2007;**93**(7): 976–979.

[37] Parsons BJ, Newbury HJ, Jackson MT, Ford-Lloyd BV. Contrasting genetic diversity relationships are revealed in rice (*Oryza sativa* L.) using different marker types. Molecular Breeding. 1997;**3**: 115–125

[38] Raghunathchari P, Khanna VK. RAPD analysis of genetic variability in Indian scented rice (Oryza sativa L.) germplasm. Current Science. 2000;**79**: 994–998.

[39] Fracaro F, Zacaria J, Echeverrigaray S. RAPD based genetic relationships between populations of three chemotypes of *Cunila galioides* Benth. Biochemical Systematics and Ecology, 2005;**33(4)**:409–417.

[40] Yuan XF, Dai ZH, Wang XD, Zhao B. Assessment of genetic stability in tissue-cultured products and seedlings of *Saussurea involucrata* by RAPD and ISSR markers. Biotechnology Letters. 2009;**31(8)**: 1279–1287.

[41] Manica-Cattani MF, Zacaria J, Pauletti G, Atti-Serafini L, Echeverrigaray S. Genetic variation among South Brazilian accessions of Lippia alba Mill. (Verbenaceae) detected by ISSR and RAPD markers. Brazilian Journal of Biology. 2009;**69**: 2.

[42] Loarce Y, Gallego R, Ferrer E. A comparative analysis of genetic relationships between rye cultivars using RFLP and RAPD markers. Euphytica. 1996;**88**: 107–115.

[43] Souframanien J and Gopalakrishna T. A comparative analysis of genetic diversity in blackgram genotypes using RAPD and ISSR markers. Theoretical and Applied Genetics. 2004;**109**: 1687–1693.

[44] Fernandez M, Figueiras A, Benito C. The use of RAPD and ISSR markers for detecting DNA polymorphism, genotyping identification and genetic diversity among barley cultivars with known origin. Theoretical and Applied Genetics. 2002;**104**: 845–851.

[45] Arif M, Zaidi NW, Singh YP, Haq QMR. A comparative analysis of ISSR and RAPD markers for study of genetic diversity in shisham (*Dalbergia sissoo*). Plant Molecular Biology Reports. 2009;**27**: 488–495.

[46] Sehgal D, Raina SN. Genotyping safflower (*Carthamus tinctorius*) cultivars by DNA fingerprints. Euphytica. 2005;**146**: 67–76.

[47] Padmesh P, Sadu KK, Seeni S, Pushpangadan P. The use of RAPD in assessing genetics variability in *Andrographis paniculata* Nees, a hepatoprotective drug. Current Science. 1999;**76**: 833–835.

[48] Chen JM, Gituru WR, Wang YH, Wang QF. The extent of clonality and genetic diversity in the rare *Caldesia grandis* (Alismataceae): comparative results for RAPD and ISSR markers. Quaternary Botany. 2006;**84**: 301–307.

[49] Kumar P, Singh K, Vikal Y, Randhawa LS, Chahal GS. Genetic diversity studies of elite cotton germplasm lines Using RAPD markers and morphological characters. Indian Journal of Genetics. 2003;**63**(1): 5–10.

[50] Bachmann K. Nuclear DNA markers in plant biosystematics research. Opera Botany. 1997;**32**: 137–148.

[51] Landergott U, Holderegger R, Kozlowski G and Schneller JJ. Historical bottlenecks decrease genetic diversity in natural populations of *Dryopteris cristata*. Heredity 2001;**87**: 344–355.

[52] Penner GA. RAPD Analysis of Plant Genomes. In: Methods of Genome Analysis in Plants. Jauhar PP (ed.). CRC, Boca Raton, 1996; 251–268.

[53] Penner GA, Bush A, Wise R, Kim W, Domier L, Kasha K, Laroch A, Scoles GS, Gedak G. Reproducibility of random amplified polymorphic DNA (RAPD) analysis among laboratories. PCR Methods and Applications. 1993;**2**:341–345.

[54] Mattioni C, Casasoli M, Gonzalez M, Ipinza R, Villani F. Comparison of ISSR and RAPD markers to characterize three Chilean Nothofagus species. Theoretical and Applied Genetics. 2002;**43**: 224–231.

[55] Dai A, Guo, Zhang L, Chang. Application of random amplified polymorphic DNA and inter-simple sequence repeat markers in the genus *Crataegus*. Annals of Applied Biology. 2009;**154**: 175–181.

[56] Mattioni C, Casasoli M, Gonzalez M Ipinza R, Villani F. Comparison of ISSR and RAPD markers to characterize three Chilean Nothofagus species. Theoretical and Applied Genetics 2002;**104**: 1064–1070.

[57] Zhao WG, Zhang JQ, Wangi YH, Chen TT. Analysis of genetic diversity in wild populations of mulberry from Western Part of Northeast China determined by ISSR markers. Genetics Molecular Biology. 2007;7: 196–203.

[58] Huang J & Sun SM. Genetic diversity and relationships of sweet potato and its wild relatives in Ipomoea series Batatas (Convolvulaceae) as revealed by inter-simple sequence repeat (ISSR) and restriction analysis of chloroplast DNA. Theoretical and Applied Genetics 2009;**100**: 1050–1060.

[59] Gupta M, Chyi YS, Romero-Severson J, Owen JL. Amplification of DNA markers from evolutionarily diverse genomes using single primers of simple-sequence repeats. Theoretical and Applied Genetics. 1994;**89**: 998–1006.

[60] Alam MA, Naik K, Mishra GP. Congruence of RAPD and ISSR markers for evaluation of genomic relationship among 28 populations of *Podophyllum hexandrum* Royle from Himachal Pradesh, India. Turkish Journal of Botany. 2009;33: 1–12

[61] Kumar M, Mishra GP, Singh R, Kumar J, Naik PK, SB. Singh SB. Correspondence of ISSR and RAPD markers for comparative analysis of genetic diversity among different apricot genotypes from cold arid deserts of trans-Himalayas. Physiology and Molecular Biology of Plants. 2009;**15**:225–236.

[62] Torres, E., Iriondo, J. M. and Perez, C. (2003). Genetic structure of an endangered plant, Antirrhinum microphyllum (Scrophulariaceae): allozyme and RAPD analysis. American Journal of Botany. 203;**90**(1): 85–92.

[63] Patra NK, Tanveer H, Khanuja SPS, Shasany AK, Singh HP, Singh VR, Kumar S. A unique interspecific hybrid spearmint clone with growth properties of *Mentha arvensis* L. and oil qualities of *Mentha spicata* L. Theoretical and Applied Genetics. 2001;**102**: 471–476.

[64] Collins D, Mill RR, Moller M. Species separation of *Taxus baccata, T. cannadensis and T. cuspidate* (Taxaceae) and origins of their reputed hybrids inferred from RAPD and cpDNA data. American Journal of Botany. 2003;**90**: 175–182.

[65] Dhanaraj AL, Rao EVB, Swamy KRM, Bhat MG, Prasad DT, Sounder SN. Using RAPDs to assess the diversity in Indian cashew (*Anarcardium occidentale* L.) germplasm. Journal of Horticultural Science and Biotechnology. 2002;77: 41–47.

[66] Shashidhara G, Hema MV, Binu Koshy Farooqi AA. Assessment of genetic diversity and identification of core collection in sandalwood germplasm using RAPDs. Journal of Horticultural Science & Biotechnology. 2003;**78**(4): 528–536.

7

Oregano Essential Oil in Animal Production

Alma Delia Alarcon-Rojo,
Hector Janacua-Vidales and
Ana Renteria-Monterrubio

Abstract

There is an increasing interest in the use of natural additives in food production such as the use of phytogenic feed additives especially for use in swine and poultry. Essential oils are a natural alternative that can be used in animal feed due to their potential health benefits, improved performance and meat production. Oregano essential oil minimises meat downgrading due to transport stress or the modification of the ruminal microorganisms. This review suggested a promising development of food natural preservative against spoilage microorganisms in food systems by the use of oregano essential oil. The addition of oregano essential oil is a good way of preserving meat and could replace the synthetic antioxidants. Moreover, oregano oil and modified atmosphere packaging exhibit an additive preservation effect in fresh meat. Oregano essential oil is effective for controlling the growth of microorganisms. However, for meat quality, special attention should be put on the optimal oregano essential oil dose and meat handling to control or improve the physical, chemical and sensory properties of meat.

Keywords: oregano essential oil, animal production, meat, animal health, packaging, pathogens, sensory, meat quality

1. Introduction

Antimicrobial growth promoters (AGP) were used for decades to increase performance in animal production. However, the link between them and the development of antibiotic resistant microorganisms added to consumer pressure caused major changes. In January 2006, the European Union banned AGP in animal production, which in turn emphasised the importance of researching alternative compounds to promote general health and increase performance in animals [1, 2]. Due to their natural origin and reduced side effects, studies have been mainly focused on herbs, spices and their extracts [3]. The effect of the aromatic plants is primarily based on their essential oils (EO) and other metabolites [4], for example, vitamins, flavonoids, terpenoids, carotenoids, phytoestrogens, minerals, etc. [6]. Among the activities and applications of EO reported in animal and meat production are antioxidant, preservative, antimicrobial and coccidiostatic and they enhance production of digestive enzymes, stimulate blood circulation and improve immune status. [5, 6–9]. Even though there are 3000 estimated EOs, only 300 of them are of commercial use [10]. However, the EO from oregano (OEO) has been one of the most widely studied due to its content of carvacrol and thymol, and to a lesser extent y-terpinene, p-cymene and myrcene [11]. Some *in vitro* and *in vivo* properties of OEO are antioxidant, antimicrobial, digestive stimulant, etc. [12–14].

2. Oregano essential oil in animal production

2.1. Poultry and egg production

Results of the effect of OEO in poultry and egg production cannot be considered conclusive or consistent, as they can differ even within researches of the same authors [15, 16]. Studies supporting the positive effects of OEO suggest that they increase performance [17], daily and final body weight in broilers [18] and laying hens [15, 19], nutrient utilisation [20, 21], egg weight and production [15, 19, 22] and feed intake [23]. Improvement in feed efficiency and growth performance might be related with changes in the intestinal morphology, like the increment in villus height to crept depth ratio [18] or enzyme activity as in the protein digestibility due to the chymotrypsin role [21] and the prevention of coccidiosis [24]. It has been implied that antioxidants from the OEO might transfer into the body of the laying hen, which in turn inhibit the chain reaction associated with lipid oxidation and thus reducing the oxidation in egg yolk [11]. In contrast, several authors have suggested that OEO have no effect on animal performance [21, 25, 26]. For example, Arpášová et al. [16] reported that the addition of thyme and OEO did not significantly influence the body weight, feed consumption and conversion, egg production, mass and weight in laying hens.

2.2. Pig production

As in poultry production, results of the effects of the inclusion of OEO in the diets are contradictory in terms of productive performance [27, 28]. However, positive effects link to dietary inclusion of OEO might be clearer in other areas, for example, immunmodulation [28] and changes in blood counts [29]; in sows, it increases their reproductive performance [30] and causes a reduction in the oxidative stress status and enhances the performance of their litters [31]. Oregano essential oil can be used as well to alleviate stress due to transportation as it improved the antioxidant status [32, 33]. Finally, animals fed 1000 ppm of OEO produced meat of good quality with minimum lipid oxidation [34].

2.3. Milk production and ruminant nutrition

The use of EOs in ruminants and milk production is lightly documented and many of these studies are laboratory based [35]. Several essential oils and their components display antimicrobial properties that may affect rumen metabolism [36] and influence milk production parameters. Many of these compounds (e.g. flavonoids) have distinct flavours and aromas, which if fed to animals, might change the sensory characteristics of the milk; however, this effect might be temporal [37]. The organoleptic quality of the milk can be affected by feeding EO due to a direct transfer of aromatic compounds from the feed (and environment) to the milk [37], formation of aromatic compounds during digestion of the feed [38] and excretion of the EO in the milk. Ruminal microorganisms utilise nutrients to produce volatile fatty acids; however, this process has energy and protein losses, which render the performance inefficient. These losses might be controlled with the inclusion of EO in the diet to limit the growth of Gram-positive and Gram-negative bacteria [39].

3. Oregano essential oil in the meat industry

3.1. Introduction

This section provides an overview of the applications of OEO in raw and processed meat and fish products. It is well known that raw and minimally processed meat is easily targeted by spoilage microorganisms. Moreover, the interest of the industry to replace synthetic chemicals by natural products with bioactive properties is increasing. The need to reduce the use of additives in foods has highlighted the importance of natural antimicrobials such as essential oils. A wide range of antimicrobial agents derived from essential oils have the potential to be used in food processing and preservation since their antimicrobial activity is well recognised.

3.2. Antioxidant activity

The effects of OEO to extend shelf life by controlling lipid oxidation and improving the sensory qualities of meat and meat products are well documented. Kodal Coskun et al. [40] studied the effectiveness of soy-based edible films incorporated with essential oils from oregano or thyme applied on oxidative stability of ground beef patties. The incorporation of OEO or thyme into the edible films reduced the redness value to an acceptable level, but within the appropriate range. The authors concluded that the addition of OEO and thyme EO into edible films retarded the oxidative changes in meats. The potential application of EOs as natural antioxidants has been studied as well in meat products. OEO (alone or in combination) added to fermented meat products as, according to Tunisian [41] and Spanish [42], sausages did not affect proteolysis and rendered a higher unsaturated fatty acid content without affecting the lipolysis. Even more, OEO-added sausages have a better texture due to an increased hardness. Sausages showed a lower number of enterobacteriaceae, coliforms, *Staphylococcus aureus* and moulds. As in beef, the colour of ground poultry meat (breast and thigh) is stabilised due to the effect of OEO [43]. The combination of (200 ppm) and tannic acid (10 ppm) had the highest effect on TBARS, total carbonyl and off-odours volatiles. Hence, OEO might be a proper replacement for synthetic antioxidants in several types of ground meat [44]. The antioxidant effect of OEO included as well cooked meat. Nieto et al. [45] demonstrated that OEO and rosemary EO retarded the loss of thiols under modified atmosphere packaging (MAP, 70% O_2: 20% CO_2:10% N_2) and aerobic conditions. However, this effect was not observed with garlic essential oil. Even though the antimicrobial activity against pathogens is well reported, flavour changes have been reported. However, these changes are acceptable [46].

3.3. Bioactive films

Antimicrobial-releasing edible films in food packaging are a form of bioactive packaging. A large number of studies have been focused on this topic. Oregano essential oil has been used in active packaging systems to protect foods from microbial contamination. Studies have shown that OEO in milk protein-based is highly effective against pathogen and spoilage bacteria even when compared with other EOs [47]. OEO not only helps control the growth of microorganisms but it can modify positively the characteristics of the bioactive film [48]. The best balance of mechanical, barrier, thermal, antioxidant and antimicrobial properties is achieved when 9% of OEO is incorporated in poly (lactic acid)/polytrimenthylene carbonate films. OEO on alginate-based edible films have the potential to limit lipid oxidation, decrease shear forces, colour and water losses Oregano added bioactive films also modify consumer perception in terms of odour, flavour and overall acceptance [49–51]. OEO not necessarily need to be included in the wrapping film, as it can be spray in meat exudate absorbent pads to extend shelf life for two more days [52]. Studies showed that oregano essential oil-blend film was an effective antimicrobial suitable for the potential food packaging applications. It has also been demonstrated the effectiveness of oregano oil containing whey protein films to increase the shelf life of fresh beef [53]. They incorporated different levels of oregano oil (0.5, 1.0 and 1.5% w/w in the film forming solution) into sorbitol-plasticised whey protein isolate films and evaluated beef quality. Wrapping of beef cuts with the antimicrobial films resulted in smaller changes in colour in chilled storage. The maximum specific growth rate of total flora and pseudomonads were significantly reduced by a factor of 2 with the use of antimicrobial films (1.5% w/w), while the growth of lactic acid bacteria was completely inhibited. However, interesting results were obtained by Emiroğlu et al. [54] who did not find significant effects on total viable counts, lactic acid bacteria and *Staphylococcus* spp. when oregano was applied on ground beef patties. They evaluated the antibacterial activity of soy protein edible films incorporated with 1, 2, 3, 4 and 5% oregano or thyme essential oils against *Escherichia coli, E. coli* O157:H7, *S. aureus, Pseudomonas aeruginosa* and *Lactobacillus plantarum. E. coli, E. coli* O157:H7 and *S. aureus* were significantly susceptible to antimicrobial films; meanwhile, *L. plantarum* and *P. aeruginosa* were more resistant. In the study of Seydim and Sarikus [55], antimicrobial properties of whey protein isolate films containing 1.0–4.0% (wt/vol) ratios of oregano, rosemary and garlic essential oils were tested against *E. coli* O157:H7, *S. aureus, Salmonella enteritidis, Listeria monocytogenes* and *L. plantarum*. As mentioned before, films containing OEO are more effective than those containing other EOs.

3.4. Antimicrobial effects in packaged raw meat

Foodborne pathogens are commonly associated with raw meats. EOs of spices can be used as biopreservatives due to their antimicrobial properties [56]. Authors have demonstrated that OEO might be more effective against pathogens when used in combination with other natural compounds and technologies. Examples of these combinations include OEO and N,O-carboxymethyl chitosan [57], caprylic acid and vacuum packaging (VP) [58], VP [59] and MAP [60–62]. These treatments might extend shelf life of up to 8 days in different types of raw and cooked meat [59–61]. The treatments also control the growth of Gram-positive and Gram-negative bacteria, and pathogens, such as *L. monocytogenes* and *Salmonella typhimurium* [58, 59, 61, 62]. The minimum inhibitory concentration for OEO against *S. enteritidis* has been reported as 3.90 μl/ml [63]. A longer shelf life (9 days) than the previously reported was observed in the combination MAP and OEO and thyme EOs [64]. Mixed treatment (OEO, orange dietary fibre and MAP) caused a decrease in TBA values and in microbial counts. This combination did not affect the sensory attributes [65]. OEO and sodium lactate not only reduces the number of microbes but render them more susceptible to heat treatments [66]. These studies showed that OEO, by itself or in combination can be used in raw and processed meats to control pathogens and extend shelf life during chill storage.

3.5. Antimicrobial effects in fish products

The demand for natural alternatives to synthetic additives increases also includes raw and minimally processed fish. The effect of VP and OEO in Mediterranean octopus increases as the concentration of EO increased. The highest concentration of EO increases the shelf life to 20 days, meanwhile half the concentration had only an 11-day shelf life or 3 days when VP was by itself [67]. The effect of EOs is also observed with other EOs, as clove. Clove essential oil incorporated in a gelatin-chitosan film decreased the numbers of Gram-negative bacteria, mainly enterobacteriaceae in chilled-stored fish [68]. In rainbow trout fillets, as in other meats, OEO in combination with MAP decreased the numbers of lactic acid bacteria, H_2S-producing bacteria, enterobacteriacea and *Pseudomonas* spp. This combination avoided lipid oxidation, however, in contrast with other meats, the highest concentration of OEO impact negatively the sensory traits [69]. The concentration of OEO must be considered in order to balance microbial inhibition and sensory characteristics, because in order to obtain the highest inhibition the sensory traits might be negatively affected [70].

4. Conclusions

Even though some results are contradictory, it seems that the use of OEO as a feedstuff in live animals and production has a positive effect. Some of the effects are indirect or might not be evident, as the use of OEO to minimise meat downgrading due to transport stress or the modification of the ruminal microorganisms. The use of EO is still very much under review, as the doses are not fully developed; however, the antimicrobial action of these compounds is fully studied *in vivo* and *in vitro*. It might be of relevance to study not only the inclusion of EO, but also the inclusion of by-products that result from the production of EO. This review suggested a promising development of food natural preservative against spoilage microorganisms in food systems by the use of oregano essential oil. The effectiveness of oregano essential oil in retarding oxidative changes in meats has been widely demonstrated. The addition of oregano essential oil is a good way of preserving meat and could replace the synthetic antioxidants. Also, oregano oil and modified atmosphere packaging exhibit an additive preservation effect in fresh meat. The oregano essential oil is effective by controlling the growth of microorganisms without detrimental changes in sensory and acceptability attributes.

Author details

Alma Delia Alarcon-Rojo[1]*, Hector Janacua-Vidales[2] and Ana Renteria-Monterrubio[1]

*Address all correspondence to: aalarcon@uach.mx

1 Autonomous University of Chihuahua, Chihuahua, Mexico

2 Autonomous University of Ciudad Juarez, Ciudad Juarez, Mexico

References

[1] Barug D, De Jong J, Kies AK, Verstegen MWA. Antimicrobial growth promoters: Where do we go from here? 1st ed. Wageningen: Wageningen Academic Publishers; 2006. 196 p. DOI: 10.3920/978-90-8686-570-3

[2] Yan F, Azizi A, Janke S, Schwarz M, Zeller S, Honermeier B. Antioxidant capacity variation in the oregano (*Origanum vulgare* L.) collection of the German National Genebank. Industrial Crops and Products. 2016;92:19–25.

[3] Fatima A, Agrawal P, Singh PP. Herbal option for diabetes: An overview. Asian Pacific Journal of Tropical Diseases. 2012;2(suppl 1): S536–S544.

[4] Brenes A, Roura E. Essential oils in poultry nutrition: Main effects and modes of action. Animal Feed Science and Technology. 2010;158(1–2):1–14. http://dx.doi.org.etechconricyt.idm.oclc.org/10.1016

[5] Calucci L, Pinzono C, Zandomeneghi M, Capocchi A. Effects of gamma-irradiation on the free radical and antioxidant contents in nine aromatic herbs and spices. Journal of Agriculture and Food Chemistry. 2013;51:927–934.

[6] Balandrin MF, Klocke JA. Natural plant chemicals: Sources of industrial and medicinal materials. Science. 1985;228:1154–1160.

[7] Langhout P. New additives for broiler chickens. World Poultry. 2000;16: 22–27.

[8] Losa R. The use of essential oils in animal nutrition. In: Feed Manufacturing in the Mediterranean Region. Improving Safety: From Feed to Food. In Proceeding 3rd Conf. Feed Manufacture Mediterranean. Reus, Spain. 2001; pp. 39–44.

[9] Wenk C. Herbs and botanicals as feed additives in monogastric animals. Asian-Australasian Journal of Animal Science. 2003;16:282–289.

[10] Burt S. Essential oils: Their antibacterial properties and potential applications in foods—a review. International Journal of Food Microbiology. 2004;94:223–253.

[11] Florou-Paneri P, Dostas D, Mitsopoulos I, Dostas V, Botsoglou E, Nikolakakis I, Botsoglou N. Effect of feeding rosemary and α-tocopheryl acetate on hen performance and egg quality. Poultry Science. 2006;465:143–149.

[12] Ertas ON, Güler TC, DalkIlIç B, Simsek ÜG. The effect of an essential oil mix derived from oregano, clove and anise on broiler performance. International Journal of Poultry Science. 2005;4:879–884.

[13] Tomaino A, Cimino F, Zimbalatti V, Venuti V, Sulfaro V, De Pasquale A, Saija A. Influence of heating on antioxidant activity and the chemical composition of some spice essential oils. Food Chemistry. 2005;89:549–554.

[14] Ebani VV, Nardoni S, Bertelloni F, Giovanelli S, Rocchigiani G, Pistelli L, Mancianti F. Antibacterial and antifungal activity of essential oils against some pathogenic bacteria and yeasts shed from poultry. Flavour and Fragance Journal. 2016;31:302–309. DOI: 10.1002/ffj.3318

[15] Arpášová H. 2011. Phytobiotics to replace antibiotic growth promoters and their impact on the usefulness and quality of the eggs of laying hens type. Nitra : SPU, 2011. 101 s. ISBN 978-80-552-0555-7.

[16] Arpášová H, Branislav G, Hrnčár C, Fik M, Herkel R, Pistová V. The effect of essential oils on performance of laying hens. Animal Science and Biotechnologies. 2015;48:8–14.

[17] Khattak F, Ronchi A, Castelli P, Sparks N. Effects of natural blend of essential oil on growth performance blood biochemistry, cecal morphology, and carcass quality of broiler chickens. Poultry Science. 2014;93:132–137.

[18] Peng QY, Li JD, Li Z, Duanb ZY, Wua YP. Effects of dietary supplementation with oregano essential oil on growth performance, carcass traits and jejunal morphology in broiler chickens. Animal Feed Science and Technology. 2016;214:148–153.

[19] Suchý P, Strakova E, Mas N, Serman V, Vecerek V, Bedrica L, Lukac Z, Horvat Z. The effect of a herbal additive on performance parameters in layers. Tierarztliche Umschau. 2010;65:74–78.

[20] Amrik B, Bilkei G. Influence of farm application of oregano on performances of sows. Canadian Veterinary Journal. 2004;45:674–677.

[21] Basmacioğlu MH, Baysal S, Misirlioğlu Z, Polat M, Yilmaz H, Turan N. Effects of oregano essential oil with or without feed enzymes on growth performance, digestive enzyme, nutrient digestibility, lipid metabolism and immune response of broilers fed on wheat-soybean meal diets. British Poultry Science. 2010;51(1):67–80.

[22] Abd EL, Motaal AM, Ahmed AMH, Bahakaim ASA, Fathi MM. Productive performance and immunocompetence of commercial laying hens given diets supplemeted with eucalyptus. International Journal of Poultry Science. 2008;7:445–449.

[23] Angelovičová M, Kačaniová M, Angelovič M, Lopašovský, Ľ. 2010. Per os use of Thymi aetheroleum for growth performance of the broiler chickens. Scientific Journal for Food Industry. Special Issue 2010,4:127–132.

[24] Mohiti-Asli M, Ghanaatparast-Rashti M. Dietary oregano essential oil alleviates experimentally induced coccidiosis in broilers. Preventive Veterinary Medicine 2015;120(2):195–202.

[25] Jang IS, Ko YH, Kang SY, Lee CY. Effect of a commercial essential oil on growth performance, digestive enzyme activity and intestinal microflora population in broiler chickens. Animal Feed Science and Technology. 2007;134:304–315.

[26] Lee KW, Everts H, Lankhorst AE, Kappert HJ, Beynen AC. Addition of β-ionone to the diet fails to affect growth performance in female broiler chickens Animal Feed Science and Technology. 2003;106:219–223.

[27] Simitzis PE, Symeon GK, Charismiadou MA, Bizelis JA, Deligeorgis SG. The effects of dietary oregano oil supplementation on pig meat characteristics. Meat Science. 2010;84(4):670–676. DOI: 10.1016/j.meatsci.2009.11.001

[28] Zeng Z, Xu X, Zhang Q, Li P, Zhao P, Li Q, Liu J, Piao X. Effects of essential oil supplementation of a low-energy diet on performance, intestinal morphology and microflora, immune properties and antioxidant activities in weaned pigs. Animal Science Journal. 2015;86:279–285. DOI: 10.1111/asj.12277

[29] Stelter K, Frahm J, Paulsen J, Berk A, Kleinwächter M, Selmar D, Dänicke S. Effects of oregano on performance and immunmodulating factors in weaned piglets. Archives of Animal Nutrition. 2013;67(6):461–476.

[30] Allan P, Bilkei G. 2005. Oregano improves reproductive performance of sows. Theriogenology. 2005;63(3):716–721. DOI: 10.1016

[31] Tan Ch, Wei H, Sun H, Ao J, Long G, Jiang S, Peng J. Effects of dietary supplementation of oregano essential oil to sows on oxidative stress status, lactation feed intake of sows, and piglet performance. Journal of Nutrition. 2015;1:1–9.

[32] Zhang T, Zhou YF, Zou Y, Hu XM, Zheng LF, Wei HK, Giannenas I, Jinc LZ, Peng J, Jiang SW. Effects of dietary oregano essential oil supplementation on the stress response, antioxidative capacity, and HSPs mRNA expression of transported pigs. Livestock Science 2015;180:143–149.

[33] Zou Y, Xiang Q, Wang J, Wei H, Peng J. Effects of oregano essential oil or quercetin supplementation on body weight loss, carcass characteristics, meat quality and antioxidant status in finishing pigs under transport stress. Livestock Science. 2016;192:33–38. DOI: 10.1016/j.livsci.2016.08.005

[34] Alarcón-Rojo AD, Peña-Gonzalez E, Janacua-Vidales H, Santana V, Ortega JA. Meat quality and lipid oxidation of pork after dietary supplementation with oregano essential oil. World Applied Sciences Journal. 2013;21(5):665–673.

[35] Benchaar C, Calsamiglia S, Chaves AV, Fraser GR, Colombatto D, McAllister TA, Beauchemin KA. A review of plant-derived essential oils in ruminant nutrition and production. Animal Feed Science and Technology. 2008;145(1–4):209–228.

[36] Newbold CJ, McIntosh FM, Williams P, Losa R, Wallace RJ. Effects of a specific blend of essential oil compounds on rumen fermentation. Animal Feed Science and Technology. 2004;114(1–4):105–112.

[37] Lejonklev J, Kidmose U, Jensen S, Petersen MA, Helwing ALF, Mortensen G, Peters,en MA, Helwing ALF, Mortensen G, Weisbjerg MR, Larsen MK. Short communication: Effect of oregano and caraway essential oils on the production and flavor of cow milk. Journal of Dairy Science. 2016;99:7898–7903.

[38] Carpino S, Horne J, Melilli C, Licitra G, Barbano DM, Van Soest PJ. Contribution of native pasture to the sensory properties of Ragusano cheese. Journal of Dairy Science. 2004;87:308–315.

[39] Calsamiglia S, Busquet M, Cardozo PW, Castillejos L, Ferret A. Essential Oils as modifiers of rumen microbial fermentation. Journal of Dairy Science. 2007;90(6):2580–2595.

[40] Kodal Coskun B, Çalikoğlu E, Karagöz Emiroğlu Z Candoğan K. Antioxidant active packaging with soy edible films and oregano or thyme essential oils for oxidative stability of ground beef patties. Journal of Food Quality. 2014;37:203–212.

[41] El Adab S, Hassouna M. Proteolysis, lipolysis and sensory characteristics of a tunisian dry fermented poultry meat sausage with oregano and thyme essential oils. Journal of Food Safety. 2016;36:19–32. DOI: 10.1111/jfs.12209

[42] Martín-Sánchez AM, Chaves-López C, Sendra E, Sayas E, Fenández-López J, Pérez-Álvarez JA. Lipolysis, proteolysis and sensory characteristics of a Spanish fermented dry-cured meat product (salchichón) with oregano essential oil used as surface mold inhibitor. Meat Science. 2011;89(1):35–44. DOI: 10.1016/j.meatsci.2011.03.018

[43] Alhijazeen M. Effect of oregano essential oil and tannic acid on storage stability and quality of ground chicken meat [thesis]. Ames, Iowa. Iowa State University; 2014.

[44] Fasseas MK, Mountzouris KC, Tarantilis PA, Polissiou M, Zervas G. Antioxidant activity in meat treated with oregano and sage essential oils. Food Chemistry. 2008;106(3):1188–1194.

[45] Nieto G, Jongberg S, Andersen ML, Skibsted LH. Thiol oxidation and protein cross-link formation during chill storage of pork patties added essential oil of oregano, rosemary, or garlic. Meat Science. 2013;95(2):177–184. DOI: 10.1016/j.meatsci.2013.05.016

[46] Pesavento G, Calonico C, Bilia AR, Barnabei M, Calesini F, Addona R, Mencarellia L, Carmagnini L, Di Martino MC, Lo Nostro A. Antibacterial activity of oregano, rosmarinus and thymus essential oils against *Staphylococcus aureus* and *Listeria monocytogenes* in beef meatballs. Food Control. 2015;54:188–199. DOI: 10.1016/j.foodcont.2015.01.045

[47] Oussalah M, Caillet S, Salmiéri S, Saucier L, Lacroix M. Antimicrobial and antioxidant effects of milk protein-based film containing essential oils for the preservation of whole beef muscle. Journal of Agriculture and Food Chemistry. 2004;52(18): 5598–5605. DOI: 10.1021/jf049389q

[48] Dong L, Hongli L, Lin J, Yongming C, Minglong Y, Haiyun C. Characterization of active packaging films made from poly(lactic acid)/poly(trimethylene carbonate) incorporated with oregano essential oil. Molecules. 2016;21(6):1–14. DOI:10.3390/molecules21060695

[49] Vital AC, Guerrero A, Monteschio JdeO, Valero MV, Carvalho CB, de Abreu Filho BA, Madrona GS, do Prado IN. Effect of edible and active coating (with rosemary and oregano essential oils) on beef characteristics and consumer acceptability. Plos One. 2016;11(8):1–15. DOI: 10.1371/journal.pone.0160535

[50] Benavides S, Villalobos-Carvajal R, Reyes JE. Physical, mechanical and antibacterial properties of alginate film: Effect of the crosslinking degree and oregano essential oil concentration. Journal of Food Engineering. 2012;110(2):232–239. DOI: 10.1016/j.jfoodeng.2011.05.023

[51] Kazemi SM. Rezaei M. Antimicrobial effectiveness of gelatin—alginate film containing oregano essential oil for fish preservation. Journal of Food Safety. 2015;35:482–490. DOI: 10.1111/jfs.12198

[52] Oral N, Vatansever L, Sezer Ç, Aydın B, Güven A, Gülmez M; Baser KHC, Kürkçüoğlu M. Effect of absorbent pads containing oregano essential oil on the shelf life extension of overwrap packed chicken drumsticks stored at four degrees Celsius. Poultry Science. 2009;88(7):1459–1465.

[53] Zinoviadou KG, Koutsoumanis KP, Biliaderis CG. Physico-chemical properties of whey protein isolate films containing oregano oil and their antimicrobial action against spoilage flora of fresh beef. Meat Science. 2009;82(3):338–345. DOI: 10.1016/j.meatsci.2009.02.004

[54] Emiroğlu ZK, Yemis GP, Coskun BK, Candoğan K. Antimicrobial activity of soy edible films incorporated with thyme and oregano essential oils on fresh ground beef patties. Meat Science. 2010;86(2):283–288.

[55] Seydim AC, Sarikus G. Antimicrobial activity of whey protein based edible films incorporated with oregano, rosemary and garlic essential oils. Food Research International. 2006;39(5):639–644. DOI: 10.1016/j.foodres.2006.01.013

[56] Marques JL, Volcão LM, Funck GD, Schneid Kroning I, Padilha da Silva W, Fiorentini ÂM, Ribeiro GA. Antimicrobial activity of essential oils of *Origanum vulgare* L. and *Origanum majorana* L. against *Staphylococcus aureus* isolated from poultry meat. Industrial Crops and Products. 2015;77(23):444–450. DOI: 10.1016/j.indcrop.2015.09.013

[57] Khanjaria A, Karabagias IK, Kontominas MG. Combined effect of N, O-carboxymethyl chitosan and oregano essential oil to extend shelf life and control *Listeria monocytogenes* in raw chicken meat fillets. LWT—Food Science and Technology. 2013;53(1):94–99. DOI: 10.1016/j.lwt.2013.02.012

[58] Hulankova R, Borilova G, Steinhauserova I. Combined antimicrobial effect of oregano essential oil and caprylic acid in minced beef. Meat Science. 2013;95(2):190–194. DOI: 10.1016/j.meatsci.2013.05.003

[59] Ntzimani AG, Giatrakou VI, Savvaidis IN. Combined natural antimicrobial treatments (EDTA, lysozyme, rosemary and oregano oil) on semi cooked coated chicken meat stored in vacuum packages at 4°C: Microbiological and sensory evaluation. Innovative Food Science & Emerging Technologies. 2010;11(1):187–196.

[60] Chouliara E, Karatapanis A, Savvaidis IN, Kontominas MG. Combined effect of oregano essential oil and modified atmosphere packaging on shelf-life extension of fresh chicken breast meat, stored at 4°C. Food Microbiology. 2007;24(6):607–617. DOI: 10.1016/j.fm.2006.12.005

[61] Tsigarida E, Skandamis P, Nychas GJE. Behaviour of *Listeria monocytogenes* and autochthonous flora on meat stored under aerobic, vacuum and modified atmosphere packaging conditions with or without the presence of oregano essential oil at 5°C. Journal of Applied Microbiology. 2000;89:901–909. DOI: 10.1046/j.1365-2672.2000.01170.x

[62] Skandamis P, Tsigarida E, Nychas GJE. The effect of oregano essential oil on survival/death of *Salmonella typhimurium* in meat stored at 5°C under aerobic, VP/MAP conditions. Food Microbiology. 2002;19(1): 97–103.

[63] Coutinho de Oliveira TL, de Araújo SR, Hilsdorf PR. A Weibull model to describe antimicrobial kinetics of oregano and lemongrass essential oils against *Salmonella enteritidis* in ground beef during refrigerated storage. Meat Science. 2013;93(3):645–651. DOI: 10.1016/j.meatsci.2012.11.004

[64] Karabagias I, Badeka A, Kontominas MG. Shelf life extension of lamb meat using thyme or oregano essential oils and modified atmosphere packaging. Meat Science. 2011;88(1): 109–116. DOI: 10.1016/j.meatsci.2010.12.010

[65] Viuda-Martos M, Ruiz-Navajas Y, Fernández-López J, Pérez-Álvarez JA. Effect of orange dietary fibre, oregano essential oil and packaging conditions on shelf-life of bologna sausages. Food Control. 2010;21(4):436–443. DOI: 10.1016/j.foodcont.2009.07.004

[66] Juneja VK, Hwang CA, Friedman M. Thermal inactivation and postthermal treatment growth during storage of multiple Salmonella serotypes in ground beef as affected by sodium lactate and oregano oil. Journal of Food Science. 2010;75:M1–M6. DOI: 10.1111/j.1750-3841.2009.01395.x

[67] Atrea I, Papavergou A, Amvrosiadis I, Savvaidis IN. Combined effect of vacuum-packaging and oregano essential oil on the shelf-life of Mediterranean octopus (Octopus vulgaris) from the Aegean Sea stored at 4°C. Food Microbiology. 2008;26(2):166–172. DOI: 10.1016/j.fm.2008.10.005

[68] Gómez-Estaca J, López de Lacey A, López-Caballero ME, Gómez-Guillén MC, Montero P. Biodegradable gelatin—chitosan films incorporated with essential oils as antimicrobial agents for fish preservation. Food Microbiology. 2010;27(7):889–896. DOI: 10.1016/j.fm.2010.05.012

[69] Pyrgotou N, Giatrakou V, Ntzimani A, Savvaidis IN. Quality assessment of salted, modified atmosphere packaged rainbow trout under treatment with oregano essential oil. Journal of Food Science. 2010;75:M406–M411.

[70] Van Haute S, Raes K, Van der Meeren P, Sampers I. The effect of cinnamon, oregano and thyme essential oils in marinade on the microbial shelf life of fish and meat products. Food Control. 2016;68:30–39. DOI: 10.1016/j.foodcont.2016.03.025

8

Tahitian Vanilla (*Vanilla ×tahitensis*): A Vanilla Species with Unique Features

Christel Brunschwig, François-Xavier Collard,
Sandra Lepers-Andrzejewski and
Phila Raharivelomanana

Abstract

This chapter reviews the main findings on Tahitian vanilla (*Vanilla ×tahitensis*) over the last 10 years. It brings new insights into the hybrid origin of *V. ×tahitensis* and its diversification in French Polynesia. It details then the different analytical methods used to characterize the flavour properties and the aroma impact compounds of Tahitian vanilla, with a special emphasis on how they can be used to differentiate Tahitian vanilla from other vanillas. Finally, the effect of the curing process on the chemical composition and the sensory properties is discussed. These results highlight the need to include some of the key volatile compounds into a more adapted quality control, in order to describe the characteristic sensory properties of Tahitian vanilla but also those from other origins.

Keywords: *V. ×tahitensis*, Tahitian vanilla, genetic biodiversity, aroma chemistry, high performance liquid chromatography, gas chromatography, sensory properties, quality control, curing process

1. Introduction

Though Tahitian vanilla production represents less than 1% of the world vanilla production [1], it possesses a unique aura, due to an original anise flavour, highly prized especially in gastronomy and perfumery. In order to better develop and organize the vanilla sector and to promote Tahitian vanilla specificities abroad, a dedicated institute "Vanille de Tahiti" was created in 2003 in French Polynesia [2]. One of its main objectives is to provide support to local actors and help controlling pests and diseases threatening vanilla vines, with the sponsored supply of insect-proof shade houses for instance. A research department was also established in order to characterize Tahitian vanilla in comparison to other vanilla species, through the study of the flavour composition and genetic diversity. The institute has been part of a larger project, which focused on characterizing, protecting and promoting the sustainable use and valorisation of vanilla biodiversity (VaBiome 2012–2015). This chapter aims at capturing the most significant results that have been acquired over the last 10 years at the institute "Vanille de Tahiti" through different collaborations inside and outside French Polynesia, with a particular focus on genetic diversity and aroma chemistry.

2. Origins and diversification of *Vanilla ×tahitensis*

The introduction of vanilla in French Polynesia is estimated to have occurred during the mid-nineteenth century. The elucidation of the origin of Tahitian vanilla is difficult due to different reports of at least three introduction events from various origins (Philippines, France and West Indies) [3–5]. On top of that, the origin of *Vanilla* introduced in the Philippines was not solved and believed to be in Central America [5, 6]. Furthermore, the number of different vanilla morphotypes or species that were introduced is unknown, as authors described the introduction of *Vanilla planifolia* or *Vanilla pompona*, and even used different names (*Vanilla aromatic* and *Vanilla sativa*) [3, 4] for species known today as synonymous of *V. planifolia*. So it remains unclear, whether the Tahitian vanilla specificities appeared before its introduction in a still indeterminate cultivation area, or after through cultivation in French Polynesia.

Even if the origin of Tahitian vanilla is still confused, it is obvious that Tahitian vanilla, as we know it today, is different from other vanillas and in particular *V. planifolia*, the most cultivated species in the world. Since 1915, about 60 years after the first well-documented introduction events, various new vanilla morphotypes were described in French Polynesia [7]. Four morphotypes were early distinguished as "Tahiti", "Haapape", "Tiarei" and "Potiti" [3, 5, 7, 8]. Based on morphological differences between vanillas found in French Polynesia and other cultivated vanillas, Moore went a step further and claimed that Tahitian vanilla was a new species and therefore called it *Vanilla tahitensis* [9]. Indeed, Tahitian vanilla differs morphologically by having thinner stems, narrower leaves and shorter pods when compared to *V. planifolia* [5, 9] (**Figure 1**).

In 1951, Porteres suggested that Tahitian vanilla could be a hybrid offspring between *V. planifolia* and a complex *V. pompona* – *V. odorata* [10]. More recent assessment of the Tahitian vanilla genetic diversity gave new insight into its hybrid origin. A genetic analysis based on universal markers widely dispersed through the genome [amplified fragment length polymorphism (AFLP)] was carried out to compare the presence/absence of a set of AFLP markers. It showed that 31% of *V. ×tahitensis* AFLP markers were shared only with *V. planifolia*, while 6% of them were shared only with *V. odorata*, and other markers were shared with more than two other *Vanill*a species [11, 12] (**Figure 2**). Another study based on the analy-

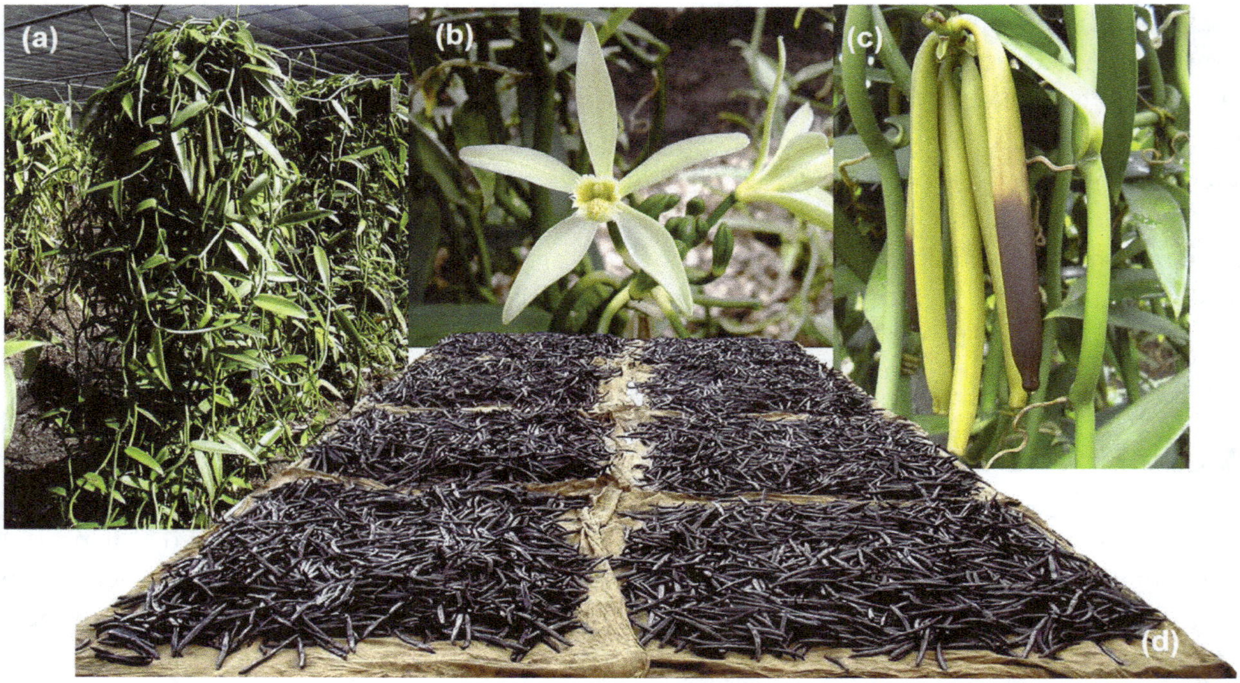

Figure 1. *Vanilla ×tahitensis* from French Polynesia: (a) vine in an insect-proof shade house, (b) flower, (c) mature pods and (d) cured vanilla pods.

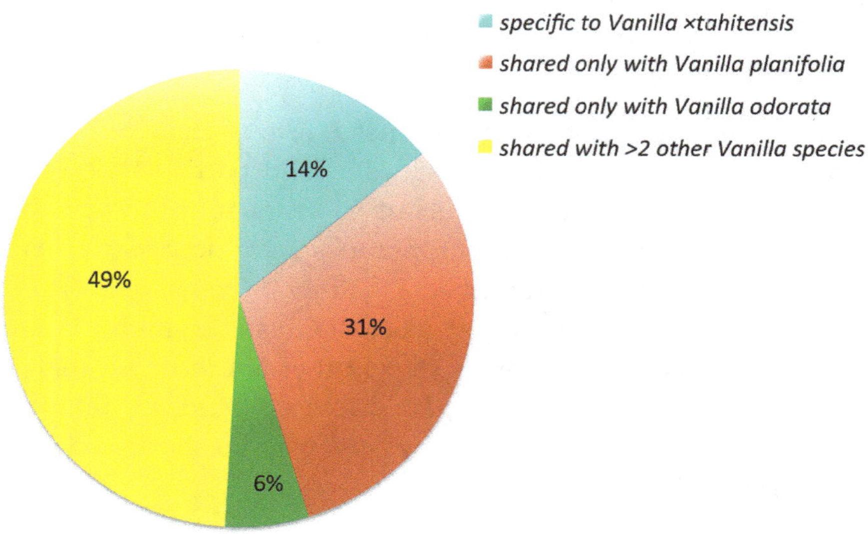

Figure 2. Specificity of the AFLP markers amplified from Tahitian vanilla accessions (*Vanilla ×tahitensis*) compared to other *Vanilla* species.

sis of a part of the genome preferentially inherited from the maternal parent (non-coding region of chloroplast DNA trnH-psbA) confirmed that *V. planifolia* was the maternal parent of Tahitian vanilla [6]. Since then, Tahitian vanilla is called *Vanilla ×tahitensis*; the "×" referring to its hybrid nature [13].

Coming back to the analysis of genetic diversity based on AFLP patterns, all Tahitian morphotypes were (i) distinct from the other *Vanilla* species studied (*V. planifolia*, *V. pompona* and *V. odorata*), (ii) genetically close to each other (mean dissimilarity index D = 0.0596) [11] and strongly grouped (**Figure 3**). Amongst Tahitian vanilla cultivars, the genetic diversity was higher than expected. While only 16 vanilla morphotypes were distinguished, more than 30 AFLP patterns were found. "Parahurahu" was the morphotype most genetically different from "Tahiti". It also differentiated by its morphological traits such as leaf size, pod shape and its aromatic composition. The genetic diversity amongst Tahitian vanilla was also explained by ploidy level differences. Indeed, the two mainly cultivated Tahitian vanilla morphotypes "Tahiti" and "Haapape" shared the same AFLP pattern, however "Tahiti" appeared to be diploid while "Haapape" was tetraploid [14]. Since vanilla is mainly propagated by stem cuttings, such variability was unexpected. The comparison of molecular markers patterns led to suggest that the recent genetic diversification in French Polynesia originated from self-pollination rather than from mutation events.

Biodiversity of Tahitian vanilla is preserved in the Genetic Resources Centre "Vanille de Tahiti" created on the island of Raiatea. About 140 accessions of *V. ×tahitensis* collected on different Polynesian islands are grown under insect-proof shade houses. These accessions, which are part of a vanilla-breeding programme, can be diffused on demand to scientists from any research institute for genetic or new flavour sourcing projects. Accessions are continuously assessed for various agronomical traits, resistance to diseases and aroma composition of their pods for further improvement.

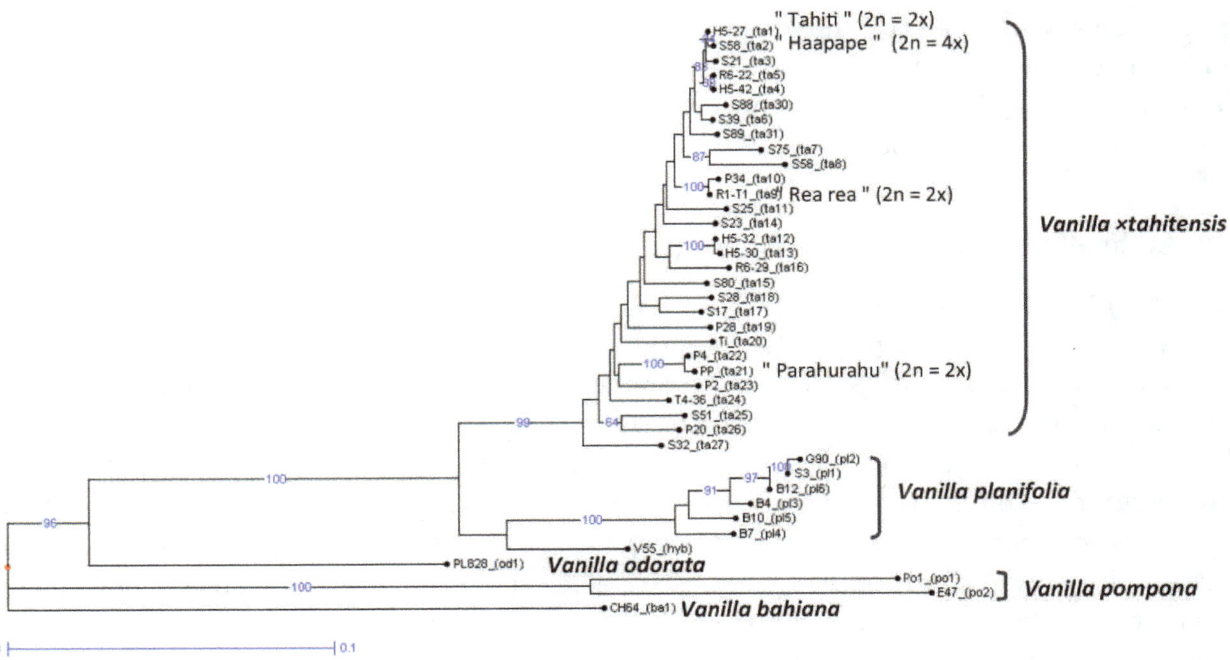

Figure 3. Phylogenetic tree of *Vanilla* species based on AFLP markers. Obtained from the Sokal and Michener genetic dissimilarity index and neighbour joining clustering; bootstrap values are expressed in percentage.

3. Tahitian vanilla flavour and differentiation from other vanillas

V. ×tahitensis is mainly cultivated in French Polynesia but is also found, together with *V. planifolia*, in New Guinea (Papua New Guinea and Indonesia). The origin of the introduction of *V. ×tahitensis* is unknown and the cultivar(s) grown have not been identified. Moreover the pods are sometimes not differentiated according to their species and commercialized as a mixture of *V. planifolia* and *V. ×tahitensis* [15]. It results in products with sensory properties completely different, when compared to those of Tahitian vanilla (see Section 3.2).

In French Polynesia, the quality of Tahitian vanilla is guaranteed by the training of different actors of the sector and several controls, after harvest and before exportation, are realized by sworn experts, as specified in the designation of origin "Vanille de Tahiti" recently released [16, 17]. Until 2014, there were no official analytical criteria to authenticate Tahitian vanilla in the international trade context, which would enable to differentiate it with vanilla from Papua New Guinea.

In order to determine what specifically differentiates Tahitian vanilla from other vanillas (*V. planifolia* the most cultivated in the world, *V. pompona* and vanilla from Papua New Guinea), in terms of flavour properties, the content of some chemical compounds of interest was assessed using different analytical techniques. Due to ease of implementation, the analysis by high performance liquid chromatography (HPLC) of vanilla extracts is still a method of reference. However, other analytical methods developed to assess the olfactory (gas chromatography-olfactometry) and gustative properties of vanilla, appear more appropriate to characterize the sensory properties of the pods. In order to correlate sensory properties and chemical composition, gas chromatography/mass spectrometry (GC/MS) analysis was also considered because of its ability to quantify a much larger number of compounds, when compared to HPLC.

3.1. Authentication based on HPLC profile

To authenticate natural vanilla (i.e. *V. planifolia*), quality control is usually based on the analysis by HPLC of some characteristic compounds (vanillyl and p-hydroxybenzyl derivatives) (**Figure 4**) extracted with ethanol as recommended by the International Organization for Standardization and the AOAC International [18, 19]. The ratios between those compounds are quite stable for the different origins of *V. planifolia* and throughout years of production, and are therefore recommended as quality markers by the Direction Générale de la Concurrence, de la Consommation et de la Répression des Fraudes (DGCCRF) guidelines [20]. However, these ratios are not appropriate to authenticate Tahitian vanilla, as data fall without ranges. It is worth noting that typical chromatograms obtained from Tahitian vanilla analysis are composed not only of p-hydroxybenzyl or vanillyl derivatives but also and predominantly of anisyl derivatives, which are actually not taken into account for those criteria (for compound structures see **Figure 4**).

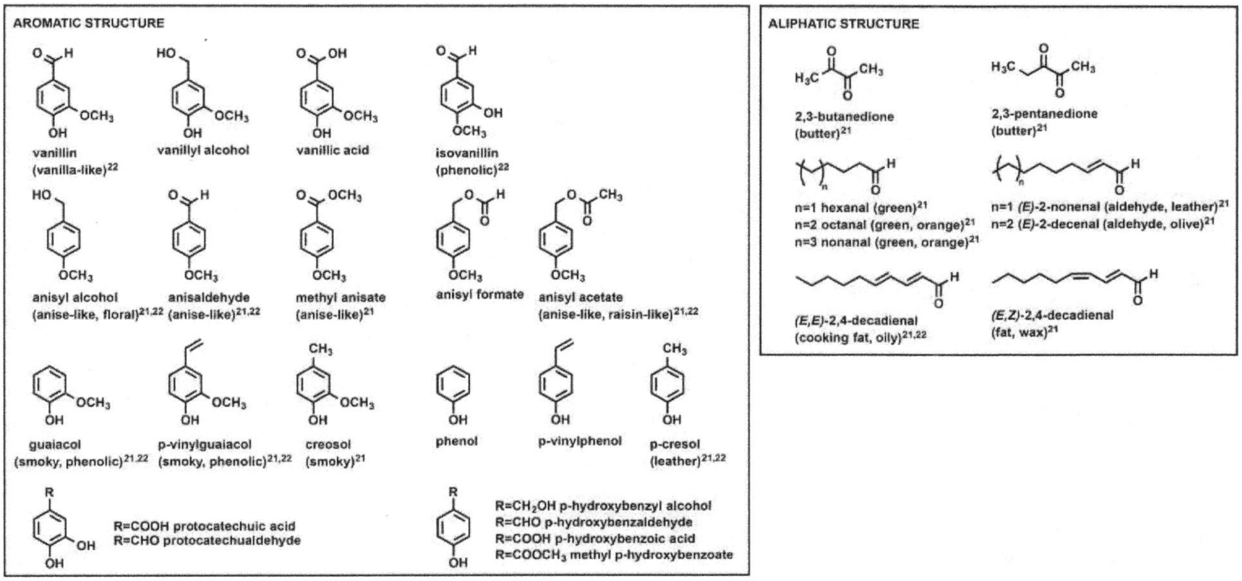

Figure 4. Structure of key compounds in the aroma chemistry of Tahitian vanilla (*V. ×tahitensis*). Odour descriptors are specified into brackets when compounds have been detected by GC-olfactometry in Refs. [21, 22].

This is exemplified by a study carried out between 2005 and 2007 at the Institute "Vanille de Tahiti". More than 300 vanilla samples, collected from vanilla curers based on the islands of Tahaa and Raiatea, where most of the vanilla was produced in French Polynesia at that time, were analysed by HPLC, together with 22 samples of *V. planifolia* and 9 samples from Papua New Guinea. The results showed that contrary to *V. planifolia,* which was composed almost only of vanillin (80% of the total quantified), Tahitian vanilla was characterized by a more subtle distribution: vanillin (25%), anisyl alcohol (30%), anisic acid (15%) as well as p-hydroxybenzyl compounds (20%) and protocatechuyl derivatives (5%) for a total content of 47,000 ppm (**Figure 5**), which exceeded the values typically reported for *V. planifolia* (40,000 ppm) [23–25].

The HPLC composition of Tahitian vanilla was homogeneous between the three years of production, for compounds whose concentration was higher than 1000 ppm (relative standard deviation <15%). As a result of this, low variability shown by principal component analysis using the HPLC composition and vanilla samples from various origins, it was possible to differentiate a set of Tahitian vanilla samples from *V. planifolia* of different origins and also from vanilla of Papua New Guinea, independently of the species (**Figure 6**).

The HPLC compositions of "Tahiti" and "Haapape" cultivars, which are the two main cultivars produced in French Polynesia, were found to be very close. The slight variations consisted in more vanillin and less p-hydroxybenzyl compounds in "Tahiti" pods. Consequently to this study, recommendations based on the contents of characteristic HPLC aroma compounds and their ratios have been made to assess Tahitian vanilla quality in French Polynesia. They have been integrated into official decrees published recently

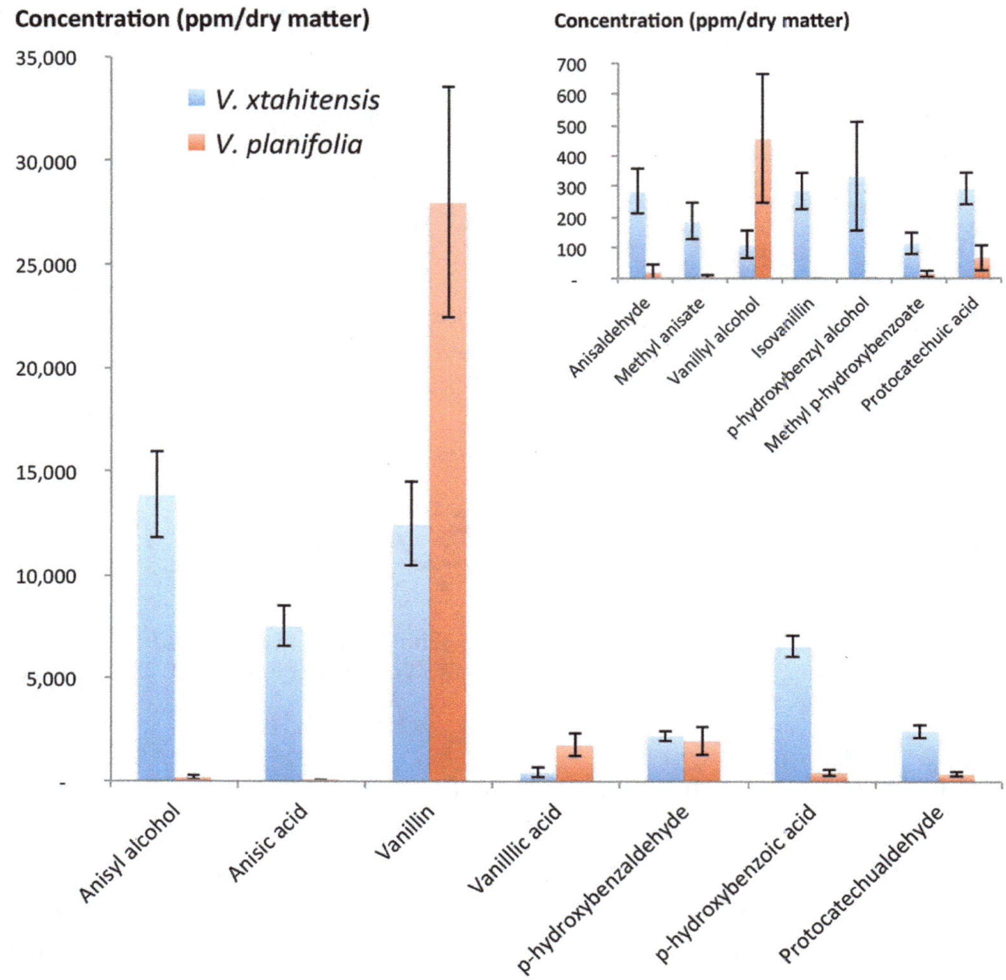

Figure 5. HPLC composition of Tahitian vanilla (*V. ×tahitensis* from French Polynesia; *n* = 300 samples over 3 years of production 2005–2007) and *V. planifolia* (20 samples from various origins: Madagascar, la Réunion, Mexico, Costa Rica).

[16, 17]. These decrees define the Tahitian vanilla's designation of origin ("Vanille de Tahiti"), its production area, the cultivars to be produced ("Tahiti" and "Haapape") with their genetic characteristics, the production and the curing process methods, as well as the pods quality based on moisture content (45–50%), aroma content and characteristic ratios using the concentrations of anisyl, vanillyl, p-hydroxybenzyl and protocatechuyl compounds determined by HPLC. These criteria can also be used to authenticate Tahitian vanilla abroad.

3.2. Towards a better authentication based on the relevant flavour compounds

Though HPLC is a reliable analytical technique to analyse some characteristic compounds of the vanilla pods, it appears as more convenient to use complementary analytical and sensory techniques to quantify more compounds, in particular those likely to contribute/to affect the vanilla flavour. The perception of a flavour is due to the detection of a complex mixture of

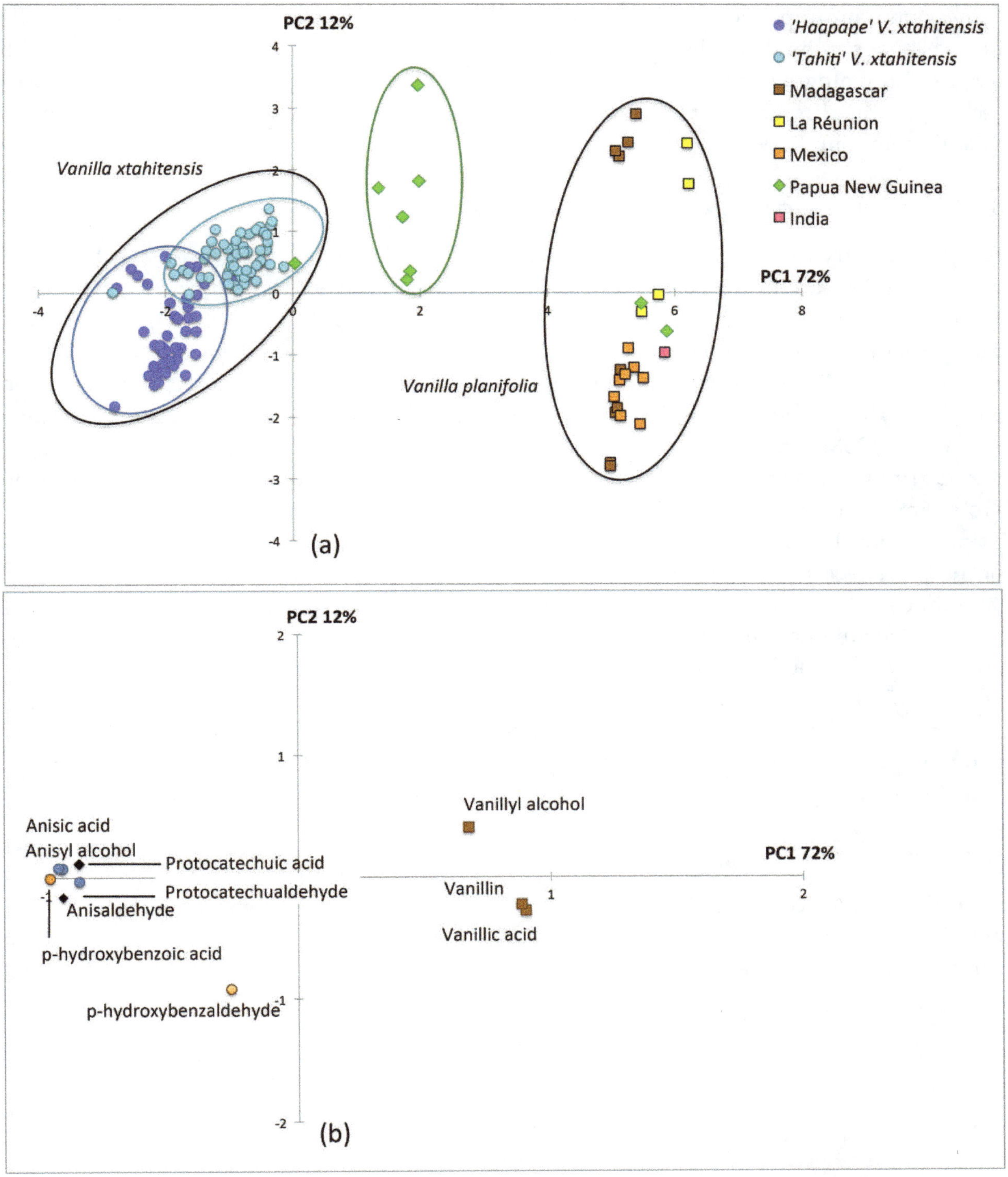

Figure 6. Projection plots on Principal Components of (a) observations scores (dataset of vanilla samples from different origins and (b) variables coefficients (compound concentrations analysed by HPLC). PC1 and PC2 explained, respectively, 72% and 12% of the total variance in the data.

compounds having various physico-chemical properties. Non-volatile (or less volatile) compounds, like essential fatty acids, have the ability to fix some non-polar aroma constituents. Volatile compounds, which have various odour-detection thresholds, can sometimes have a preponderant impact on the aroma, even when present in low amounts. Tahitian vanilla aroma chemistry has been therefore investigated using additional analytical techniques, such as gas chromatography-mass spectrometry (GC-MS), sensory analysis and a hyphenated technique, gas chromatography coupled with olfactometry (GC-O) designed to detect more volatile compounds.

3.2.1. Gas chomatography-olfactometry and volatile compounds

GC-olfactometry enables to decompose the individual odours of an aroma extract and attribute these odours to specific compounds, which are called aroma impact compounds. GC-olfactometry was applied to the analysis of different vanilla extracts: *V. planifolia* from Mexico [26], *V. planifolia* from Madagascar and Uganda [27], *V. ×tahitensis* from French Polynesia [21, 22] and *V. pompona* from Mexico [28]. The unique sensory fingerprint of Tahitian vanilla was highlighted by the detection of about 60 notes using the odour-specific magnitude estimation (OSME) method for both cultivars "Tahiti" and "Haapape" [21]. Amongst them, 38 were attributed to a specific compound. Anisaldehyde and guaiacol were found to be the main aroma impact compounds of Tahitian vanilla. These two compounds were also found to be primary impact aroma compounds of *V. pompona*, although the overall aroma characteristics of the two species were quite different. Main aroma impact compounds of *V. planifolia* were vanillin derivatives and phenolic compounds such as guaiacol, creosol, p-cresol or phenol. It is noteworthy that despite a relatively low content in the pods, anisyl compounds such as anisaldehyde and anisylalcohol were also identified as odour-impact compounds in *V. planifolia* [26, 27]. The GC-O profile of *V. ×tahitensis* was more balanced compared to other species; enabling the co-expression of multiple notes such as phenolic-vanilla like notes, anise-spicy and floral notes, while *V. planifolia* flavour was mainly characterized by phenolic-vanilla notes and *V. pompona* by floral notes (**Figure 7**).

3.2.2. Sensory properties and volatile compounds

In addition to the compounds analysed by HPLC, various volatile compounds such as phenolic compounds, aliphatic aldehydes, ketones and esters contributing to the flavour of Tahitian vanilla were identified and quantified by GC-MS [29]. Still, this method highlighted

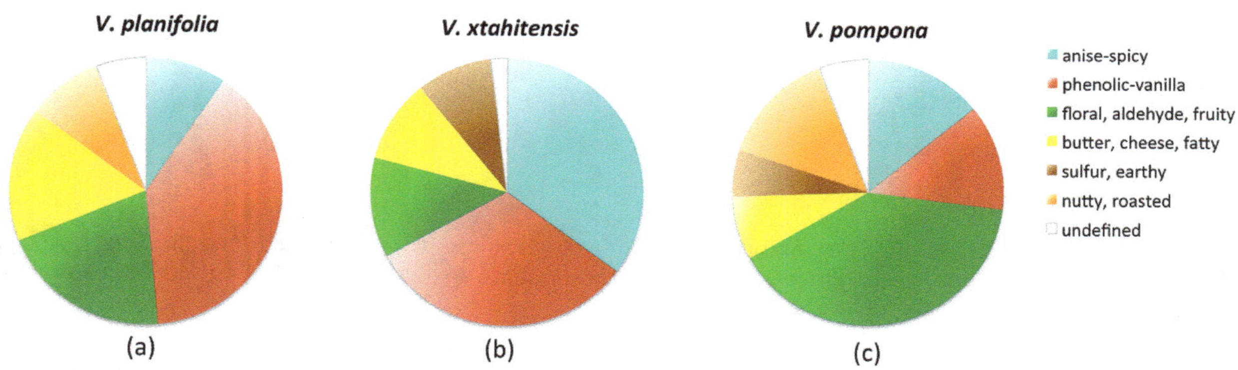

Figure 7. Distribution of odour vanilla notes based on the analysis by GC olfactometry of the impact aroma compounds of (a) *V. planifolia*, (b) *V. xtahitensis*, and (c) *V. pompona* (adapted with permission from Ref. [21, 27, 28]).

that compared to *V. planifolia*, *V. ×tahitensis* had a higher content of anisyl compounds, which represented 70% of the total volatile content against 7% for *V. planifolia*; amongst them anisyl alcohol, anisaldehyde, methyl anisate and anisyl acetate were the major ones (for compound structures see **Figure 4**). The other characteristics of *V. ×tahitensis* were a much lower vanillin content than *V. planifolia* (5–10% against 30%, respectively), as well as lower contents of phenolic compounds and aliphatic aldehydes (less than 10% against more than 40% and 0.5–1% against 2%, respectively). The volatile composition of Papua New Guinea vanilla showed some similarities to that of Tahitian vanilla especially regarding anisyl compounds, but some key compounds could differentiate them such as methyl esters, anisyl formate, p-cresol or p-vinylguaiacol [29].

In relation to their volatile composition, it was also possible to clearly differentiate the sensory properties of Tahitian vanilla from *V. planifolia* and also from vanilla from Papua New Guinea. The method used, called quantitative descriptive analysis, consisted in a panel of judges who tasted aroma extracts. Compared to the other vanillas, Tahitian vanilla displayed more intense anise, caramel and vanilla notes despite a relatively low vanillin content. *V. planifolia* was characterized by more intense phenolic, woody and smoky notes (**Figure 8**) [29]. Similarly, another sensory study depicted Tahitian vanilla aroma as less resinous, less dried fruit-like and more floral compared to *V. planifolia* from Madagascar [22]. The sensory profile of vanilla from Papua New Guinea was well differentiated from that of Tahitian vanilla with strong fruity, spicy and brown rum notes [29], the latter being probably related to the curing method as those were found to become stronger throughout the curing process (see Section 4).

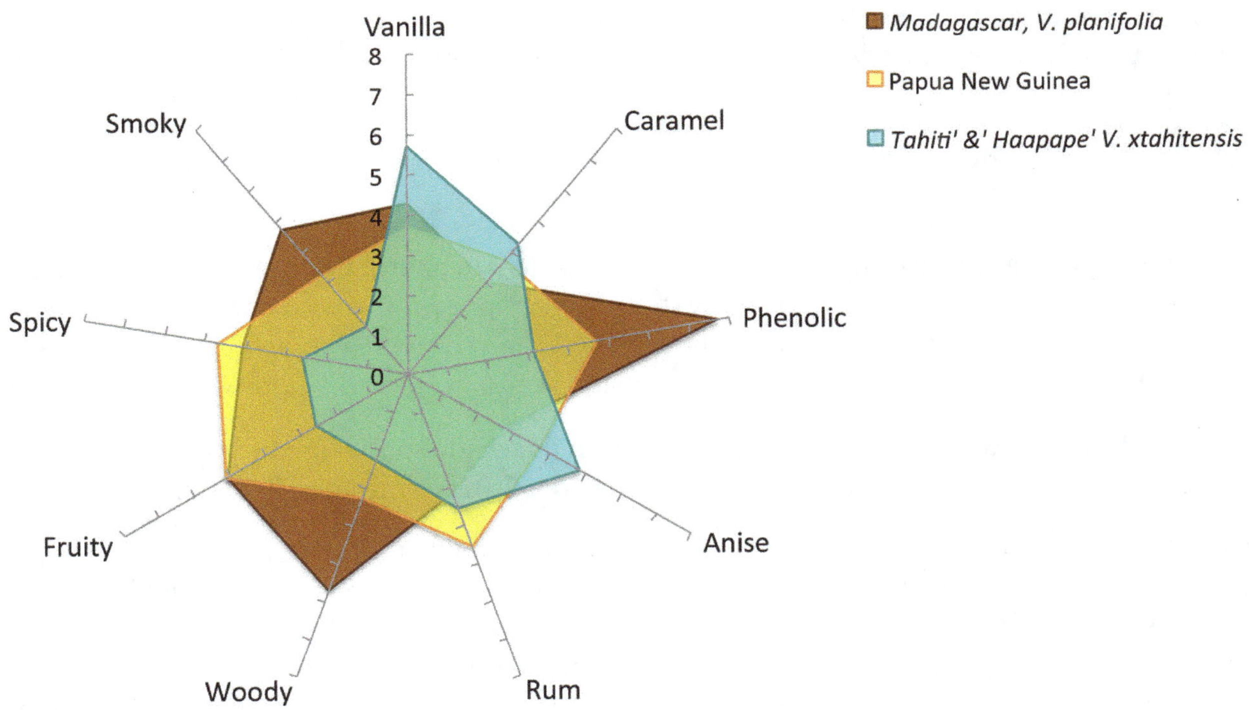

Figure 8. Sensory profiles of Tahitian vanilla (*V. ×tahitensis,* mix of "Tahiti" and "Haapape" cultivars) compared to vanilla from other origins (adapted with permission from Ref. [29]).

As we tried to correlate the sensory properties of vanilla from different origins to their volatile composition, it remained difficult to link single volatile compounds to specific notes, as there are many interactions between volatile and non-volatile compounds. However, we were able to show that the strongest correlations were between phenolic, woody, smoky notes and a pool of phenolic compounds such as guaiacol and creosol. Such correlation between guaiacol and woody notes has also been highlighted for *V. planifolia* [25] and led to the development of more appropriate analysis methods to characterize vanilla flavour also based on the detection of negative compounds such as guaiacol [30]. Anisyl compounds, especially methyl anisate were well correlated with anise notes. p-Vinylguaiacol was another compound of interest, as

differentiated the two origins [29]. These results stressed the need to integrate volatile compounds belonging to the phenolic series (guaiacol, creosol, p-cresol and p-vinylguaiacol) and to the anisyl series (anisyl alcohol, anisaldehyde and methyl anisate but also anisyl formate and anisyl acetate) in a more appropriate quality control, be it to authenticate *V. ×tahitensis* or more generally to assess vanilla quality independently of its origin.

4. The effect of curing process on vanilla flavour

Since we started our journey studying Tahitian vanilla characteristics, there was a question that needed to be answered: how much of the aroma is inherent to the vanilla species and what is the influence of the curing process on the aroma development? To get an answer, we first have to go back to the curing process as it is performed in French Polynesia. First, Tahitian vanilla pods are harvested when fully ripe, then they are cured following three main steps [31]:

(1) Shade browning: vanilla pods have 80% moisture and are exposed on the shade until being entirely brown.

(2) Sun drying and sweating: for several weeks, pods are alternatively exposed for a short period of time (2–4 h) in the sun every day, then wrapped into a cotton fabric and leave to sweat overnight in closed wooden cases. As pods become increasingly flexible and glossy due to water loss, they are massaged to ensure seeds are spread lengthwise.

(3) Air drying and refining: finally pods are left in the shade so that the moisture and aroma contents stabilize in order to obtain homogeneous batches (around 50% moisture).

Unlike other vanilla species, *V. ×tahitensis* pods do not split when fully ripe. It means they can be kept on the vine until full maturity when aroma content is at its optimum. Late harvest is also likely to limit the risk of mould formation during storage. Another consequence is that there is no need for any initial heat treatment in hot water or in an oven, as it is performed commonly in the Indian Ocean region, in Central America or in New Guinea. During curing, many biotransformations take place due to the presence of intrinsic enzymes located in the pods and/or the action of colonizing microorganisms on the surface as evidenced by the latest findings on *V. planifolia* [32]. Even if the different biotransformations involved are still unclear, they will definitely contribute to the development of the final vanilla flavour that one can experience when smelling cured vanilla pods.

4.1. Effect of curing on aroma composition using HPLC

The evolution of the aroma composition of Tahitian vanilla pods was monitored by HPLC analysis of "Tahiti" and "Haapape" samples collected at various steps of the curing process. It was observed that through drying, the aroma content of the pods decreased by around 30%, from around 70,000 ppm at 80% moisture content to 50,000 ppm for a final moisture content of 50–55% (**Figure 9**). This loss could be attributed to co-evaporation of the compounds with water while sun drying and/or loss in liquid form during pod sweating, as evidenced by the oily substance observed at the surface of the fabric wrap.

Within a same compound series, acids concentrations (in red) remained stable during the curing process; while alcohols concentrations (in blue) tended to decrease linearly over time. The fate of aldehydes (in black) varied across the series, as anisaldehyde concentration remained stable, while vanillin concentration decreased linearly. These different trends were related to many interdependent factors such as the oxidation state of the compounds (alcohols can be oxidized into aldehydes then into acids within a series), their physico-chemical properties (volatility and lipophilicity), and the fact that the compounds can be potential substrates or

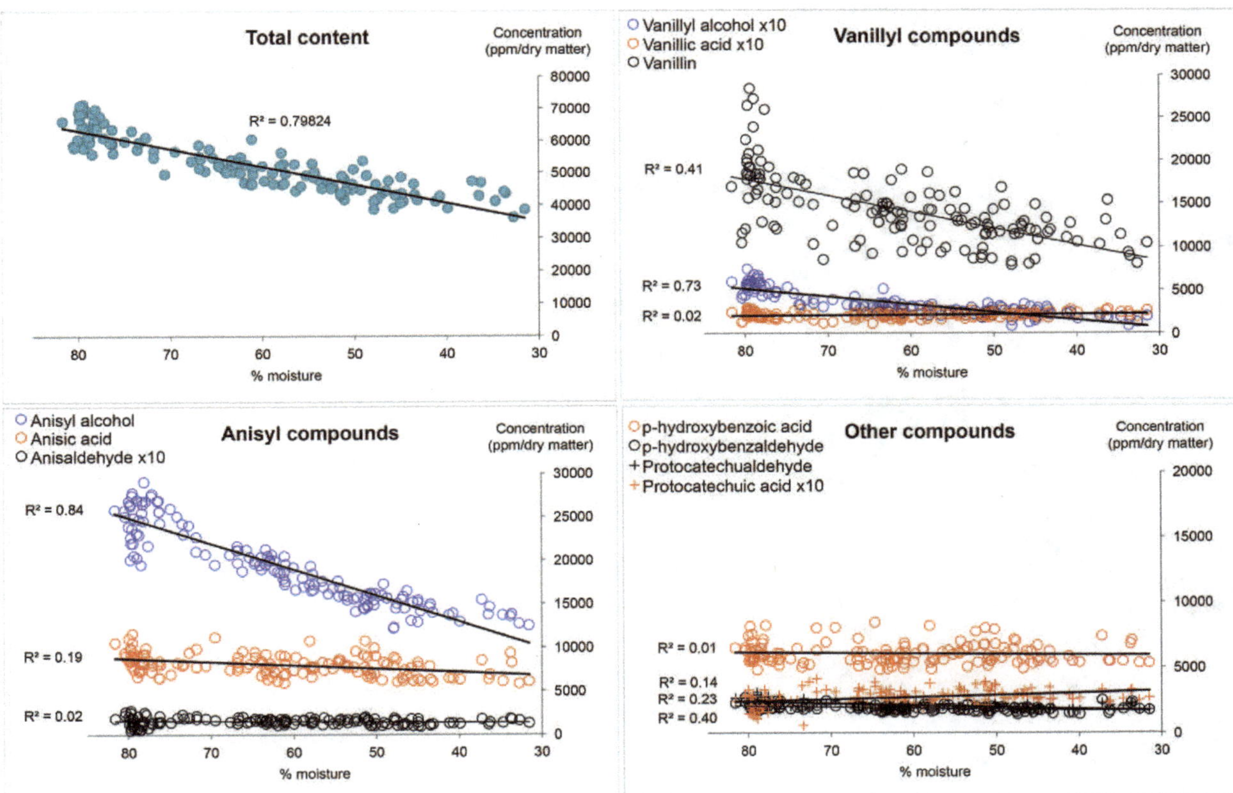

Figure 9. Variations of Tahitian vanilla composition obtained by HPLC during the curing process (*V. ×tahitensis*, "Tahiti" and "Haapape" cultivars).

metabolites of intrinsic enzymes or colonizing microorganisms. The relatively high variability of the compounds concentration, especially vanillin, observed at the beginning of the curing process progressively decreased, resulting in more homogeneous vanilla batches at the end of the curing process.

4.2. Effect of curing on sensory properties and volatile compounds

In order to get a better understanding of how the pod aroma was developed, we studied the evolution of sensory properties by quantitative descriptive analysis and of relative volatile compounds concentration by GC-MS at different steps during the curing process: (i) step S1—shade browning (80% moisture), (ii) step S2—sun drying (60–65%, pods are wrinkled); (iii) step S3—air drying (50–55% moisture); (iv) step S3*—enhanced drying: sun drying was extended to mimic curing methods of vanillas from other origins and obtain vanilla pods at 40% moisture.

Some of the sensory notes of "Tahiti" cultivar varied significantly during the curing process (**Figure 10**), while the variations for "Haapape" were not significant (data not shown). Regarding the "Tahiti" cultivar, vanilla, anise, rum and caramel notes remained as intense as they were initially or slightly decreased while woody, phenolic, smoky, spicy and fruity notes progressively (and significantly for most of them) built up during the curing process. It is noteworthy that even when *V. ×tahitensis* pods were taken to the enhanced drying step until

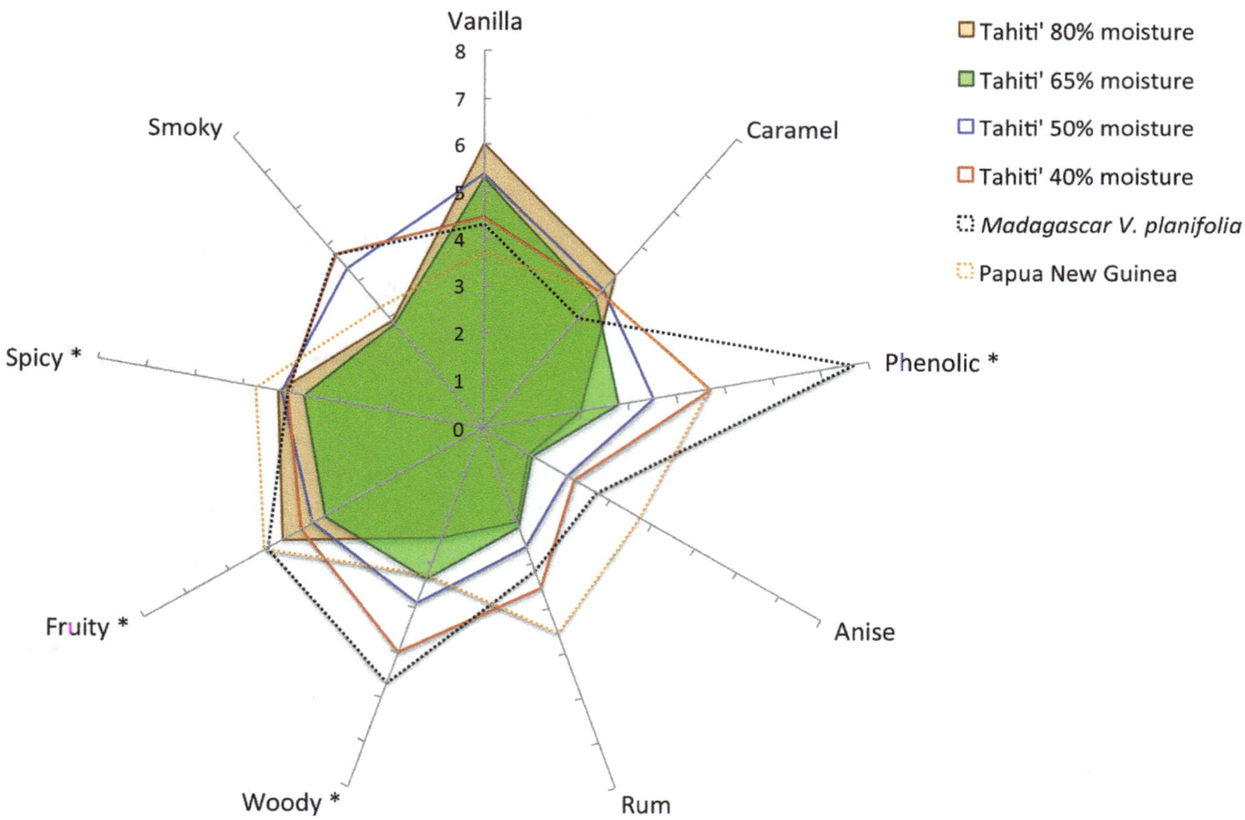

Figure 10. Sensory scores of Tahitian vanilla (*V. ×tahitensis*, "Tahiti" cultivar) at different moisture contents during the curing process compared to other vanillas. *indicate that sensory scores were significantly different between Tahitian vanilla samples during the curing process ($p < 0.05$).

reaching 40% moisture, they still had a sensory profile different from other vanillas. However, some sensory characteristics, especially phenolic, woody, fruity and spicy notes tended towards to that of *V. planifolia* or vanilla from Papua New Guinea, which is not required as the development of such notes is not seen as an improvement. Based on these findings, curing should be processed judiciously in order to enable the perfect balance of phenolic and anise-floral notes to develop. Drying up to 50% appeared to be the optimal conditions in order to retain as much as possible the initial organoleptic properties of Tahitian vanilla (vanilla and caramel) while limiting the woody, smoky and phenolic notes.

The curing method induced variations in the volatile composition, which impacted greatly the final flavour. Despite a relatively low concentration in the Tahitian vanilla extracts, some aliphatic aldehydes and ketones played a pivotal role by GC-olfactometry [21] due to a low odour threshold [29]. They originate from the oxidation of essential fatty acids such as linoleic and oleic acids, the major fatty acids in Tahitian vanilla pods [33]. Indeed, the fatty acid content was found to decrease from 2.7% of dry matter to 1.6% during the curing process (cultivar "Tahiti"). The increase in the concentration of saturated aldehydes (hexanal, heptanal, octanal and nonanal) linked to fruity notes was seen as positive, contrary to the increase of monounsaturated (heptenal, octenal, nonenal and decenal) and diunsaturated aldehydes (2,4 decadienal) (**Figure 11a**), which displayed less pleasant notes like leather, olive, wax and cooking fat by GC-O [21]. Thus, drying the pods until 40% moisture is not recommended. Similar variations of aliphatic aldehydes were observed during the curing process of *V. planifolia* [34]. Aliphatic ketones, such as 2,3 butanedione and 2,3 pentanedione perceived as butter, were found to have an optimal content at 50% moisture, while 3-hydroxybutanone decreased, being metabolized by bacili bacteria into 2,3-butanediol as suggested for cocoa [35].

The overall content of odour-active anisyl compounds was stable during the curing process of Tahitian vanilla, even though individual compounds contents varied (**Figure 11b**). When comparing the evolution between steps S1 and S3*, anisyl alcohol and methyl anisate contents were found to decrease, while anisaldehyde, anisyl acetate and anisyl formate contents slightly increased. The overall content of phenolic compounds (guaiacol, p-cresol, creosol, phenol, p-vinyl-phenol and p-vinyl guaiacol) increased during the curing process, in tune with the development of phenolic notes. Particularly, there was a dramatic increase of p-vinyl guaiacol by five-fold (**Figure 11c**). The increase of such phenolic compounds was also observed when Tahitian vanilla was stored for a long period of time (five years, data not shown). Overdrying vanilla pods to 40% moisture, as usually performed in other countries, was not beneficial to the Tahitian vanilla aroma, due to the concomitant increase of phenolic compounds concentration and the development of phenolic notes. The higher levels of p-vinylguaiacol and other phenolic compounds detected in vanilla from Papua New Guinea can find its roots in the way the curing process is performed.

Single compounds variations such as anisaldehyde, methyl anisate, guaiacol or p-vinyl guaiacol could not explain all the variations observed while monitoring sensory properties during the curing process, as aroma compounds also interact with less volatile components and between them. However, they were found to be overall good indicators of the development of the targeted sensory properties and it would be advisable to monitor their concentrations.

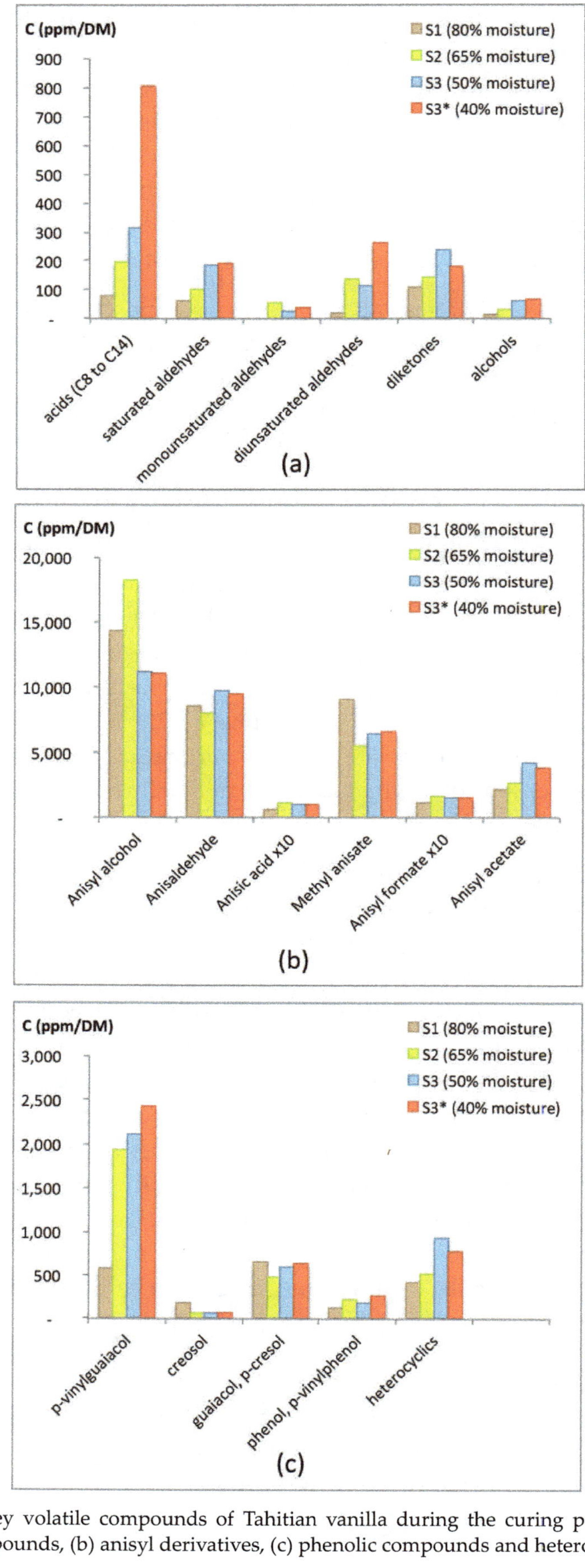

Figure 11. Evolution of key volatile compounds of Tahitian vanilla during the curing process (*V. ×tahitensis,* Tahiti cultivar) (a) aliphatic compounds, (b) anisyl derivatives, (c) phenolic compounds and heterocyclics. DM: dry matter.

5. Conclusion

Tahitian vanilla has come a long way to be as it is known today. Various vanilla vines from different species have travelled around the world and been introduced in French Polynesia, to give the hybrid *V. ×tahitensis,* which is currently grown in French Polynesia. Polynesian vanilla growers have selected over time the best cultivars to be produced, "Tahiti" and "Haapape" and have refined the curing method according to the specificity of Tahitian vanilla. This study showed that HPLC analysis and vanillin content of the pods were not always appropriate to assess the flavour properties of the pods. Modern analytical techniques have highlighted the subtle aroma chemistry of Tahitian vanilla. The use of sensory techniques has enabled to show that the flavour of Tahitian vanilla differentiated from other vanilla by stronger anise, vanilla and caramel notes. The weaker phenolic and woody notes appeared to be linked to the curing process, which plays a very important role in the development of volatile compounds. Curing vanilla pods at 50% moisture seems to be the optimal content so that Tahitian vanilla aroma develops fully and keeps its distinctive characteristics compared to other origins.

New authentication criteria of Tahitian vanilla based on HPLC profiles and specific anisyl compounds have been published recently in French Polynesia and could be used to certify its origin. In order to maintain Tahitian vanilla originality, quality control should also be orientated towards odour-active compounds, which impact definitely the aroma. This will help protecting the specificities of this unique spice.

Author details

Christel Brunschwig[1,2]*, François-Xavier Collard[2], Sandra Lepers-Andrzejewski[2] and Phila Raharivelomanana[1]

*Address all correspondence to: christel.brunschwig@gmail.com

1 Integrated Study of Secondary Metabolites (EIMS), Research Unit UMR 241 Insular Ocean Ecosystems (EIO), University of French Polynesia, Faaa, Tahiti, French Polynesia

2 Research and Development Department, Institute "Vanille de Tahiti", Raiatea, French Polynesia

References

[1] FAOSTAT. Vanilla production in French Polynesia between 2000 and 2013 [Internet]. 2015. Available from: http://faostat3.fao.org/browse [Accessed: 2016–10–25]

[2] Institute "Vanille de Tahiti". About us [Internet]. 2015. Available from: http://vanilledetahiti.com [Accessed: 2016–10–25]

[3] Chevalier A. La systématique du genre Vanilla et l'amélioration des plants de vanille [Systematics of Vanilla genus and improvement of vanilla seedlings]. Revue de botanique appliquée et d'agriculture tropicale. 1946;26(281):107–111.

[4] Cuzent G. Archipel de Tahiti: recherches sur les productions végétales [Tahiti archipelago: research on plant production], 2nd edition (1860 reed. 1983), Papeete: Eds Haere po no Tahiti, 1983. 208 p.

[5] Henry C. Caractères généraux des différents vanilliers cultivés à Tahiti [Systemic characteristics of various vanilla plants cultivated in Tahiti]. L'agronomie tropicale. 1924;79:133–136.

[6] Lubinsky P, Cameron KM, Molina MC, Wong M, Lepers-Andrzejewski S, Gomez-Pompa A, et al. Neotropical roots of a polynesian spice: the hybrid origin of Tahitian vanilla, *Vanilla tahitensis* (Orchidaceae). American Journal of Botany. 2008;95(8):1040–1047. DOI:10.3732/ajb.0800067

[7] Costantin J, Bois D. Note sur trois types de vanilles commerciales de Tahiti [Note on three commercial vanilla types from Tahiti]. Compte rendu de l'académie des Sciences de Paris. 1915;61:196–202.

[8] Bouriquet G, Hibon E. Quelques vanilliers cultivés dans les établissements français d'Océanie [Some vanilla plants cultivated in the french settlements in Oceania]. L'agronomie tropicale. 1950;1–2:54–61.

[9] Moore JW. New and critical plants from Raiatea. Bernice P Bishop Museum Bulletin. 1933;102:25.

[10] Portères R. Nouvelles espèces de vanilliers [New vanilla plant species]. Bulletin de la Société Botanique de France. 1951;98(4–6):92–95. DOI:10.1080/00378941.1951.10834884

[11] Lepers-Andrzejewski S, Causse S, Caromel B, Wong M, Dron M. Genetic linkage map and diversity analysis of Tahitian vanilla (*Vanilla ×tahitensis*, Orchidaceae). Crop Science. 2012;52:795–806. DOI:10.2135/cropsci2010.11.0634

[12] Duval MF, Bory S, Andrzejewski S, Grisoni M, Besse P, Causse S, et al. Diversité génétique des vanilliers dans leurs zones de dispersion secondaire [Genetic diversity of vanilla plants observed in secondary dispersal areas]. Les Actes du Bureau des Ressources Génétiques. 2006;6:181–196.

[13] Soto Arenas MA, Dressler RL. A revision of the Mexican and Central American species of *Vanilla* Plumier ex Miller with a characterisation of their ITS region of the nuclear ribosomal DNA. Lankesteriana. 2010;9(3):285–354. DOI:10.15517/lank.v0i0.12065

[14] Lepers-Andrzejewski S, Siljak-Yakovlev S, Brown S, Wong M, Dron M. Diversity and dynamics of plant genome size: an example of polysomaty from a cytogenetic study of Tahitian vanilla (*Vanilla ×tahitensis*, Orchidaceae). American Journal of Botany. 2011;98(6):1–12. DOI:10.3732/ajb.1000415

[15] Ranadive AS. Vanilla cultivation. Vanilla First International Congress, East Brunswick. 2003, 25–32.

[16] Conseil des Ministres de la Polynésie française. Arrêté n° 960 du 26 juin 2014 portant définition de l'appellation d'origine "Vanille de Tahiti" [Order n° 960 from the Executive Council, June 26th 2014, defining the designation of origin "Vanille de Tahiti"]. Journal Officiel de la Polynésie française. 2014:8210–8214.

[17] Conseil des Ministres de la Polynésie française. Arrêté n°1111 CM du 10 août 2016 portant définition de l'appellation d'origine "Vanille de Tahiti" [Order n° 1111 from the Executive Council, August 10th 2016, defining the designation of origin "Vanille de Tahiti"]. Journal Officiel de la Polynésie française. 2016:9169–9175.

[18] The International Organization for Standardization. ISO 5565–2 Vanilla (Vanilla fragrans (Salisbury) Ames)—Part 2: tests methods. 1999. Geneva : ISO. 11 p.

[19] AOAC International. AOAC Official method 990:25—Vanillin, vanillic acid, p-hydroxybenzaldehyde, and p-hydroxybenzoic acid and ethyl vanillin in vanilla extract and artificial vanilla flavor. Liquid chromatographic method. 2013. AOAC Official Methods of Analysis AOAC: Rockville, MD.

[20] Ministère de l'Economie, des Finances et de l'Industrie, République Francaise. Direction Générale de la Concurrence de la Consommation et de la Répression des Fraudes. Note d'information n°2003–61 sur la vanille: Définition des critères analytiques d'authenticité de la vanille, des extraits et des arômes naturels vanille [Information note n°2003–61 on vanilla: Definition of analytical criteria of authenticity of vanilla, vanilla extracts, and natural vanilla flavours]. 2003. 6 p.

[21] Brunschwig C, Senger-Emonnot P, Aubanel ML, Pierrat A, George G, Rochard S, et al. Odor-active compounds of Tahitian vanilla flavor. Food Research International. 2012;46(1):148–157. DOI:10.1016/j.foodres.2011.12.006

[22] Takahashi M, Inai Y, Miyazawa N, Kurobayashi Y, Fujita A. Identification of the key odorants in Tahitian cured vanilla beans (Vanilla tahitensis) by GC-MS and an aroma extract dilution analysis. Bioscience, Biotechnology, and Biochemistry. 2013;77(3):601–605. DOI:10.1271/bbb.120840

[23] Fayet B, Tisse C, Guérère M, Estienne J. Nouveaux critères analytiques dans l'étude des gousses de vanille. Analusis [New analytical criteria for the study of vanilla pods]. 1987;15(5):217–226.

[24] Derbesy M. Gousses de vanille Comores. Banque de données pour la récolte 1987 [Vanilla pods from Comoros. Database from harvest year 1987]. Parfums, cosmétiques, arômes. 1989;87:77–90.

[25] Gassenmeier K, Riesen B, Magyar B. Commercial quality and analytical parameters of cured vanilla beans (*Vanilla planifolia*) from different origins from the 2006–2007 crop. Flavour and Fragrance Journal. 2008;23:194–201. DOI:10.1002/ffj.1874

[26] Pérez-Silva A, Odoux E, Brat P, Ribeyre F, Rodriguez-Jimenes G, Robles-Olvera V, et al. GC-MS and GC-olfactometry analysis of aroma compounds in a representative organic aroma extract from cured vanilla (*Vanilla planifolia* G. Jackson) beans. Food Chemistry. 2006;99:728–735. DOI:10.1016/j.foodchem.2005.08.050

[27] Zhang S, Mueller C. Comparative analysis of volatiles in traditionally cured Bourbon and Ugandan vanilla bean (*Vanilla planifolia*) extracts. Journal of Agricultural and Food Chemistry. 2012;60(42):10433–10444. DOI:10.1021/jf302615s

[28] Del Pilar Galeas M. Gas-chromatography-mass spectrometry and gas-chromatography-olfactometry analysis of aroma compounds of *Vanilla pompona* Schiede. Master thesis. Graduate School-New Brunswick, Rutgers, The State University of New Jersey. 2015.

[29] Brunschwig C, Rochard S, Pierrat A, Rouger A, Senger-Emonnot P, George G, et al. Volatile composition and sensory properties of *V. ×tahitensis* bring new insights for vanilla quality control. Journal of the Science of Food and Agriculture. 2016;96:848–858. DOI:10.1002/jsfa.7157

[30] Takahashi M, Sakamaki S, Fujita A. Simultaneous analysis of guaiacol and vanillin in a vanilla extract by using high-performance liquid chromatography with electro-chemical detection. Bioscience, Biotechnology, and Biochemistry. 2013;77(3):595–600. DOI:10.1271/bbb.120835

[31] Lepers-Andrzejewski S, Brunschwig C, Collard F-X, Dron M. Morphological, chemical, sensory and genetic specificities of Tahitian vanilla. In: Grisoni M, Odoux E, editors. Vanilla, medicinal and aromatic plants-industrial profiles. CRC Press, Taylor and Francis: Boca Raton, USA. 2011. pp. 205–228.

[32] Chen Y, Gu F, Li J, He S, Xu F, Fang Y. Involvement of colonizing *Bacillus* isolates in glucovanillin hydrolysis during the curing of *Vanilla planifolia* Andrews. Applied and Environmental Microbiology. 2015;81(15):4947–4954. DOI:10.1128/AEM.00458–15

[33] Brunschwig C, Collard F-X, Bianchini J-P, Raharivelomanana P. Evaluation of chemical variability of cured vanilla beans (*Vanilla tahitensis* and *Vanilla planifolia*). Natural Product Communications. 2009;4(10):1393–1400.

[34] Pérez-Silva A, Günata Z, Lepoutre J-P, Odoux E. New insight on the genesis and fate of odor-active compounds in vanilla beans (*Vanilla planifolia* G. Jackson) during traditional curing. Food Research International. 2011;44(9):2930–2937. DOI:10.1016/j.foodres.2011.06.048

[35] Rodriguez-Campos J, Escalona-Buendía HB, Orozco-Avila I, Lugo-Cervantes E, Jaramillo-Flores ME. Dynamics of volatile and non-volatile compounds in cocoa (*Theobroma cacao* L.) during fermentation and drying processes using principal components analysis. Food Research International. 2011;44(1):250–258. DOI:10.1016/j.foodres.2010.10.028

9

Dietary Administration of Animal Diets with Aromatic and Medicinal Plants: Influence on Meat Quality

Gema Nieto and Gaspar Ros

Abstract

Aromatic plants are gaining importance in recent years as potential sources of natural food preservatives due to the growing interest in the development of safe and effective natural food preservation. The use of vegetal substances with antimicrobial and antioxidant properties to increase the shelf life in meat and meat products is a promising technology. Taking into account that the diet with antioxidant may be absorbed and prevent lipid oxidation and colour deterioration, the possibility of feeding animal diets contains aromatic and medicinal plant (as thyme leaf, rosemary and sage) as natural antioxidants and antimicrobials represent a very interesting opportunity to replace synthetic antioxidants. In this sense, herbs of the Labiatae family, such as rosemary and sage, have been extensively studied for antioxidant and antimicrobial activities in a variety of systems. This review gives an overview of the current knowledge and recent trends in the use of plant-derived compounds from aromatic and medicinal as antimicrobials and antioxidant in animal diet and its effect on meat quality, their potentials and challenges.

Keywords: aromatic plants, meat, animal diet, antioxidant, antimicrobial, meat quality

1. Introduction

Animal scientists have been interested in improving meat quality and product composition through the modification of the diet of animals. The possible use of nutritional strategies to improve quality of food products from livestock is a new approach that emerges at the interface of food science and animal science. These strategies have emphasized in the improvement of the oxidative stability, such as supplementation of animal with natural antioxidants to minimize pigment and lipid oxidation in meat or the alteration of nutritional profile, increasing the content of polyunsaturated fatty acid (PUFA). The consumption of meat (rich in saturated fatty acid) is related with diseases such as some types of cancers and cardiovascular diseases (especially in developed countries).

In this sense, in recent years, consumers' pressure to reduce the composition and quality of fat in meat has led to attempts to modify meat by dietary strategies [1]. The modification of fatty acid profile of meat is to decrease saturated fatty acid and increase the ratio n-3: n-6 and PUFA: SFA (>4).

Between the strategies used, meat can be modified by external addition in the elaboration of meat or by the addition in the animal diet of ingredients considered beneficial for health, where these ingredients are able to eliminate or reduce components that are considered harmful. In this sense, several studies have shown that animal diet can strongly influence the quality of the meat.

For example, the stability of muscle foods further improves after the addition of food ingredients in diet of animals than the direct addition to the meat products, because the antioxidants are deposited where it is most needed. In order to alter the oxidative stability of intact muscle foods, the only technology available is the use of food ingredients in the diet. In these products, where natural antioxidants are added to the diet producing a nutritional alteration of muscle composition, no additive declarations are required and are more label-friendly.

Taking into account all these considerations, recent changes in legislation controlling the use of animal feed additives and the increasing demand of consumers for healthier meat products, if possible free of chemical additives, have stimulated interest in bioactive secondary metabolites as alternative performance enhancers.

2. Production of functional meat products

2.1. Functional meat products

Meat and meat products are essential for a balanced diet, although it must also be remembered that they are susceptible to modifications to give them a 'healthier' appearance. Numerous studies have demonstrated the possibility of changing the image of meat and meat products from the traditionally accepted image to one of healthy living thanks to the modification of animal diet, addition (vegetables, extracts, fibres, herbs, spices, etc.), elimination (fats) and reduction (saturated fatty acid, additives) of different ingredients. The object of including functional ingredients in the case of meat is not only concerned with providing it with certain desirable properties but also an attempt to change its image in these health-conscious days.

However, meat has beneficial health effects, for example, regarding obesity, and it also has satiating properties. This aspect is very important in the development of tasty and satiating functional meat products.

Therefore, in meat, the modifications to which it may be subjected to confer functional properties on it are based on modifications to the feed an animal receives or on postmortem manipulation of the carcass. Therefore, through the modification of animal diet, the lipid, fatty acid, and vitamin E content can be changed [2].

In the market of functional food, rapid progress has been made in the development of this kind of food, based on the results of studies on food components providing positive health benefits over and above normal nutritional benefits. Although many books and reviews on functional foods have been published, few of them have emphasized in the functional properties of meat and meat products (examples of functional properties of foods are anticarcinogenicity, antimutagenicity, antioxidative activity and antiaging activity). By modification of animal diet with the introduction of bioactive compounds, it should be possible to develop new meat products with potential health benefits. Such meat products would open up a new market in the meat industry.

2.2. Dietary supplementation of functional ingredients

2.2.1. Natural antioxidants

Fresh meat is mainly packed unprocessed and refrigerated. Currently the most widely used method in the marketing of fresh meat is packaging under modified atmosphere, both in the form of vacuum packaging and gas mixtures of known composition. The short shelf life of packed fresh meat is one of the principal concerns for its marketing. Lipid composition is a major determinant in the susceptibility of meat to oxidative changes and rancidity, leading to warmed-over flavours [3]. The quality attributes of meat products deteriorate due to the lipid oxidation during processing and storage. Lipid oxidation is responsible for development of primary and secondary oxidation products (short-chain aldehydes and ketones), reduction in nutritional quality, as well as changes in flavour, which can precipitate economic losses in terms of inferior product quality. The compounds formed after oxidation may adversely affect the overall quality and acceptability of meat and meat products (changes in flavour, texture and nutritional value).

In addition, the oxidative stability also affects the meat proteins. Specifically, the oxidation of indispensable amino acid reduces their digestibility and availability, and the tenderness of meat [4]. In addition, the oxidizable components of meat need to be protected from damages caused by the reactive oxygen species (ROS). The protection could be provided naturally through the deposition of antioxidant compounds derived from the feeds into the animal tissues.

Regarding meat storage stability can be extended with opportune packaging systems, by the exogenous addition of antioxidants or by adopting feeding systems able to improve the antioxidant status of muscle [4].

The rate of lipid oxidation can be effectively retarded by restricting the access to oxygen during storage vacuum-packaging and by the use of antioxidants that can be synthetic or natural: synthetic antioxidants were widely used in the meat industry, but consumer concerns over safety and toxicity pressed the food industry to find natural sources [5].

As alternative, synthetic antioxidants can be used natural extract from plant as grape, olives, sesame seed, tea, soybean, rosemary, thyme, etc with antioxidant properties [6]. Phenolic-rich plant materials or extracts used as dietary supplement or added to meat products exerted antioxidant properties by inhibiting lipid and protein oxidation in meat [7–9]. Studies reported that dietary antioxidant prevents colour deterioration and lipid oxidation [10–11].

Antioxidant compounds are usually added at a moderate dosage level since high level of inclusion may mechanistically cause adverse effects through pro-oxidative action [12].

Several studies have indicated that the modification of animal diet alters the oxidation of the meat (e.g. studies with lambs). The value of lambs lies in their ability to use low-quality feeds, in a sense upgrading low-quality inputs to high-quality outputs [13]. Santé-Lhoutellier et al. [14] studied the influence of diet on lamb meat oxidation and founds that the oxidative stability of lamb meat clearly depends on diet.

Scerra et al. [15] compared ewe's diet with pasture or concentrated and showed an increase in the PUFA content in intramuscular fat lamb fed with pastures. Nieto et al. [16] showed an increase in PUFA content of lamb meat fed with thyme compared with control diets. Elmore et al. [17] reported the same increase of PUFA in lamb meat after inclusion of diet fish in the diet. Similarly, Bas et al. [18] and Ponnampalam et al. [19] reported increases in the content of long-chain n-3 fatty acids in lamb meat with the diet of linseed or fish oil, respectively.

Including herb distillates into livestock diets can have positive effects. Moñino and others [13] reported that inclusion of herb distillates (distilled rosemary leaves) into pregnant ewes diet increased carbonic acid, carnosol and rosmarinic acid in the lamb meat. Fresh lamb meat from distilled rosemary diet presented lower DPPH values and higher total ferric reducing antioxidant power, indicating that rosemary reduced lipid oxidation. Another studies in pigs reported similar results [20].

In addition, Simitzis et al. [21] found that meat from lambs fed a feed that had been sprayed with oregano essential oil (1 mL/kg) was much more stable to lipid oxidation during both refrigerated and frozen storage than that from controls. Boler et al. [22] found that feeding vitamin E to pigs increased pork stability during storage. Gobert et al. [23] reported a synergism effect in the combination of plant extract rich in polyphenols and vitamin E.

2.2.2. Conjugated linoleic acid

Interests in conjugated linoleic acid (CLA) have increased in the last decades as a result of its potential effects on human health-related benefits and animal production, as a result of the effects of dietary CLA to increase the animal performance, improve meat quality and provide meat products with high amounts of CLA.

Inconsistent results have been reported about the effects of dietary CLA on the growth, body composition and meat quality. Different animal species, different breeds, age, duration and levels of CLA, husbandry conditions and the composition of feed could explain these conflicting results [24].

Conjugated linoleic acid has been studied in many animal models to determine its effects on lipid metabolism, as trans-10, cis-12 is known to reduce adipose deposition. In the mouse model, CLA in the diet has been found to increase metabolic rate and fatty acid oxidation while reducing fatty acid synthesis, lipoprotein lipase activity and division and differentiation of adipocytes [25]. Study by Wynn et al. [26] found a 36-fold increase in muscle trans-10, cis-12 CLA when a source of CLA (containing similar amounts of cis-9, trans-11 and trans-10, cis-12 isomers) was fed to growing lambs at 100 g/kg DM (approximately 50 g/kg DM of each isomer). They also found a 2- to 5-fold increase in cis-9, trans-11 CLA and a 3- to 20-fold increase of trans-10, cis-12 CLA in liver and adipose tissues.

It is generally accepted that dietary CLA can improve the body composition through reducing fat deposition and backfat thickness. In pigs, the fat deposition was reduced and the ratio of lean to fat increased linearly as the dietary CLA increased [27]. Dietary CLA not only reduced fat deposition but also altered the fatty acid composition of tissue lipids. In the study of Szymczyk et al. [28], the proportion of saturated fatty acids such as palmitic and stearic acids increased significantly, while that of monounsaturated and polyunsaturated fatty acids including palmitoleic, oleic, linoleic and arachidonic acid in broiler chickens decreased significantly.

In addition, other studies have shown that dietary CLA could increase the concentration of CLA in muscle and adipose tissues of chicken. Du and Ahn [29] reported that the amount of total CLA increased from 0 to 10.51 and 17.75 mg/g lipids in broiler breast muscle after 5 weeks of feeding 2 and 3% CLA. Therefore, feed nonruminant animal with synthesized CLA changes the fatty profile. These studies show that supplementation of CLA in the diet could be a strategy for developing a value-added meat product.

2.2.3. *Vitamin E*

Supplementation with vitamin E in animal diet improves meat quality by limiting lipid and protein oxidation [30–32]. Guidera et al. [32] reported an improvement in colour stability in lambs receiving with 1000 mg α-tocopherol/kg feed compared with non-supplemented feeds.

Rowe et al. [33] showed that dietary vitamin E decreased the levels of protein oxidation and its influence on beef tenderization. Other study about texture of meat reported that the diet supplementation with 1000 IU vitamin E caused lower shear force in beef steaks from longissimus dorsi after 14 day of postmortem storage [34].

In addition, the effects of dietary vitamin E on drip loss were inconsistent: in poultry, dietary vitamin E inhibited the development of PSE conditions induced by heat stress resulting in improved meat quality [35].

Some studies have indicated a possible role for high doses of vitamin E in preventing shifts in PUFA biohydrogenation pathways [36, 37], thus minimizing any negative effect of plant oil on milk production, milk fat yield and/or milk fatty acid composition. Vitamin E could act either as an inhibitor of bacteria producing trans-10 C18:1 [37] or affect the accumulation of biohydrogenation intermediates in rumen fluid and CLA content [38].

The supplementation of ewes and lamb diet with Vitamin E [39, 40] is usually carried out by using a synthetic source of α-tocopherol (all-rac-α-tocopheryl-acetate), due to its stability and lower cost in animal feeds [41]. Another vitamin E source is RRR-α-tocopheryl-acetate, which is a derivate from vegetable oils and exhibits higher biological activity than synthetic vitamin

E [42]. Recent studies in dairy cows have estimated that the relative bioavailability of vitamin E from natural sources is 1.36 times greater than that of synthetic vitamin E [43].

2.2.4. Omega-3 (ω3) fatty acids

Omega-3 PUFA consumption reduces the risk of cardiovascular disease [44] and inhibits the growth of mammary and prostate gland tumours [45]. It also delays the loss of immunological functions and is required for the normal foetal development of the brain [46].

PUFA is essential constituents for the development and growth of animal. In this group, docosahexaenoic acid (DHA, 22:6), docosapentaenoic acid (DPA, 22:5) and eicosapentaenoic acid (EPA, 20:5) are included.

It is possible to obtain enhanced n-3 PUFA meat, including the diet different raw materials such as linseed, chia (*Salvia hispanica*) or its oils and fish meal or other sea products [47].

One of the most important strategies in nonruminants is the inclusion of marine sources of n-3 PUFA and the study of product quality. For example, fed pigs or poultry with cereal-based diet increase n-3 PUFA and n-6 PUFA.

Coates et al. [48] reported that regular consumption of ω3 fatty acid-enriched pork can decrease the content of serum triglycerides and increase the production of serum thromboxane, and thus, it can reduce cardiovascular diseases. There are many other alternative food sources rich in long-chain PUFA available, and they include meat, milk and eggs from animals fed with ω3-enriched diets [49].

Crespo and Esteve-García [50] studied the inclusion of 10% olive oil, sunflower oil and linseed oil in broiler chickens for 20 days before slaughter. They showed highest n-3 PUFA and more favourable n-6:n-3 ratio in broilers fed with linseed oil, highest C18:1 in chicken fed with olive oil and highest proportion of linoleic acid in chicken fed with sunflower oil. Therefore, poultry diet with plant oils reported significant changes in the SFA, PUFA and MUFA content of abdominal fat of chicken. Similarly, Lu et al. [51] reported significant increase in C18:2 and C18:3 content in meat from pigs fed with soybean oil and linseed oil, respectively.

In addition, duration of feeding and time influences in the transfer of n-3 long-chain polyunsaturated fatty acids were found to be influenced by time and duration of feeding and the presence of other oil supplements. Haak et al. [52] studied the effect of inclusion of linseed or fish oil into the diet of pigs and concluded that a direct dietary source of DHA was required to increase DHA in animal muscle and that levels in pork could not be substantially influenced by dietary supply of precursors.

In addition, Lopez-Ferrer et al. [53] demonstrated that inclusion of rapeseed oil and linseed oil into the diet increased linoleic acid (used to synthesize w-3 PUFA).

Few studies have demonstrated that the oxidation of muscle from animal-derived enriched in n-3 PUFA is higher: for example, studies are made in rabbit meat [54–57], lamb meat [58], poultry [59] and pigs [60].

In order to avoid the higher tendency to oxidation in meat rich-PUFA, is recommended adding antioxidant in animal diet [61]. Therefore, the incorporation of the natural ingredients with antioxidant properties into the feed could be an interesting strategy to prevent oxidation of the meat [62–67].

2.2.5. *Selenium*

In many countries, there is a deficiency of selenium intake. The recommendations for selenium (60 and 75 μg/day for adult female and male in UK) are not covered by diet. Thus, the strategies to improve human selenium intake are the production of selenium-rich foods (eggs, milk and meat) with selenium supplementation in the animal diet or intake of selenium supplement capsular form.

Particular interest in selenium has been generated as a result of clinical studies showing that dietary supplementation with organic selenium, in the form of yeast grown on a media enriched with this trace element, decreased cancer mortality twofold [68]. Selenium is an essential trace mineral for human and animal because it is involved in regulating various physiological functions as an integral part of selenoproteins. Additionally, inadequate selenium consumption is associated with decreased fertility, genetic defects and poor health [69].

Various types of meat are important natural sources of selenium in human nutrition [70]. The selenium concentration in meats depends of selenium supplements used and geographical origin [71, 72]. Indeed, it is well established that selenite or selenate dietary supplementation is not effective in increasing selenium concentration in the meat. The main form of selenium in muscles of animals fed on grain-based diet is Se-Met, animals cannot produce this form of selenium Se-Met, and it must be in the diet. The form of selenium found in breast and muscle of chicken fed with high doses of selenium yeast is Se-Met. Therefore, only the organic selenium (in the form Se-Met) in cattle, pigs or chicken can increase the selenium concentration in the meat.

Pork: Producing selenium-enriched pork is reported in several studies. Kim and Mahan [73] compared the effects of supplementation dietary of inorganic and organic selenium in pork. These authors shown that selenium concentration in loin increased from 0.154 to 3.375 mg/kg with organic selenium supplementation. In addition, to increased selenium level, good colour, low drip loss, reduced pig odour, chewy and tender improved in final meat [74]. This selenium pork is available in Korea and Canada.

Beef: It is considered the major source of dietary selenium. However, there is a variation of concentration depending on country. For example, in USA, the selenium content in beef is higher than in Europe. This content of selenium can be increased with the addition of organic form into the diet of cattle [75].

Lamb: It can also be enriched with organic selenium into the diet. In this sense, Bierla et al. [76] reported that 100 g of selenium lamb reported 50% of recommendation of selenium per day.

Chicken: As in the case of beef and pork, the inclusion of selenite increases moderately the selenium level. Therefore, the use of organic selenium into the diet is necessary in order to increase the levels in meat [77]. There is a commercial option of chicken-enriched selenium called 'Selen Chicken' in Korea. In Ukraine, a combination of selenium and Vitamin E is added to commercial chicken meat [78] in order to produce selenium-enriched meat and improves meat quality during storage.

Turkey: The option of producing selenium-enriched turkey meat is available in USA where the high levels (around 34 g/100 g) are obtained by using organic selenium in the diet and the soil rich in selenium [79].

These increased selenium contents in meat products can be an excellent way to improve selenium status and safe for people living in selenium-deficient areas.

2.2.6. Plants, fruits, herbs and spices

As alternative, synthetic antioxidants can be used for plants, fruit, herbs or spices as carob, citrus pulp, algae, grape, olives, sesame seed, tea, soybean, rosemary, thyme, etc. Phenolic-rich plant materials or extracts are used as dietary supplement or added to meat products exerted antimicrobial and antioxidant properties.

Carob: Gravador et al. [80] studied the modification of fatty acids and oxidative stability of meat from lambs fed carob-containing diets. Previous studies showed that growth performance in lamb is compromised when a level of carob higher than 45% is administered into the animal diet [81]. Therefore, in this study, either 24 or 35% carob pulp was used in the diets in the current study in order to assure similar lamb growth performances compared to a conventional barley-based diet.

Citrus pulp: Several studies have reported an improvement of meat oxidative stability in response to the administration of citrus-pulp diets. Taking into accounts that citrus fruits can be processed to obtain juices, a substantial amount of by-products originates. Among these, the dried citrus pulp is widely used for ruminant feeding, and for its favourable nutrient composition, it can replace high proportions of cereal concentrates in the diet with no detrimental effects on animal productivity. Citrus fruits contain high levels of bioactive compounds, including polyphenols, terpenes, carotenoids and ascorbic acid, which exhibit antioxidant properties [82]. Therefore, the study of Inserra et al. [7] studied the effect of inclusion dried citrus pulp in the diet of lamb on the meat oxidative stability. These authors concluded that including high levels of dried citrus pulp in diets for intensively reared lambs might represent a feasible strategy to decrease the amount of cereal concentrates without compromising animal performances and to naturally improve meat oxidative stability.

The bioactive compounds (phenolic compounds) originating from the citrus fruits may cause the protective effects of dietary citrus pulp, against oxidation of lipid and meat proteins. Gladine et al. [83] showed that, after the dietary administration of a citrus extract to sheep, naringenin was detected in plasma and was able to increase its resistance to lipid peroxidation. Therefore, some of bioactive compounds in citrus are bioavailable in ruminants. Citrus pulp, which otherwise is just an agricultural waste, could find a valuable application in small ruminant feeding as a natural and cheap alternative to cereal concentrate feedstuffs with an ultimate positive impact on meat protein oxidative stability.

Algae are the original sources of DHA [84]. Several studies reported the inclusion of algae in animal feed in order to improve DHA content in eggs [85, 86] and chicken meat [87].

In this sense, the study of Delles et al. [88] investigated the influence of dietary algae and selenium (organic or inorganic) on quality of chicken meat. The results indicate that feeding diets with high-oxidized oil increased the vulnerability of lipids and proteins to oxidation and reduced the activities of tissue antioxidant defence enzymes. However, the dietary supplementation with an algae-based Se yeast and organic mineral antioxidant blend negated these effects. Furthermore, dietary antioxidant supplementation imparted a protective barrier against oxidation of broiler breast meat under HiOx, PVC, and SK packaging conditions throughout retail display. The improved oxidative stability appears to be associated with enhanced cellular antioxidant enzymatic activity and reduced ROS propagation in vivo. A more limited number of studies have looked into the effects of dietary supplementation with DHA-rich marine algae on the fatty acid composition of muscle tissue of pigs [89, 90].

Herbs and spices: Some herbs of the *Labiatae* family, particularly rosemary and sage, have been extensively studied for their antioxidative and antimicrobial activity. The vegetation in Southeast Spain is richer in aromatic plants than any other place in Europe. The province of Murcia is a major importer and processor of medicinal herbs. Rosemary and thyme are the most exploited, and their use mainly being the extraction of essential oils, a process that generates an excess of distilled leaves. These products are currently underused but could be used as potential sources of natural antioxidants and antimicrobials in the food industry.

Rosemary is the only spice commercially available for use as an antioxidant in Europe and the United States. Its extract contains antioxidant compounds, the most active being phenolic diterpenes such as carnosic acid, carnosol, rosmanol, epirosmanol, isorosmanol, methylcarnosate and rosmarinic acid [91]. These compounds have been shown to help prevent oxidation.

Thyme essential oil (*EO*) contains more than 60 ingredients, most of which posses important beneficial effects, for example, antiseptic, carminative, antioxidant and antimicrobial properties. The most important compounds of thyme *EO* are the phenols thymol (68.1%) and carvacrol (3.5%), which constitute the major and most active constituents, as well as the monoterpene hydrocarbons *p*-cymene (11.2%) and γ-terpinene (4.8%), which are known to have antioxidant properties and slow antimicrobial activity. The antibacterial properties of these compounds are in part associated with their lipophilic character, leading to their accumulation in membranes and to subsequent membrane-associated events such as energy depletion. Moreover, the (poly)phenolic compounds are characterized by having redox properties, which allow them to act as reducing agents, hydrogen donors, singlet oxygen quenchers and also as metal chelators.

Essential oil and extracts from *Labiatae* herbs have been successfully used in a wide variety of foods with good results as far as oxidative deterioration is concerned: for example, in turkey products [92], beef [93], pork [94], chicken [95], hens [96], lamb [13, 97–99] and in vitro system [100]. In contrast, unsatisfactory results have been obtained in others cases. For example, Galobart et al. [101] and O'Grady et al. [102] concluded that a diet supplemented with rosemary did not affect the lipid stability of eggs or fresh meat.

3. Current status on the consumers acceptance and market for functional meat products

Regarding diversity in enriched poultry products, it is interesting to note that selenium-enriched eggs are already commonly seen on supermarket shelves in the Ukraine and Belarus. Selenium enrichment of eggs, meat and milk may be viewed as merely production of naturally designed food ingredients.

Indeed, production and commercialization of functional meat products have already opened a new era in supplementation of animals and have provided a real chance for producers to differentiate and add value to meat poultry products and to meet the increasingly diverse requirements of consumers.

There is a lack of studies on the effect on human health and safety of these meats. By that reason, the European food authorities are reluctant to promote the consumption of functional foods. However, the consumers have been accepted the link between health and food, and the responsibility of researcher and food authorities is to ensure that new functional meat products and products are healthy and safe. Promoted studies in this sense could lead to the development of differentiated meat products and meat with potential human health benefits, for example, promote the use of antioxidants that are components with nutraceutical and maintain the product safety of foods.

4. Conclusion and future prospects

The possibility to produce new animal-derived products with specific nutrients that promote health and improve the diet of consumers is a real target.

These animal-derived products are development with the same sensory characteristics that the only difference is the amount of specific nutrients. No modifications of traditions or eating habits of poblations are produced, and these foods are cooked and consumed as usual. Therefore, without any modification of consumer's habits, problem related with deficit of various nutrients (e.g. selenium) can be solved.

The main difficulties in the market of functional meat products are consumer's idea that consumption of meat is unhealthy. However, consumers of many countries accept other animal-derived products as healthy food (e.g. milk and dairy products). Thus, more studies are necessary to demonstrate and afterwards inform consumers the functional value of meat.

Author details

Gema Nieto* and Gaspar Ros

*Address all correspondence to: gnieto@um.es

Department of Food Technology and Science and Human Nutrition, Veterinary Faculty, University of Murcia, Espinardo, Murcia, Spain

References

[1] Wood, JD., Richardson, RI., Nute, GR., Fisher, AV., Campo, MM., Kasapidou, E., Sheard, PR., Enser, M. (2003). Effects of fatty acids on meat quality: A review. Meat Sci. 66, 21–32.

[2] Jiménez-Colmenero, F., Carballo, J., Cofrades, S. (2001). Healthier meat and meat products: their role as functional foods. Meat Sci. 59, 5–13.

[3] Jeremiah, LE. (2001). Packaging alternatives to deliver fresh meats using short- or long-term distribution. Food Res Int, 34, 749–772.

[4] Descalzo, AM., Sancho, AM. (2008). A review of natural antioxidant and their effects on oxidative status, odor and quality of fresh beef produced in Argentina. Meat Sci, 79, 423–436.

[5] Coronado, SA., Trout, GT., Dunshea, FR., Shah, NP. (2002). Antioxidant effects of rosemary extract and whey powder on the oxidative stability of wiener sausages during 10 months frozen storage. Meat Sci, 62, 217–24.

[6] Tang, S., Kerry, JP., Sheehan, D., Joe Bukley, D., Morrissey, PA. (2001). Antioxidative effect of added tea catechins on susceptibility of cooked red meat, poultry and fish patties to lipid oxidation. Food Res Int, 34, 651–7.

[7] Inserra, L., Priolo, A., Biondi, L., Lanza, M., Bognanno, M., Gravador, RS., Luciano, G. (2014). Dietary citrus pulp reduces lipid oxidation in lamb meat. Meat Sci. 96(4), 1489–1493.

[8] Gravador, RS., Jongberg, S., Andersen, ML., Luciano, G., Priolo, A. Marianne N. Lund, MN. (2014). Dietary citrus pulp improves protein stability in lamb meat stored under aerobic conditions. Meat Sci. 97(2), 231–236.

[9] Nieto, G., Díaz, P., Bañon, S., Garrido, MD. (2010). Dietary administration of ewe diets with a distillate from rosemary leaves (*Rosmarinus officinalis* L.): influence on lamb meat quality. Meat Sci. 84, 23–29.

[10] Botsoglou, NA., Govaris, A., Giannenas, I., Botsoglou, E., Papageorgiou, G. (2007). The incorporation of dehydrated rosemary leaves in the rations of turkeys and their impact

on the oxidative stability of the produced raw and cooked meat. Int J Food Sci Nutr. 58(4), 312–320.

[11] Luciano, G., Monahan, FJ., Vasta, V., Pennisi, P., Bella, M., Priolo, A. (2009). Lipid and colour stability of meat from lambs fed fresh herbage or concentrate. Meat Sci. 82(2), 193–199.

[12] Moyo, B., Oyedemi, S., Masika, PJ., Muchenje, V. (2012). Polyphenolic content and antioxidant properties of *Moringa oleifera* leaf extracts and enzymatic activity of liver from goats supplemented with *Moringa oleifera* leaves/sunflower seed cake. Meat Sci. 91, 441–447.

[13] Moñino, I., Martinez, C., Sotomayor, JA., Lafuente, A., Jordan, MJ. (2008). Polyphenolic transmission to Segureno lamb meat from ewes' diets supplemented with the distillate from rosemary (*Rosmarinus officinalis*) leaves. J Agric Food Chem. 56(9), 3363–7.

[14] Santé-Lhoutellier, V., Engel, E., Gatellier, Ph. (2008). Assessment of the influence of diet on lamb meat oxidation. Food Chem. 109(3), 573–579.

[15] Scerra, M., Caparra, P., Foti, F., Galofaro, V., Sinatra, MC., Scerra, V. (2007). Influence of ewe feeding systems on fatty acid composition of suckling lambs. Meat Sci. 76, 390–394.

[16] Nieto, G., Bañon, S., Garrido, MD. (2012a). Incorporation of thyme leaves in the diet of pregnant and lactating ewes: Effect on the fatty acid profile of lamb. Small Ruminant Res. 105, 140–147.

[17] Elmore, JS., Cooper, SL., Enser, M., Mottram, DS., Sinclair, LA., Wilkinson, RG., Wood, JD. (2005). Dietary manipulation of fatty acid composition in lamb meat and its effect on the volatile aroma compounds of grilled lamb. Meat Sci. 69, 233–242.

[18] Bas, P., Berthelot, E., Pottier, E., Normand, J. (2007). Effect of level of linseed on fatty acid composition of muscles and adipose tissues of lambs with emphasis on trans fatty acids. Meat Sci. 77, 678–688.

[19] Ponnampalam, EN., Trout, GR., Sinclair, AJ., Egan, AR., Leury, BJ. (2001). Comparison of the color stability and lipid oxidative stability of fresh and vacuum packaged lamb muscle containing elevated omega-3 and omega-6 fatty acid levels from dietary manipulation. Meat Sci. 58, 151–161.

[20] McCarthy, TL., Kerry, JP., Kerry, JF., Lynch, PB., Buckley, DJ. (2001). Evaluation of the antioxidant potential of natural food/plant extracts as compared with synthetic antioxidants and vitamin E in raw and cooked pork patties. Meat Sci. 58(1), 45–52.

[21] Simitzis, PE., Deligeorgis, SG., Bizelis, JA., Dardamani, A., Theodosiou, I., Fegeros, K. (2008). Effect of dietary oregano oil supplementation on lamb meat characteristics. Meat Sci. 79(2), 217–23.

[22] Boler, DD., Gabriel, SR., Yang, H., Balsbaugh, R., Mahan, DC., Brewer, MS., McKeith, FK., Killefer, J. (2009). Effect of different dietary levels of natural-source vitamin E in grow-finish pigs on pork quality and shelf life. Meat Sci. 83(4), 723–30.

[23] Gobert, M., Gruffat, D., Habeanu, M., Parafita, E., Bauchart, D., Durand, D. (2010). Plant extracts combined with vitamin E in PUFA-rich diets of cull cows protect processed beef against lipid oxidation. Meat Sci. 85(4), 676–83.

[24] Zhang, W., Xiao, S., Samaraweera, H., Lee, EJ., Ahn, DU. (2010). Improving functional value of meat products. Meat Sci. 86(1), 15–31.

[25] Wahle, KWJ., Stevens, SD., Rotondo, D. (2004). Conjugated linoleic acids: are they beneficial or detrimental to health? Prog Lipid Res. 43, 553–87.

[26] Wynn, RJ., Daniel, ZCTR., Flux, CL., Craigon, J., Salter, AM., Buttery, PJ. (2006). Effect of feeding rumen-protected conjugated linoleic acid on carcass characteristics and fatty acid composition of sheep tissues. J Anim Sci. 84, 3440–50.

[27] Ostrowska, E., Muralitharan, M., Cross, RF., Bauman, DE., Dunshea, FR. (1999). Dietary conjugated linoleic acids increase lean tissue and decrease fat deposition in growing pigs. J Nutr. 129, 2037–2042.

[28] Szymczyk, B., Pisulewski, PM., Szczurek, W., Hanczakowski, P. (2001). Effects of conjugated linoleic acid on growth performance, feed conversion and subsequent carcass quality in broiler chickens. Br J Nutr. 85, 465–473.

[29] Du, M., Ahn, DU. (2002). Effect of dietary conjugated linoleic acid on the growth rate of live birds and on the abdominal fat content and quality of broiler meat. Poultry Sci, 81, 428–433.

[30] Chan, WKM., Hakkarainen, K., Faustman, C., Schaefer, DM., Scheller, KK., Liu, Q. (1996). Dietary vitamin E effect on color stability and sensory assessment of spoilage in three beef muscles. Meat Sci. 42, 387–399.

[31] Lanari, MC., Schaefer, DM., Scheller, KK. (1995). Dietary vitamin E supplementation and discoloration of pork bone and muscle following modified atmosphere packaging. Meat Sci. 41, 237–250.

[32] Guidera, J., Kerry, JP., Buckley, DJ., Lynch, PB., Morrissey, PA. (1997). The effect of dietary vitamin E supplementation on the quality of fresh and frozen lamb meat. Meat Sci. 45, 33–43.

[33] Rowe, LJ., Maddock, KR., Lonergan, SM., Huff-Lonergan, E. (2004). Oxidation environments decrease tenderization of beef steaks through inactivation of μ-calpain. J Anim Sci. 82, 3254–3266.

[34] Carnagey, KM., Huff-Lonergan, EJ., Trenkle, A., Wertz-Lutz, AE., Horst, RL., Beitz, DC. (2008). Use of 25-hydroxyvitamin D3 and vitamin E to improve tenderness of beef form longissimus dorsi of heifers. J Anim Sci. 86, 1649–1657.

[35] Olivo, R., Soares, AL., Ida, EI., Shimokomaki, M. (2001). Dietary vitamin E inhibits poultry PSE and improves meat functional properties. J Muscle Food. 25, 271–283.

[36] Juárez, M., Dugan, MER., Aalhus, JL., Aldai, N., Basarab, JA., Baron, VS., McAllister, TA. (2011). Effects of vitamin E and flaxseed on rumen-derived fatty acid intermediates in beef intramuscular fat. Meat Sci. 88, 434–440.

[37] Pottier, J., Focant, M., Debier, C., De Buysser, G., Goffe, C., Mignolet, E., Froidmont, E., Larondelle, Y. (2006). Effect of dietary vitamin E on rumen biohydrogenation pathways and milk fat depression in dairy cows fed high-fat diets. J Dairy Sci. 89, 685–692.

[38] Hou, J., Wang, F., Wang, Y., Liu, F. (2013). Effects of vitamin E on the concentration of conjugated linoleic acids and accumulation of intermediates of ruminal biohydrogenation in vitro. Small Rumin Res. 111, 63–70.

[39] Capper, JL., Wilkinson, RG., Kasapidou, E., Pattinson, SE., Mackenzie, AM., Sinclair, LA. (2005). The effect of dietary vitamin E and fatty acid supplementation of pregnant and lactating ewes on placental and mammary transfer of vitamin E to the lamb. Br J Nutr. 93, 549–557.

[40] Kasapidou, E., Wood, JD., Richardson, RI., Sinclair, LA., Wilkinson, RG., Enser, M. (2012). Effect of vitamin E supplementation and diet on fatty acid composition and on meat colour and lipid oxidation of lamb leg steaks displayed in modified atmosphere packs. Meat Sci. 90, 908–916.

[41] Vagni, S., Saccone, F., Pinotti, L., Baldi, A. (2011). Vitamin E bioavailability: past and present insights. Food Nutr Sci. 2, 1088–1096.

[42] Lauridsen, C., Engel, H., Craig, AM., Traber, MG. (2002). Relative bioactivity of dietary RRR- and all-rac-alpha-tocopheryl acetates in swine assessed with deuterium-labeled vitamin E. J Anim Sci, 80, 702–707.

[43] Weiss, WP., Hogan, JS., Wyatt, DJ. (2009). Relative bioavailability of all-rac and RRR vitamin E based on neutrophil function and total α-tocopherol and isomer concentration in periparturient dairy cows and their calves. J Dairy Sci. 92, 720–731.

[44] Temple, NJ. (1996). Dietary fats and coronary heart disease. Biomed Pharmacother. 50(6–7), 261–268.

[45] Rose, DP. (1997). Dietary fatty acids and prevention of hormone-responsive cancer. Proc Soc Exp Biol Med, 216(2), 224–233.

[46] Leung, IYF., Sandstrom, MM., Zucker, CL., Neuringer, M., Max Snodderly, D. (2005). Nutritional manipulation of primate retinas. IV. Effects of n-3 fatty acids, lutein, and zeaxanthin on S-cones and rods in the foveal region. Exp Eye Res. 81(5), 513–529.

[47] Ayerza, R., Coates, W., Lauria, M. (2002). Chia seed (*Salvia hispanica L.*) as an omega-3 fatty acid source for broilers: Influence on fatty acid composition, cholesterol and fat content of white and dark meats, growth performance, and sensory characteristics. Poult Sci. 81(6), 826–837.

[48] Coates, AM., Sioutis, S., Buckley, JD., Howe, PRC. (2009). Regular consumption of n-3 fatty acid-enriched pork modifies cardiovascular risk factors. Br J Nutr. 101, 592–597.

[49] Simopoulos, AP. (1999). New products from the agri-food industry: The return of n-3 fatty acids into the food supply. Lipids 34, 297–301.

[50] Crespo, N., Esteve-García, E. (2002). Nutrient and fatty acid deposition in broilers fed different dietary fatty acid profiles. Poult Sci. 81, 1533–1542.

[51] Lu, P., Zhang, LY., Yin, JD., Everts, AKR., Li, DF. (2008). Effects of soybean oil and linseed oil on fatty acid compositions of muscle lipids and cooked pork flavour. Meat Sci. 80, 910–918.

[52] Haak, L., De Smeet, A., Fremaut, D., Van Walleghem, K., Raes, K. (2008). Fatty acid profile and oxidative stability of pork influence by duration and time of dietary linseed or fish oil supplementation. J Anim Sci. 86, 1418–1425.

[53] Lopez-Ferrer, S., Baucells, MD., Barroeta, AC., Grashorn, MA. (2001). n-3 Enrichment of chicken meat. 1. Use of very long-chain fatty acids in chicken diets and their influence on meat quality: Fish oil. Poult Sci. 80, 741–752.

[54] Kouba, M., Benatmane, F., Blochet, JE., Mourot, J. (2008). Effect of a linseed diet on lipid oxidation, fatty acid composition of muscle, perirenal fat, and raw and cooked rabbit meat. Meat Sci. 77(80), 829–834.

[55] Castellini, C., Dal Bosco, A., Bernardini, M., Cyril, HW. (1998). Effect of dietary vitamin E on the oxidative stability of raw and cooked rabbit meat. Meat Sci. 50, 153–161.

[56] Dal Bosco, A., Castellini, C., Bianchi, L., Mugnai, C. (2004). Effect of dietary alinolenic acid and vitamin E on the fatty acid composition, storage stability and sensory traits of rabbit meat. Meat Sci. 66, 407–413.

[57] Oriani, G., Salvatori, G., Pastorelli, G., Pantaelo, L., Ritieni, A., Corino, C. (2001). Oxidative status of plasma and muscle in rabbits supplemented with dietary vitamin E. J. Nutr Biochem. 12, 138–143.

[58] Berthelot, V., Bas, P., Pottier, E., Normand, J. (2012). The effect of maternal linseed supplementation and/or lamb linseed supplementation on muscle and subcutaneous adipose tissue fatty acid composition of indoor lambs. Meat Sci, 90, 548–557.

[59] Lin, CF., Asghar, A., Gray, JI., Buckley, DJ., Booren, AM., Crackel, RL., et al. (1989). Effects of oxidised dietary oil and antioxidant supplementation on broiler growth and meat stability. Br Poult Sci. 30, 855–864.

[60] Monahan, FJ., Buckley, DJ., Morrissey, PA., Lynch, PB., Gray, JI. (1992). Influence of dietary fat and a-tocopherol supplementation on lipid oxidation in pork. Meat Sci. 31, 229–241.

[61] Díaz, MT., Cañeque, V., Sánchez, S., Lauzurica, C., Pérez, C., Fernández, C., Àlvarez, I., De la Fuente, J. (2011). Nutritional and sensory aspects of light lamb meat enriched in n-3 fatty acids during refrigerated storage. Food Chem.124, 147–155.

[62] Joo, ST., Lee, JI., Ha, YL., Park, GB. (2002). Effects of dietary conjugated linoleic acid on fatty acid composition, lipid oxidation, color, and water-holding capacity of pork loin. J Anim Sci. 80, 108–112.

[63] You, KM., Jong, HG., Kim, HP. (1999). Inhibition of cyclooxygenase/lipoxygenase from human platelets by polyhydroxylated/methoxylated flavonoids isolated from medicinal plants. Arch Pharm Res. 22(1), 18–24.

[64] Vasta, V., Pennisi, M., Lanza, D., Barbagallo, M., Bella, A., Priolo, A. (2007). Intramuscular fatty acid composition of lambs given a tanniniferous diet with or without polyethylene glycol supplementation. Meat Sci. 76, 739–745.

[65] Youdim, KA., Deans, SG. (2000). Effect of thyme oil and thymol dietary supplementation on the antioxidant status and fatty acid composition of the ageing rat brain. Br J Nutr. 83, 878.

[66] Lee, KW., Everts, H., Kappert, HJ., Frehner, M., Losa, R., Beynen, AC. (2003). Effects of dietary essential oil components on growth performance, digestive enzymes and lipid metabolism in female broiler chickens. Br Poult Sci. 44, 450.

[67] Govaris, A., Botsoglou, E., Florou-Paneri, P., Moulas, A., Papageorgiou, G. (2005). Dietary supplementation of oregano essential oil and α-tocopheryl acetate on microbial growth and lipid oxidation of turkey breast fillets during storage. Int J Poult Sci. 4, 969.

[68] Clark, LC., Combs, GF. Jr, Turnbull, BW., Slate, EH., Chalker, DK., Chow, J., Davis, LS., Glover, RA., Graham, GF., Gross, EG, Krongrad, A., Lesher, JL. Jr, Park, HK., Sanders, BB. Jr, Smith, CL., Taylor, JR. (1996). Effects of selenium supplementation for cancer prevention in patients with carcinoma of the skin. A randomized controlled trial. Nutritional Prevention of Cancer Study Group. J Am Med Assoc. 276, 1957–1963.

[69] Surai, PF., Karadas, F., Pappas, AC., Sparks, NH. (2006). Effect of organic selenium in quail diet on its accumulation in tissues and transfer to the progeny. Br Poult Sci. 47, 65–72.

[70] Lawler, TL., Taylor, JB, Finley, JW., Caton, JS. (2004). Effect of supranutritional and organically bound selenium on performance, carcass characteristics, and selenium distribution in finishing beef steers. J Anim Sci. 82, 1488–1493.

[71] McNaughton, SA., Marks, GC. (2002). Selenium content of Australian foods: a review of literature values. J Food Compos Anal. 15, 169–182.

[72] Daun, C., Johansson, M., Onning, G., Akesson, B. (2001). Glutathione peroxidase activity, tissue and soluble selenium content in beef and pork in relation to meat ageing and pig RN phenotype. Food Chem. 73, 313–319.

[73] Kim, YY., Mahan, DC. (2001). Comparative effects of high dietary levels of organic and inorganic selenium on selenium toxicity of growing–finishing pigs. J Anim Sci. 79, 942–948.

[74] Cole, DJA. (2000). Selenium, the pig and the human diet. In: T.P. Lyons and D.J.A. Cole (Eds.), *Conc. Pig Sci. 2000*. Nottingham University Press, Nottingham, pp. 149–158.

[75] Simek, J., Chladek, G., Koutnik, V., Steinhauser, L. (2002). Selenium content of beef and its effect on drip and fluid losses. Anim Sci Pap Rep. 20(Suppl. 1), 49–53.

[76] Bierla, K., Dernovics, M., Vacchina, V., Szpunar, J., Bertin, G., Lobinski, R. (2008). Determination of selenocysteine and selenomethionine in edible animal tissues by 2D size-exclusion reversed-phase HPLC-ICP MS following carbamidomethylation and proteolytic extraction. Analyt Bioanalyt Chem. 390, 1789–1798.

[77] Arnold, RL., Olson, OE., Carlson, CW. (1973). Dietary selenium and arsenic additions and their effects on tissue and egg selenium. Poult Sci. 52, 847–854.

[78] Yaroshenko, FO., Surai, PF., Yaroshenko, YF., Karadas, F., Sparks, NHC. (2004). Theoretical background and commercial application of production of Se-enriched chicken. Proceedings of the XXII World's Poultry Congress, Turkey, p. 410.

[79] Schubert, A., Holden, JM., Wolf, WR., (1987). Selenium content of a core group of foods based on a critical evaluation of published analytical data. J Am Dietetic Assoc. 87, 285–299.

[80] Gravador, RS., Luciano, G., Jongberg, S., Bognanno, M., Scerra, M., Andersen, ML., Marianne, N., Lund, MN., Priolo, A. (2015). Fatty acids and oxidative stability of meat from lambs fed carob-containing diets. Food Chem. 182(1), 27–34.

[81] Vasta, V., Pennisi, P., Lanza, M., Barbagallo, D., Bella, M., Priolo, A. (2007). Intramuscular fatty acid composition of lambs given a tanniniferous diet with or without polyethylene glycol supplementation. Meat Sci. 76, 739–745.

[82] Abeysinghe, DC., Li, X., Sun, CD., Zhang, W., Zhou, C., Chen, K. (2007). Bioactive compounds and antioxidant capacities in different edible tissues of citrus fruit of four species. Food Chem. 104, 1338–1344.

[83] Gladine, C., Rock, E., Morand, C., Bauchart, D., Durand, D. (2007). Bioavailability and antioxidant capacity of plant extracts rich in polyphenols, given as a single acute dose, in sheep made highly susceptible to lipoperoxidation. Br J Nutr. 98, 691–701.

[84] Abril, R., Garret, J., Zeller, SG., Sande, WJ., Mast, RW. (2003). Safety assessment of DHA-rich microalgae from *Schizochytrium* sp.: Part V. Target animal safety/toxicity in growing swine. Regul Toxicol Pharmacol. 37,73–82.

[85] Van Elswyk, ME. (1997). Comparison of n-3 fatty acid sources in laying hen rations for improvement of whole egg nutritional quality. A review. Br J Nutr. 78(Suppl. 1), 61–69.

[86] Meluzzi, A., Sirri, F., Tallarico, N., Franchini, A. (2001). Effect of different vegetable lipid sources on the fatty acid composition of egg yolk and on hen performance. Arch Geflugelkd. 65, 207–213.

[87] Sirri, F., Minelli, G., Iaffaldano, N., Tallarico, N., Franchini, A. (2003). Oxidative stability and quality traits of n-3 PUFA enriched chicken meat. Italian J Anim Sci. 2(1), 450–452.

[88] Delles, RM., Xiong, YL., True, AD., Ao, T., Dawson, KA. (2014). Dietary antioxidant supplementation enhances lipid and protein oxidative stability of chicken broiler meat. Poult Sci. 93, 1561–1570.

[89] Marriott, NG., Garret, JE., Sims, MD., Abrul, JR. (2002). Composition of pigs fed a diet with docosahexaenoic acid. J Muscle Foods. 13, 265–277.

[90] Sardi, L., Martelli, G., Lambertini, L., Parisini, P., Mordenti, A. (2006). Effects of a dietary supplement of DHA-rich marine algae on Italian heavy pig production parameters. Livest Sci. 103, 95–103.

[91] Cuvelier, ME., Richard, H., Berset, C. (1996). Antioxidative activity and phenolic composition of pilot-plant and commercial extracts of sage and rosemary. J Am Oil Chem Sci. 73, 645–652.

[92] Govaris, A., Florou-Paneri, P., Botsoglou, E., Giannenas, I., Amvrosiadis, I., Botsoglou, N. (2007). The inhibitory potential of feed supplementation with rosemary and/or a-tocopheryl acetate on microbial growth and lipid oxidation of turkey breast during refrigerated storage. Food Sci Technol, LWT, 40, 331–337.

[93] Djenane, D., Sánchez-Escalante, A., Beltrán, JA., Roncalés, P. (2002). Ability of a-tocopherol, taurine and rosemary, in combination with vitamin C, to increase the oxidative stability of beef steaks displayed in modified atmosphere. Food Chem. 76, 407–415.

[94] Janz, JAM., Morel, PCH., Wilkinson, BHP., Purchas, RH. (2007). Preliminary investigation of the effects of low-level dietary inclusion of fragrant essential oils and oleoresins on pig performance and pork quality. Meat Sci. 75, 360–365.

[95] López-Bote, CJ., Gray, JI., Gomaa, EA., Flegal, CJ. (1998). Effect of dietary administration of oil extracts from rosemary and sage on lipid oxidation in broiler meat. Br Poult Sci. 39, 235–240.

[96] Parpinello, GP., Meluzzi, A., Sirri, F., Tallarico, N., Versari, A. (2006). Sensory evaluation of egg products and eggs laid from hens fed diets with different fatty acid composition and supplemented with antioxidants. Food Res Int. 39, 47–52.

[97] Nieto, G., Estrada, M., Jordán, M.J., Garrido, M.D., Bañon, S. (2011). Effects in ewe diet of rosemary by-product on lipid oxidation and the eating of cooked lamb under retail display conditions. Food Chem. 124, 1423–1429.

[98] Nieto, G., Bañon, S., Garrido, MD. (2011b). Administration of distillate Thyme leaves into the diet of Segureña ewes: effect on lamb meat quality. Anim J. 6(12), 2048–56.

[99] Nieto, G. (2013). Incorporation of by-products of rosemary and thyme in the diet of ewes: effect on the fatty acid profile of lamb. Eur Food Res Technol. 236, 379–389.

[100] Nieto, G., Huvaere, K., Skibsted, LH. (2011). Antioxidant activity of rosemary and thyme by-products and synergism with added antioxidant in a liposome system. Eur Food Res Technol. 233, 11–18.

[101] Galobart, J., Barroeta, AC., Baucells, MD., Codony, RM., Ternes, W. (2001). Effect of dietary supplementation with rosemary extract and a-tocopheryl acetate on lipid oxidation in eggs enriched with w3-fatty acids. Poult Sci. 80, 460–467.

[102] O'Grady, MN., Maher, M., Troy, DJ., Moloney, AP., Kerry, JP. (2006). An assessment of dietary supplementation with tea catechins and rosemary extract on the quality of fresh beef. Meat Sci. 73, 132–143.

10

Investigation of *Campomanesia* Components: A Fruit of Brazilian Cerrado

Nayara Vieira de Lima, Daniela Granja Arakaki,
Paula F. Saldanha Tschinkel,
Anderson Fernandes da Silva,
Rita de Cássia Avellaneda Guimarães,
Priscila Aiko Hiane and
Valter Aragão do Nascimento

Abstract

A survey of chemical composition of the fruit of *Campomanesia adamantium* used by rural and urban inhabitants of the cities of the Campo Grande, Mato Grosso do Sul State, Brazil, was carried out by inductively coupled plasma-optical emission spectroscopy (ICP-OES) aiming at the detection of minerals. Fifteen minerals were detected in the peel, pulp, and seeds of plant. The concentrations of elements K, Ca, Na, and P are found to be present at the major level in peel, pulp, and seeds of fruit. The zinc concentration is very low compared to other detected elements. The levels of some chemical elements in the fruit do not exceed the limits established by international legislation. Animal studies should be performed. The knowledge of the chemical elements in plants has economic interest, and involves global health problem.

Keywords: medicinal plants, guavira, inductively coupled plasma mass spectrometry

1. Introduction

Medicinal and aromatic plants are important source of natural wealth. It is estimated that there are about 350,000 species of existing plants. Therapeutic plants have been valued as a mode of treatment of a variety of diseases and have played a very important role in the health. So, they serve as raw materials for manufacturing several traditional and modern medicines [1, 2].

The records of medicinal plants' use for treating diseases and ailments date back to centuries ago. However, currently, more than half of the world's population still uses plants for the development of new medicines. In countries such as China, Africa, India, and Brazil, the traditional medicine is still the support of health care, and most of the drugs and cures come from plants. The World Health Organization (WHO) estimated that 80% of people worldwide rely on herbal medicines partially for their primary health care [3]. As in other countries, in Brazil increasingly, medicinal plants are used by rural and urban inhabitants, especially for treating minor ailments.

The vegetation of Brazil is richly endowed with a wide variety of plants, some of which are yet to be fully exploited. Some of the plants are cultivated and used as food or drugs while a good number of others grow wild in the Brazilian Amazon Forest. In Brazil, an effort for documenting the traditional uses of medicinal plants in several Brazilian forests reported 117 medicinal plants used in the Brazilian Amazon [4]. With the exception of the Amazon, few studies on medicinal plants have been performed in other Brazilian areas such as the Pantanal and Cerrado.

Located in South America, the Brazilian Cerrado is located mainly in the Midwest region of Brazil. The Cerrado is the second largest biome in Brazil, behind only the Amazon Rainforest. The Cerrado is rich in traditional medicine. The Midwest region of Brazil, in Mato Grosso do Sul State, in the city of Campo Grande/MS, has several medicinal plants, the *Campomanesia adamantium* (Cambess.) O. Berg and other plants species are part of the Cerrado vegetation of this city. The *C. adamantium* (Cambess.) O. Berg is also known popularly as gabiroba, guabiroba, or guavira. It is a fruit produced by gabirobeira, a wild shrub that grows in the fields and pastures of Brazil's Cerrado that develops in hot tropical climate with low rainfall. This species belongs to the family Myrtaceae. The fruits are of round-shaped, with a soft pulp, and very smooth well-appreciated taste.

There are many varieties of guavira fruit in Brazil. The differences between guavira of a same variety are often greater than the differences between two different varieties. Some varieties of guavira have different characteristics among them, and they are not as great as those among the different varieties of oranges or mandarins. Sometimes, it is impossible to distinguish one variety from the other, since the difference among the fruit of the same plant is as great as that between the fruit of different varieties. The most common species are *C. xanthocarpa* (Mart.) O. Berg, *C. corymbosa* (Cambess.) O. Berg, *C. Cambessedeana* O. Berg, *C. adamantium* (Cambess.) O. Berg, and *C. pubescens* (Mart. ex DC.) O. Berg.

The reproduction of guavira relies largely on their interaction with animal pollinators and fruit and seed dispersers. These plants are found as deciduous shrub, with a height from 0.5 to 1.5 m; flowering is usually from September to October, the flowers are lily and plentiful. Fruiting occurs from November to January and the fruits generally range from 2 to 2.5 cm in diameter (**Figure 1**); however, the morphological variation from one species to another is evident.

The fruit has 90% sweet juicy pulp and is widely appreciated by the population of the Brazilian Cerrado region. They are mature when the fruit has turned from green to yellow (see **Figure 1**). These plants have a delicate epicarp, demanding care during transport when ripe. A quick processing or freezing is recommended. Refrigerated storage recommendations are at 25°C. In nature, the guavira has low caloric value, mainly due to the high moisture content and therefore a lower concentration of sugars, lipids, and proteins in their structure. The gabiroba fruits have nutritional properties due to its high content of vitamin C, minerals, and phenolic compounds, which allows considering it as functional food [5–7]. In **Figure 1**, images represent different parts of the fruit of *C. adamantium* (Cambess.) O. Berg, popularly known as guavira, from Cerrado, Campo Grande-MS, Brazil: (a) fruits of guavira, (b) peel and pulp guavira, (c) magnified image of the fruit, and (d) seed guavira.

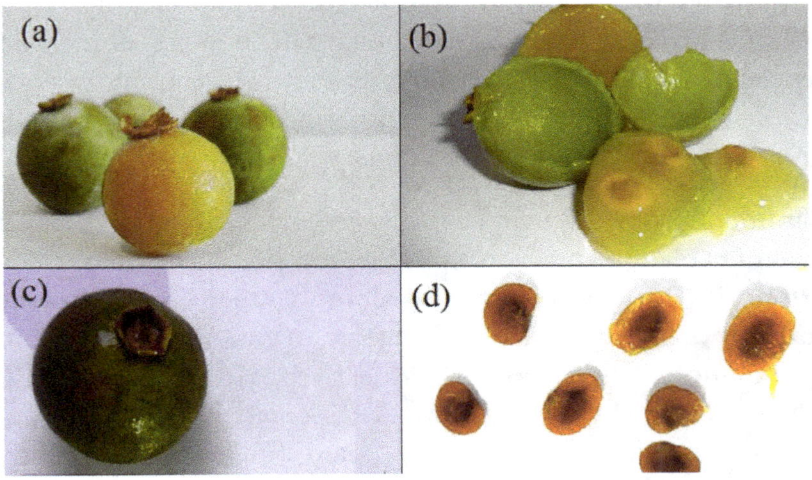

Figure 1. *Campomanesia adamantium* (Cambess.) O. Berg fruits, popularly known as guavira, from Cerrado, Campo Grande-MS, Brazil: (a) fruit of guavira, (b) peel and pulp guavira, (c) magnified image of the fruit, and (d) guavira seeds.

Several studies have shown the importance of the plant *C. xanthocarpa* Berg. (Myrtaceae) as potential effect in reducing blood cholesterol levels. In Brazil, one clinical study with hypercholesterolemic people investigated the effects of plant *C. xanthocarpa* Berg. (Myrtaceae) on inflammatory processes, oxidative stress, endothelial dysfunction, and lipid biomarkers in hypercholesterolemic individuals. According to results, the treatment reduced the blood total cholesterol (TC) and low-density lipoprotein (LDL-C) levels, reduced the oxidative stress in hypercholesterolemic individuals, and improved the levels of nitric oxide (NOx) [8]. In this work, the authors state that their results are in accordance with a previous preclinical study conducted in mice, which showed that this plant was effective in preventing gastric ulcerations and did not produce toxic symptoms [9].

Other studies on these species properties showed the effects of the aqueous extracts of these plants in rats fed on a high calorie diet. Comparing the results from the experimental group with the results of the control group, the chronic treatment with the *C. xanthocarpa* aqueous extract induced a significant reduction in weight gain in the rat. Equally, biochemical analysis showed that this treatment reduced glycemia. However, no effects on lipidic levels were observed [10]. On the other hand, one study with some species of plants used for weight loss purpose in Brazil and around the world showed that scientific data found are not sufficient to guarantee the efficacy and safety of these plants for treating obesity [11]. Consistent with the results aforementioned studies *Campomanesia* species are used in folk medicine as anti-inflammatory, antirheumatic, antidiarrheal, and hypocholesterolemic [12].

During several years, this plant is used in Brazilian folk medicine for ulcer treatment. Although there is no study in humans, the oral administration of the extract in animals proved to be effective in preventing gastric ulceration in rats and did not produce toxic symptoms [13]. The determination of groups as presence of flavonoids, saponins, and tannins has been related to antiulcer activity in other published work [14].

Studies *in vivo* evaluated the antinociceptive and anti-inflammatory activity of ethanolic extract from *C. velutina* leaves and its fractions, using male Swiss albino mice. The results of the present study demonstrated that *C. velutina* has anti-inflammatory and antinociceptive. However, the complete mechanisms of these actions remain to be elucidated [15].

Indigenous and rural populations used the leaves of *C. adamantium* (Cambess.) O. Berg and its fruits to treat inflammatory, obesity, diarrheal, and aseptic urinary tract problems. The infusion of the leaves is used for bladder problems, high blood pressure, throat infections, vomiting, indigestion, and cramps. The leaves are also used for the treatment of rheumatic diseases and as cholesterol reducers. *C. adamantium* (Myrtaceae) is an antioxidant fruit, and results showed the hepatoprotective effects of pulp or peel/seed hydroalcoholic extracts on injured liver-derived HepG2 cells by CCl_4. The results in part are associated with the presence of antioxidant compounds, especially flavonoids [16]. Researches and studies prove that the oleic and linoleic fatty acids obtained from the oil of the seeds from *C. xanthocarpa* Berg. showed amounts of bioactive compounds, and the results of fatty acid contents indicated a high degree of unsaturation. Oleic acid is included in the normal human diet as a part of animal fats and vegetable oils. It plays a key role in the synthesis of hormones [17]. Linoleic acid is found in many vegetable oils, including flaxseed oil, sunflower seed oil, and corn oil. In the traditional medicine in Brazil, the roots and leaves of *C. xanthocarpa* Berg. are used for antidiabetic effects [18].

The ingestion of such plants for medicinal purpose can have imperative side effects. Scientific surveys of these plants are necessary because many of them may have detrimental effects, such as acute or chronic toxicity, or their use may inhibit the adoption of the proper and effective treatment. Hence, with regard to the toxicological consideration of medicinal plants, the major hazard that may be associated with the use of plants is the presence of potentially toxic mineral elements such as the accumulative elements copper, lead, cadmium, mercury, arsenic, fluorine, selenium, molybdenum, and vanadium. Currently, an effort has been made by Brazilian researchers to review the elemental contents and efficacy of traditional herbal medications.

Some people believe that *C. adamantium* (Cambess.) O. Berg is rich in zinc, aluminum, potassium, calcium, phosphor, and magnesium. In this context, each chemical element has its chemical properties, health effects, and would be associated with important applications in the treatment of ailments. In the case of zinc because of its effect in the fight against infections. On the other hand the adverse effect of zinc deficiency increases the susceptibility of children to infectious diarrhea and contributes to malnutrition increases the susceptibility of children to infectious diarrhea, and contributes to zinc deficiency and malnutrition [19]. According to information popular, this species is rich in aluminum. So, *C. adamantium* is popularly used to treat ulcer disease in Mato Grosso do Sul State, in Midwest Brazil. It is logical that among the various categories of antiulcer drugs in the market, many contain aluminum. According to the elders who live in some farms, the fruit of guavira has potassium and helps maintain muscle force. In fact, several investigations have shown that the health benefits of potassium include relief from stroke, blood pressure, heart and kidney disorders, anxiety and stress, as well as enhanced muscle strength. However, there are no scientific data confirming the concentration of this element in the guavira fruit.

Knowledge of element concentrations in highly consumed plant samples is of interest. Especially of trace elements toxic as well as nontoxic in plants are very important medicinally. The diets of the world's population lack one or more essential mineral elements. This can be remedied through dietary diversification, mineral supplementation, food fortification, or increasing the concentrations and/or bioavailability of mineral elements in produce. Some medicinal plants are rich in minerals important to human. Until now, we know that each mineral has a role in human metabolism. For example, sodium is essential to humans. An adult person requires about 2.5–3.0 g per day [3]. Any extra sodium may contribute to high blood pressure. High blood pressure is a leading cause of cardiovascular disease. It accounts for two-thirds of all strokes and half of heart disease [20]. Sodium helps cells to transmit nerve signals and regulates water levels in tissues and blood. On the other hand, potassium has opposite effects on heart health, while high potassium intake can help relax blood vessels and excrete the sodium and decrease blood pressure. Our bodies need far more potassium than sodium each day [21].

Studies demonstrated that elements such as potassium, calcium, sodium, magnesium, manganese, and copper could reduce cardiovascular disease in human beings [22]. Low amount of phosphorus and calcium determined in the sample may still contribute to bone formation. Calcium plays a role in final common pathway mediating stimulus-contraction coupling in cardiac and smooth muscle [23]. Also, low potassium may till reduce the risk of stroke while low sodium content may add value in osmotic regulation of the body fluids and transmission of nerve impulse [24].

Calcium is the most abundant element in the human body. According to a study published [25], the amount of calcium that the body loses through urination increases with the amount of salt that is ingested. Other element as magnesium is abundant in intracellular fluid. Nevertheless, the mechanism involved in its regulation is still unknown. The potential uses of magnesium include the treatment of eclampsia, myocardial infarction, and arrhythmias [26]. Vegetables, nuts, seeds, and legumes are the best sources for magnesium. In contrast to the calcium and magnesium, quantities of manganese in mammalian tissue are scant. But at the same time, this mineral is essential for bone mineralization and metabolism [27]. Studies using plasma of conscious horses increased superoxide capacity in a manner related to the dose of manganese [28].

Based on the above information, the present chapter includes a preliminary study of the detection of chemical composition of medicinal plant (*C. adamantium* (Cambess.) O. Berg) used by the rural and urban communities of Campo Grande city, Mato Grosso do Sul State, Brazil. This study is necessary because to date there have been no definitive studies on the chemical composition of *C. adamantium* (Cambess) O. Berg fruits in Mato Grosso Sul State, Brazil.

Nowadays, *C. adamantium* (Cambess.) O. Berg (Myrtaceae) is used in folk medicine to treat inflammation and rheumatism. This could be used as an alternative medicine for other disease control. The literature search reveals that few studies have been done on this plant by Brazilian researchers [29, 6]. For this reason, the aim of this work is to characterize the chemical constituents of this plant species native to the Brazil. Using one inductively coupled plasma-optical emission spectroscopy (ICP-OES), we performed measurements of the chemical concentration in the peel, pulp, and seeds of the fruit.

2. Experimental background

2.1. Research area

The *C. adamantium* (Cambess.) O. Berg (Myrtaceae) fruits were collected in Campo Grande city, Mato Grosso do Sul State, Brazil, in October 2015. Fruits of *C. adamantium* in various stages of ripening were collected from various plants. **Figure 2** shows the geographic coordinates of

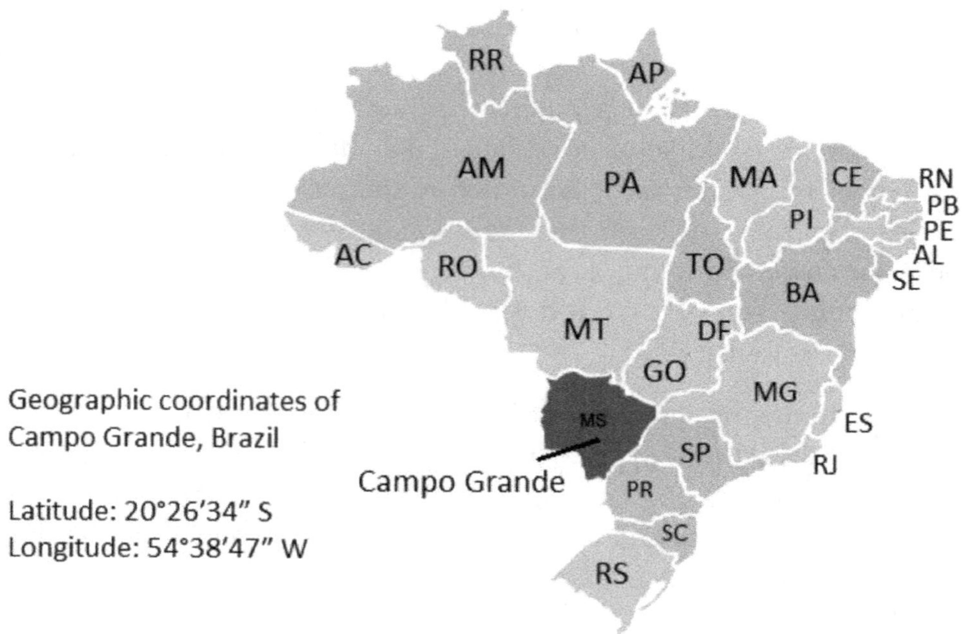

Figure 2. Geographic coordinates of Campo Grande, Mato Grosso do Sul State, Brazil.

Campo Grande, Mato Grosso do Sul State, Brazil, which is used in mapping and navigation, including GPS satellite navigation system (the global positioning system).

2.2. Elemental analysis by ICP-OES technique

All the samples of peel, pulp, and seeds of the fruit were weighed and digested in HNO_3 + H_2O_2 mixture. Samples were prepared as follows: a mixture of 0.5 g sample plus 5.0 mL HNO_3 (65% Merck) and 3.0 mL H_2O_2 (35%, Merck Millipore) was processed in the microwave digestion system Speedwave®, Berghof, Germany. After digestion, samples were diluted to 100 mL using ultrapure water. The final acid concentration of the samples was quite high (4% HNO_3).

In the present paper, the concentration of the elements (K, Ca, Na, P, Mg, Fe, Si, Mo, Mn, Z, Cr, and Cu) was determined with the use of ICP-OES technique (Thermo Scientific—iCAP 6000 Series). The concentrations of the different elements in these samples were determined using the corresponding standard calibration curves obtained by using standard solutions of the elements of interest (Merck). Triplicate analyses were performed on each sample.

The specimen has been identified by Dr. Arnildo Pott and deposited (Nº 53328) in herbarium of Federal University of Mato Grosso do Sul (UFMS)/Brazil.

3. Results and discussions

The concentrations of different mineral elements of seed, pulp, and peel of guavira fruit analyzed are listed in **Table 1**. In the present work, the concentration of elements in the peel decreases in the following order: K > Ca > Na > P > Mg > Fe > Si > Mo > Mn > Zn > Cr > Cu > Co. The pulp of the fruit decreases in the following order: K > P > Na > Ca > Mg > Si > Fe > Al > Mo > Zn > Mn > Cr > Cu > Co. The results attributed to seeds of fruit: P > K > Ca > Mg > Na > Fe > Al > Si > Zn > Mo > Cu > Mn > Cr > Cu > Co. Among the various elements, K, Ca, Na, and P are found to be present at the major level, and Cr, Cu, and Co are at minor level. Our studies demonstrated that the guavira seeds are rich in copper, iron, phosphorus, chromium, and molybdenum. However, this plant is not a good source of other elements such as nickel, zinc, potassium, magnesium, manganese, silicon, sodium, and calcium. The chemical characteristic of each chemical element obtained in this study will be described below.

Copper contents were 0.005, 0.0031, and 0.0326 mg/g for the guavira peel, pulp, and seed, respectively. In our study, the copper content of the seeds is the highest while that of the peel is the least. The present results indicate that seeds of guavira are a rich source of copper. In a recent study in Serbia, the concentration of copper in *Foeniculum vulgare* was mentioned as 0.001542 mg/g [30]. The permissible limit of copper set by Food and Agriculture Organization/World Health Organization (FAO/WHO) (1984) in edible plants is 0.003 mg/g. The WHO limit for copper in medicinal herbs has not been established yet. However, some countries had set limits for copper in medicinal plants at 20 and 0.150 mg/g, respectively [31].

Iron contents were 0.01453, 0.01089, and 0.05022 mg/g for the guavira peel, pulp, and seed, respectively. The seeds of guavira are a rich source of iron. The regulatory limits of the WHO/FAO (2005) have not been established yet for the iron in herbal medicines. The limit set by FAO/WHO (1984) in edible plants was 0.02 mg/g. The iron concentration found in Pakistani medicinal plants ranged with values between 0.18163 and 6.79688 mg/g [32]. Values of iron found in Egyptian species and medicinal plants ranged from 0.02696 to 1.046.25 mg/g [33]. Iron is necessary for several functions in the human body. However, iron toxicity has an adverse effect on various metabolic functions and cardiovascular system [34].

Elements	Peel (mg/g)	Pulp (mg/g)	Seeds (mg/g)
Cu	0.005	0.0031	0.0326
Zn	0.00118	0.00221	0.01063
Ca	0.2598	0.199	0.4608
K	2.0236	1.7515	2.5482
Na	0.2334	0.21566	0.0582
P	0.2332	0.5755	4.0652
Cd	ND	ND	ND
Fe	0.01453	0.01089	0.05022
Ni	ND	ND	0.00017
Mn	0.00269	0.00099	0.00237
Co	0.0001	0.00005	0.00013
Mg	0.15304	0.10371	0.1981
Al	ND	0.00597	0.02037
Cr	0.00101	0.00074	0.00084
Mo	0.00627	0.00434	0.00469
Si	0.01346	0.01182	0.01104

ND, non-detected.

Table 1. Levels of inorganic elements in guavira fruit.

The present study indicates that the seeds of guavira are a rich source of phosphorus (4.0652 mg/g). In an Indian plant known as *Sesbania bispinosa* (Jacq.), the lowest concentration of phosphorus found in seeds was 0.00532 mg/g followed by the concentrations in leaves 0.00292 mg/g and in roots 0.0028 [35].

Chromium contents were 0.00101, 0.00074, and 0.00084 mg/g for the guavira peel, pulp, and seed, respectively. On the other hand in the Pakistan, the range of chromium varied between 0.0012 mg/g in *Convolvulus arvensis* and 0.02949 mg/g in *Cannabis sativa* [32]. The permissible limit set by FAO/WHO (1984) in edible plants was 0.00002 mg/g. The permissible limit of chromium for plants is 0.00130 mg/g recommended by WHO. After comparison of researches of data above, the concentration of chromium in fruit peel was recorded above the permissible limit set by WHO. The beneficial effects of supplemental chromium in individuals with type 2 diabetes were observed at levels higher than the upper limit of the estimated safe and adequate daily dietary intake [36].

Molybdenum contents in the guavira peel, pulp, and seed were 0.00626, 0.00434 and 0.00469 mg/g, respectively. In 1973, the WHO experts suggested that 2 μg/kg of body weight would be appropriate to maintain normal parameters in health [37]. Representative diets of various countries showed an average concentration of molybdenum in diet 0.23 mg/kg; this corresponds to a daily intake of 100 μg of molybdenum per day for adults. The values of dietary intake of Mo are scarce in the literature reports in Brazil and other countries. This is important information required in assessing risks to human health due to their overburden. So, knowledge of the current levels of dietary intake of guavira by indigenous and rural populations is of primary importance [38].

The nickel concentration was detected by only seeds (0.00017 mg/g). According to the Food and Agriculture Organization of the United Nations (1984), the permissible limit in edible plants is 0.00163 mg/g. Until 2005, there is no permissible limit for nickel by WHO in medicinal plants. Scientific findings have shown that Ni is toxic as evidenced by lipid peroxidative damage to placental membrane; in this case, the metabolic change may be responsible for decreased placental viability, altered permeability, and potential subsequent embryotoxicity [39].

In India, the plant *Withania somnifera* known commonly as Indian ginseng has below concentration of zinc 0.0206 mg/g. In our work, in relation to guavira seeds, we obtained the amount of zinc 0.01063 mg/g. There are no limits of zinc concentration in medicinal plants by the World Health Organization (WHO, 2005). However, the zinc concentration in guavira is less than other Pakistani plants [32]. The guavira fruits are not rich in zinc, as some people claim. However, the recommendation of zinc is beneficial in the treatment of several disorders, such as several pro-inflammatory conditions and cancer [40].

The range of potassium varied between 2.023 mg/g in peel, 1.75 mg/g in pulp, and 2.54 mg/g in the seeds. These values are low when compared with other medicinal plants: *Rheum australe* (0.00622 mg/g) and *Anethum graveolens* (36.93961 mg/g). Potassium has been found in higher concentrations in *Allium cepa* (86.422 mg/g) [41]. On the other hand, minimum concentrations of Ca were observed in the pulp (0.199 mg/g) and maximum in seeds (0.4608 mg/g), which is less than 13.34 mg/g in *Brassica campestris*, Pakistani medicinal plant [32]. According to a study with several herbal medicaments, the reported tolerable upper intake level of calcium in herbs is 2500 mg/day. It has been suggested that for those athletes who may require calcium supplementation to improve bone density, building up to an intake of 1500 mg daily in doses of at least 500 mg at a time is recommended [42]; higher doses could result in adverse gastrointestinal symptoms in some people [43]. So, the guavira fruit is not a good source of potassium and calcium.

In this study, the concentration of magnesium obtained was 0.1981 mg/g. In some Pakistani medicinal plants, magnesium content ranged between 0.00333 mg/g in *Punica granatum* [44] to 2.24188 mg/g in *Convolvulus arsenis* [32]. There are no current data to establish a safe upper level for the magnesium intake.

The range of Mn varied between 0.00269 mg/g in peel and 0.00237 mg/g in seeds of guavira. According to FAO/WHO, the permissible limit set in edible plants was 0.002 mg/g [45]. Studies on medicinal plants in Nigeria obtained a concentration of manganese 0.000399 mg/g in *Fleurya aestuans* (Urticaceae). After this comparison, the concentrations of manganese in fruits of guavira are in perfect harmony with those limits of FAO/WHO. However, for manganese in medicinal plants limits have not yet been established by WHO (2005).

Silicon contents in the guavira peel, pulp, and seed were 0.01346, 0.01182 and 0.01104 mg/g, respectively. There are no guidelines to establish a permissible level of silicon in medicinal herbs. It is not certain that silicon is essential to all plants. No silicon deprivation studies have been conducted in humans. However, silicon appears to have a beneficial role in bone formation and in bone health [46].

The sodium concentrations for fruit studied ranged from 0.0582 mg/g (seed) to 0.2334 mg/g (peel). In the plant *F. aestuans* Linn. (Urticaceae) of Nigeria, the concentration of sodium obtained was 0.01225 mg/g. The minimum daily intake of sodium is 2.3 g.

In analyzed fruits, the sodium contents varied between 0.2598 mg/g (peel), 0.199 mg/g (pulp),and 0.4608 mg/g (seeds). In the reported plants [44], Na contents ranged from 0.0006 mg/g *Therminalia chebula*)) to 90.375 mg/g (*Linum usitatissimum*) [44]. The recommended daily allowance of sodium is 0.12–0.37 g/d for infants, 1.5–1.7 g/d for children, and 1.2–1.5 g/d for adults [47].

4. Conclusions

The results of the analysis showed that the guavira fruits are rich in mineral contents, especially potassium, calcium, sodium, and phosphorus.

The concentrations of elements K, Ca, Na, and P are found at the major level in peel, pulp, and seeds of fruit. The zinc concentration is very low compared to other detected elements.

The mineral composition results of the medicinal plants showed that these plants contain rich source of mineral elements; this result became so important when the usefulness of minerals such as Ca, Mg, P, K, and Na in body is considered. The knowledge of the current levels of dietary intake of guavira by indigenous and rural populations is of primary importance. The elemental analysis of the guavira showed significant variation among different elements. The analysis of Cr concentration showed the highest in peel and the lowest value was found in pulp. It was found that the highest amount of Mo was present in peel and pulp had the lowest value. The concentrations of chromium (Cr) and molybdenum (Mo) were reportedly found higher than the permissible levels.

Some minerals of guavira showed elemental contents above the permissible levels as recommended by the WHO.

Animal studies should be performed. The knowledge of the chemical elements in plants has economic interest and involves global health problem.

Author details

Nayara Vieira de Lima, Daniela Granja Arakaki, Paula F. Saldanha Tschinkel, Anderson Fernandes da Silva, Rita de Cássia Avellaneda Guimarães*, Priscila Aiko Hiane and Valter Aragão do Nascimento

*Address all correspondence to: rita.guimaraes@ufms.br

Post Graduation Program in Health and Development in the Middle West Region, Federal University of Mato Grosso do Sul—UFMS, Campo Grande, MS, Brazil

References

[1] Pan SY, Litscher G, Gao SH, Zhou SF, Yu ZL, Chen HQ, Zhang SF, Tang MK, Sun JN, Ko KM. Historical perspective of traditional indigenous medical practices: the current renaissance and conservation of herbal resources. Evidence-Based Complementary and Alternative Medicine. 2014; 2014: 20. DOI: 10.1155/2014/525340.

[2] Falodun A. Herbal medicine in Africa-distribution, standardization and prospects. Research Journal of Phytochemistry. 2010; 4: 154–161. DOI: 10.3923/rjphyto.2010.154.161.

[3] Di Stasi LC, Hiruma CA, Guimarães EM, Santos CM. Medicinal plants popularly used in Brazilian Amazon. Fitoterapia; 1994; 65: 529.

[4] Soetan KO, Olaiya CO, Oyewole OE. The importance of mineral elements for humans, domestic animals and plants: A review. African Journal of Food Science. 2010; 4: 200–222.

[5] Santos MS, Carneiro PIB, Wosiacki G, Petkowicz CLO, Carneiro EBB. Physicochemical characterization, extraction and analysis of pectins from fruit of *Campomanesia xanthocarpa* B. (Gabiroba). Ciências Agrárias, 2009; 30: 101–106. DOI: 10.5433/1679-0359.2009v30n1p101.

[6] Vallilo MI, Moreno PRH, Oliveira E, Lamardo LCA, Garbelotti ML. Chemical composition of *Campomanesia xanthocarpa* Berg-Myrtaceae Fruit, Ciência e Tecnologia de Alimentos, 2008; 28: 231–237. DOI: 10.1590/S0101-20612008000500035.

[7] Vieira RF, Agostini-Costa TS, Silva DB, Ferreira FR, Sano SM. Frutas nativas da região Centro-Oeste. Brasília: Embrapa Recursos Genéticos e Biotecnologia, 2006; 12–25.

[8] Viecili PRN, Borges DO, Kirsten K, Malheiros J, Viecili E, Melo RD, Trevisan G, Silva MA, Bochi GV, Moresco RN, Klafke JZ. Effects of Campomanesia xanthocarpa on inflammatory processes, oxidative stress, endothelial dysfunction and lipid biomarkers in hypercholesterolemic individuals. Atherosclerosis. 2014; 234: 85–92. DOI: 10.1016/j.atherosclerosis.2014.02.010.

[9] Markman BE, Bacchi EM, Kato ET. Antiulcerogenic effects of *Campomanesia xanthocarpa*. Journal of Ethnopharmacology. 2004; 94: 55–57. DOI: 10.1016/j.jep.2004.04.025.

[10] Biavatti MW, Farias C, Curtius F, Brasil LM, Hort S, Schuster L, Leite SN, Prado SRT. Preliminary studies on *Campomanesia xanthocarpa* (Berg.) and *Cuphea carthagenensis* (Jacq.) J.F. Macbr. aqueous extract: weight control and biochemical parameters. Journal of Ethnopharmacology. 2004; 93: 385–389. DOI: 10.1016/j.jep.2004.04.015.

[11] Dickel ML, Rates SMK, Ritter MR. Plants popularly used for loosing weight purposes in Porto Alegre, South Brazil. Journal of Ethnopharmacology. 2007; 109: 60–71. DOI: 10.1016/j.jep.2006.07.003.

[12] Lorenzi H, Bacher L, Lacerda M, Sartori, S. Frutas brasileiras e exóticas cultivadas (de consumo in natura). São Paulo: Plantarum; 2006. 640 p.

[13] Markman BEO, Bacchi EM, Kato ETM. Antiulcerogenic effects of *Campomanesia xanthocarpa*. Journal of Ethnopharmacology 2004; 94: 55–57. DOI: 10.1016/j.jep.2004.04.025.

[14] Hodek P, Trefil P, Stiborová M. Flavonoids-potent and versatile biologically active compounds interacting with cytochromes P450. Chemico-Biological Interactions. 2002; 139: 1–21. DOI: 10.1016/S0009-2797(01)00285-X.

[15] Michel MCP, Guimarães AG, Paula AC, Rezende SA, Sobral MEG, Guimarães DAS. Extracts from the leaves of *Campomanesia velutina* inhibits production of LPS/INF-γ induced inflammatory mediators in J774A.1 cells and exerts anti-inflammatory and antinociceptive effects in vivo. Revista Brasileira de Farmacognosia. 2013; 23: 927–936. DOI: 10.1590/S0102-695X2013000600010.

[16] Fernandes TO, Avila RI, Moura SS, Riberiro GA, Naves MMV. *Campomanesia adamantium* (Myrtaceae) fruits protect HEPG2 cells against carbon tetrachloride-induced toxicity, Toxicology Reports. 2015; 2: 184–193. DOI: 10.1016/j.toxrep.2014.11.018.

[17] Santos MS, Miguel OG, Petkowicz CLO, Cândido LMB. Antioxidant and fatty acid profile of gabiroba seed (*Campomanesia xanthocarpa* Berg). Ciência e Tecnologia de Alimentos. 2012; 32: 234–238. DOI: 10.1590/S0101-20612012005000045.

[18] Vinagre AS, Rönnau ÂDRO, Pereira SF, Silveira LU, Wiilland EDF, Suyenaga ES. Antidiabetic effects of *Campomanesia xanthocarpa* (Berg) leaf decoction. Brazilian Journal of Pharmaceutical Sciences. 2010; 46: 167–177. DOI: 10.1590/s1984-82502010000200002.

[19] Bhutta ZA, Bird SM, Black RE, Brown KH, Gardner JM, Hidayat A, Khatun F, Martorell R, Ninh NX, Penny ME, Rosado JL, Roy SK, Ruel M, Sazawal S, Shankar A. Therapeutic effects of oral zinc in acute and persistent diarrhea in children in developing countries: pooled analysis of randomized controlled trials. The American Journal of Clinical Nutrition. 2000; 72: 1516–1522.

[20] He FJ, MacGregor GA. A comprehensive review on salt and health and current experience of worldwide salt reduction programmes. Journal of Human Hypertension. 2009; 23: 363–384. DOI: 10.1038/jhh.2008.144.

[21] Dietary Guidelines for Americans Scientific Advisory Committee. Report of the Dietary Guidelines Advisory Committee on the Dietary Guidelines for Americans, 2010, to the Secretary of Agriculture and the Secretary of Health and Human Service. 2010.

[22] Anke M, Groppel B, Kronemann H, Bratter P, Schramel P, editors. Significance of newer essential trace elements (like Si, Ni, As, Li, V,) for the nutrition of man and animals. Journal of Trace Elements in Medicine and Biology. 1984; 3: 421.

[23] Gielen M, Tiekink ERT, editors. Metallo therapeutic drugs and metal-based diagnostic agents: the use of metals in medicine. 2nd ed. Chichester: Wiley; 2008. 638 p.

[24] Hassan LG, Usman BB, Kamba AS, Hassan SW. Nutritional compositions of vegetable spaghetti (*Hastala pasta*). Nigeria Food Journal. 2009; 27 (2). DOI: 10.4314/nifoj.v27i2.47471.

[25] Devine A, Criddle RA, Dick IM, Kerr DA, Prince RL. A longitudinal study of the effect of sodium and calcium intakes on regional bone density in postmenopausal women. The American Journal of Clinical Nutrition. 1995; 62: 740–745.

[26] Douglas K, Redman C. Magnesium. British Medical Journal. 1994; 309: 53–59.

[27] Keen C, Ensunsa J, Clegg M. Metal Ions Bio, Syst., 37, 89–121, 2000; Environmental Protection Agency (EPA), Drinking Water Health Advisory for Manganese, US EPA, Washington, DC, 2004.

[28] Singh R, Kooreman K, Babbs C. Potential use of simple manganese salts as antioxidant drugs in horses. American Journal of Veterinary Research. 1992; 53 (10): 1822–1829.

[29] Ferreira LC, Grabe-Guimarães A, Paula CA, Michel MCP, Guimaraes RG, Rezende SA, Souza Filho JD, Guimaraes DAS. Anti-inflammatory and antinociceptive activities of *Campomanesia adamantium*. Journal of Ethnopharmacology. 2013; 145: 100–108. DOI: 10.1016/j.jep.2012.10.037.

[30] Stanojkovic-Sebic A, Pivic R, Josic D, Dinic Z, Stanojkovic A. Heavy metals content in selected medicinal plants commonly used as components for herbal formulations. Journal of Agricultural Sciences. 2015; 21: 317–325.

[31] Ulla R, Khader JA, Hussain I, AbdElsalam NM, Talha M, Khan N. Investigation of macro and micro-nutrients in selected medicinal plants. African Journal of Pharmacy and Pharmacology. 2012; 6 (25): 1829–1832. DOI: 10.5897/AJPP12.006.

[32] Jabeen S, Shah MT, Khan S, Hayat MQ. Determination of major and trace elements in ten important folk therapeutic plants of Haripur basin, Pakistan. Journal of Medicinal Plants Research. 2010; 4 (7): 559–566. DOI: 10,5897/JMPR10.015.

[33] Dghaim R, Khatib SA, Rasool H, Khan MA. Determination of heavy metals concentration in traditional herbs commonly consumed in the United Arab Emirates. Journal of Environmental and Public Health. 2015; 2015: 6. DOI: 10.1155/2015/973878.

[34] Martin S, Griswold W. Human health effects of heavy metals. Environmental Science and Technology Briefs for Citizens. 2009; 15: 1–6.

[35] Parab N, Vaidya S. Determination of some trace elements and macro minerals. International Journal of Pharmacy and Pharmaceutical Research. 2016; 6 (2): 383–401.

[36] Anderson RA, Cheng N, Bryden NA, Polansky MM, Cheng N, Chi J, Feng J. Elevated intakes of supplemental chromium improve glucose and insulin variables in individuals with type 2 diabetes. Diabetes. 1997; 46 (11): 1786–1791. DOI: 10.2337/diab.46.11.1786.

[37] World Health Organization. Trace elements in human nutrition. Geneva: Macmillan/Ceuterick; 1973.

[38] Parr RM. An international collaborative research programme on minor and trace elements in total diets. In: Bratter P, Schramel P, editors. Trace element analytical chemistry in medicine and biology. Berlin: Walter De Gruyter Inc; 1987. p. 157–165.

[39] Chen CY, Lin TH. Nickel toxicity to human term placenta: in vitro study on lipid peroxidation. Journal of Toxicology and Environmental Health. 1998; 54 (1): 37–47. DOI: 10.1080/009841098159015.

[40] Connell P, Young VM, Toborek M, Cohen DA, Barve S, McClain CJ, Hennig B. Zinc attenuates tumor necrosis factor-mediated activation of transcription factors in endothelial cells. The Journal of the American College of Nutrition. 1997; 16: 411–417. DOI: 10.1080/07315724.1997.10718706.

[41] Khan SA, Ahmad I, Mohajir MS. Evaluation of mineral contents of some edible medicinal plants. Pakistan Journal of Pharmaceutical Sciences. 2006; 19: 141–148.

[42] Austin K, Seebohar B. Performance Nutrition: Applying the Science of Nutrient Timing. 1st ed. Champaign, IL: Human Kinetics; 2011. 200 p.

[43] Wolf SM. Worst Pills, Best Pills: A Consumer's Guide to Avoiding Drug-Induced Death or Illness. Revised ed. New York, NY: Pocket Books; 2005. 913 p.

[44] Aziz MA, Adnan M, Begum S, Azizullah A, Nazir R, Iram S. A review on the elemental contents of Pakistani medicinal plants: Implications for folk medicines. Journal of Ethnopharmacology. 2016; 188: 177–192. DOI: 10.1016/j.jep.2016.05.011.

[45] Omokehide A, Lajide L, Hammed O, Babatunde O. Trace elements and majors minerals evaluation in *Fluerya aestuans* Linn. (Urticaceae). International Journal of Pharma Sciences. 2013; 3 (5): 328–332.

[46] Carlisle EM. Silicon: an essential element for the chick. Science. 1972; 178: 619. DOI: 10.1126/science.178.4061.619.

[47] Crook MA. Clinical Chemistry and Metabolic Medicine. 7th ed. London: Holder Arnold; 2006. 426 p.

11

Thymus Plants: A Review—Micropropagation, Molecular and Antifungal Activity

Fernanda Leal, Meriem Taghouti, Fernando Nunes,
Amélia Silva, Ana Cláudia Coelho and
Manuela Matos

Abstract

Medicinal and aromatic plants are important sources for plant secondary metabolites. The genetic manipulation of plants associated with in vitro plant regeneration systems facilitates efforts to engineer secondary product metabolic pathways. The fungal infections have been increasing in recent years due to several factors, namely, the increased incidence of high-risk patients, particularly immunocompromised hosts. Aromatic plants have been empirically used as antimicrobial agents, but the mechanisms of action are still unknown. Thyme has a great interest due to the possibility of its use in different applications, in medicine, in the cosmetic industry, or as food additives. Several studies have shown that thyme oils possess antimicrobial activity. Increasingly, plant breeding has taken advantage of molecular biology developments in order to genotype the species of interest to accelerate their selection. These approaches consist in choosing desired genotypes based on molecular markers or the knowledge of the genes involved in a particular trait. The in vitro culture techniques can be used to multiply plants selected after molecular and antifungal studies. The course of the investigation and the current state in relation to micropropagation, molecular studies, and antifungal action of the *Thymus* genus plants will be presented.

Keywords: *Thymus*, micropropagation, molecular, antifungal

1. Introduction

The genus *Thymus* L. belongs to the Lamiaceae family and consists of over 400 species of herbaceous annuals and perennial plants that are extensively used, for medicinal and non-medicinal purposes. These plants are widely distributed throughout the Old World [1, 2] and have been used for many centuries in traditional medicine due to their antiseptic, carminative, antiviral, and antioxidant properties [3]. *Thymus* species are also interesting as a source of pentacyclic triterpenoids with several properties, as anti-inflammatory, hepatoprotective, antimicrobial, anti-HIV-1 activity, antiulcer, gastroprotective, hypoglycemic, antihyperlipidemic activity, and specific cytotoxicity against a variety of tumor cell lines [4–6]. By all this it becomes increasingly important to know the bioactive components of the *Thymus*.

Furthermore, interests focusing mainly on few selected chemotypes for the cosmetic and food industries, among others, lead to the loss of other species in nature, such as *Thymus cariensis* Hub.-Mor. & Jalas, *Thymus cilicicus* Boiss. & Balansa, *Thymus sipyleus* Boiss., *Thymus pulvinatus* Čelak., and *Thymus cherlerioides* Vis. [7]. These species should be preserved to make available the access to a wide range of genetic diversity. On the other hand, as the plant has a low propagation rate in nature, a suitable method to obtain a high number of plants is needed [8].

2. *Thymus* main active compounds

Among the *Lamiaceae* family, the genus *Thymus* is one of the most studied genera, due to the use of these plants as a remedy in folk medicine and as a condiment, mainly in the Mediterranean zone [1]. High bioactivity (e.g., antioxidant, anti-inflammatory, antiproliferative, and antimicrobial effects) is linked to the considerable content in phytochemicals of different *Thymus* species. Volatile compounds are extracted in essential oils (EOs), while nonvolatile compounds are found in alcoholic and aqueous extracts obtained by maceration, decoction, or infusion [9].

Noticeable interest was given to the study of EO in different *Thymus* species. High intraspecific chemical polymorphism was reported, especially in *Thymus vulgaris* L., which was shown to have a polymorphic variation in monoterpene production [10, 11]. Phenolic monoterpenes, such as carvacrol and thymol (**Figure 1**, compounds 1 and 2), seem to explain the important biological activity of the majority of *Thymus* spp. essential oils characterized by phenolic chemotypes. However, the presence of other terpenes in the EO results in the enhancement or reduction of EO bioactivity due to synergistic or antagonistic effects [12]. In the *Lamiaceae* family, EOs are produced in the glandular trichomes and stored in their cavities [13]. Several enzymes are involved in the biosynthetic pathways of terpenes, such as the terpene synthases enzyme class and the cytochrome P450s that are involved in the core terpene molecule functionalization [14].

Carvacrol and thymol have *p*-cymene as common precursor (**Figure 1**, compound 5). Carvacrol is frequent in some Lamiaceae aromatic plant genera like *Thymus*, *Origanum*, and *Satureja* [15], while thymol is mainly frequent in *Thymus* plants. Phenolic chemotypes are characteristic of *T. vulgaris* [10], *Thymus hyemalis* Lange [16], *Thymus capitatus* L. [17], *Thymus zygis* L. [18], and some populations of *Thymus pulegioides* L. [19]. Thymol's antibacterial effect is enhanced by the presence of carvacrol in the essential oil [12]. Both thymol and carvacrol have important antifungal effect; they act by causing damage in the cell membrane and interacting with ergosterol [18, 20–22]. This mechanism was also proved with other monoterpenes, namely, linalool (**Figure 1**, compound 3), which acts also by interfering with biofilm formation and stability [23].

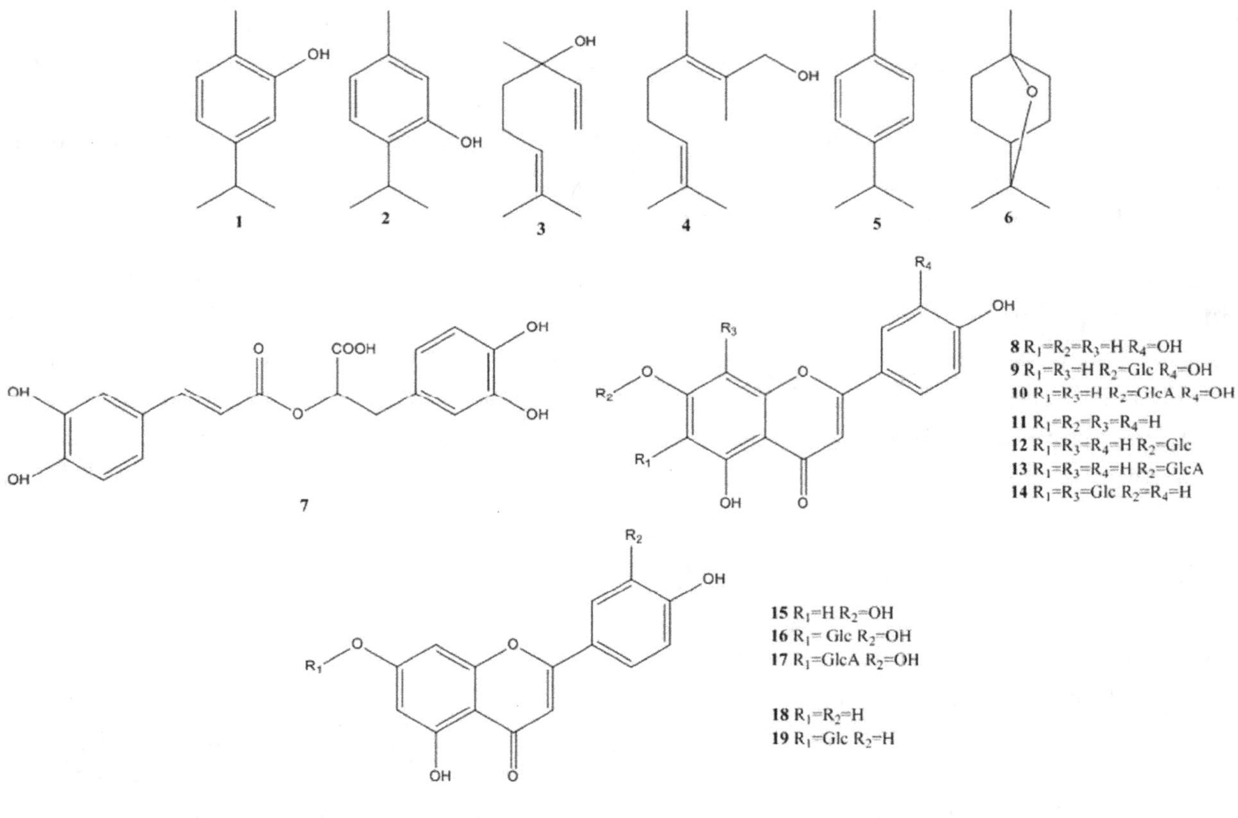

Figure 1. Chemical structure of main active compounds in *Thymus* spp. (1) carvacrol, (2) thymol, (3) linalool, (4) geraniol, (5) *p*-cymene, (6) eucalyptol, (7) rosmarinic acid, (8) luteolin, (9) luteolin-*O*-glucoside, (10) luteolin-*O*-glucuronide, (11) apigenin, (12) apigenin-7-*O*-glucoside, (13) apigenin-7-*O*-glucuronide, (14) apigenin-6,8-di-*C*-glucoside, (15) eriodictyol, (16) eriodictyol-*O*-glucoside, (17) eriodictyol-*O*-glucuronide, (18) naringenin, (19) naringenin-7-*O*-glucoside. Glc, glucoside unit; GlcA, glucuronide unit.

Linalool and geraniol (**Figure 1**, compounds 3 and 4, respectively) are monoterpene alcohols, which characterize several chemotypes of *Thymus* species such as *Thymus pulegioides*, *T. x. citriodorus* (Pers.) Schreb., *Thymus algeriensis* Boiss. & Reut., and some populations of *T. vulgaris* [11, 19, 24, 25]. Eucalyptol, or 1,8-cineole (**Figure 1**, compounds 6), a monoterpene cyclic ether monoterpene that is mainly present in *Eucalyptus* genus, is the major component of *Thymus mastichina* (L.) L. EO [26] and was also reported in populations of *T. algeriensis*, *Thymus hirtus* Raf., and *Thymus glabrescens* [27, 28].

Although more interest has been given to study thyme essential oils, nonvolatile extracts contain highly active secondary metabolites which are mainly phenolic compounds. Aromatic amino acids L-phenylalanine and L-tyrosine, produced by the shikimic acid pathway, are the precursors of the biosynthesis of polyphenols, namely, phenolic acids and flavonoids [29, 30]. Rosmarinic acid and luteolin (**Figure 1**, compounds 7 and 8, respectively) are the main frequent phenolic compounds found in thyme plants and which are related to their extracts' biological activity. Rosmarinic acid, caffeic acid esterified with 3,4-dihydroxyphenyllactic acid, is the most abundant phenolic acid in several *Thymus* species: *T. vulgaris*, *T. pulegioides*, *T. zygis*, *T. mastichina*, *T. capitatus*, *Thymus longicaulis* C. Presl, and *T. x. citriodorus* [9, 31–36].

From the class of flavones, luteolin and apigenin (**Figure 1**, compounds 8 and 11, respectively) are the most important in *Thymus*. Luteolin is frequently present also in fruits and other

Lamiaceae genera like *Mentha*. Its glycosylated derivatives such as luteolin-*O*-glucoside (**Figure 1**, compound 9) are also frequent in thyme species. Apigenin and its derivatives (**Figure 1**) are reported in some species such as *T. x. citriodorus, T. vulgaris,* and *Thymus herba-barona* Loisel. [37]. Eriodictyol and naringenin (**Figure 1**, compounds 15 and 18) are flavanones which were described as well as their glucoside and glucuronide derivatives (**Figure 1**, compounds 16 and 19 and 17, respectively) in some *Thymus* species such as *T. x. citriodorus* and *T. vulgaris* [34].

3. Micropropagation of *Thymus*

Advances in biotechnological approaches provide a set of techniques that contribute to solving problems of extinction or genetic erosion in particular of plants. Alternatives for fast multiplication, like "in vitro micropropagation" that enables propagation of plants under controlled environmental conditions, can help in multiplying selected plants after molecular and antifungal studies or subjected to excessive demand by the people.

Furthermore, it was also possible to develop techniques that allow the maintenance of germplasm for a long time, like "cryopreservation" that make available long-term storage of *Thymus* germplasm at ultra-low temperatures [8].

Species	Achievements	Growth regulators or others	References
Thymus mastichina	Propagation of thyme from mature field-grown plants	Nodal segments—MS + 0.1 mg L^{-1} BAP Roots—MS + 1 mg L^{-1} NAA	[40]
Thymus vulgaris and *Thymus longicaulis*	In vitro propagation protocol	Shoots, semisolid MS + 1 mg L^{-1} KN and 0.3 mg L^{-1} GA3; roots, MS + 0.05 mg L^{-1} 2,4-D	[41]
Thymus lotocephalus	Propagation protocol using seeds as explants	MS BAP induce high % of hyperhidric shots	[42]
Thymus caespititius	Shoots with high proliferation capacity	MS + 0.4 mg L^{-1} BA + 0.1 mg L^{-1} IBA	[43]
Thymus persicus	System for regeneration via direct organogenesis	Shoot, 8.9 μM BAP + 2.7 μM NAA; roots, 1/2 MS + 2.5 μM IBA	[44]
Thymus hyemalis	Regeneration of plants through somatic embryogenesis	MS + 4.44 μM BAP, 0.54 μM NAA, and 4.65 μM KIN	[45]
Thymus daenensis	Colloidal silver nanoparticles reduce hyperhydricity	2.5 mg L^{-1}AgNPs (silver nanoparticles)	[46]
Thymus moroderi	Propagation disinfection processDouble phase culture system	growth regulators did not improve the morphogenic response	[47]
Thymus persicus	Callus induction and micropropagation	Callus, MS + 2.0 mg L^{-1} NAA and 0.5 mg L^{-1} KN Shoot, MS + 2.0 mg L^{-1} BAP + 1.0 mg L^{-1} NAA	[48]

Table 1. Approaches in *Thymus* plant micropropagation.

Optimizations for micropropagation process involve the use of different growth regulators like cytokinins, auxins, or gibberellic acid for the induction of multiple shoots. The first works in *Thymus* micropropagation are from Furmanowa and Olszowska dated from 1980 [38] to 1992 [39]. Since that date, a lot of works for the micropropagation of different species of *Thymus* (**Table 1**), as well as the cryopreservation of the same plants, were developed (**Figure 2**).

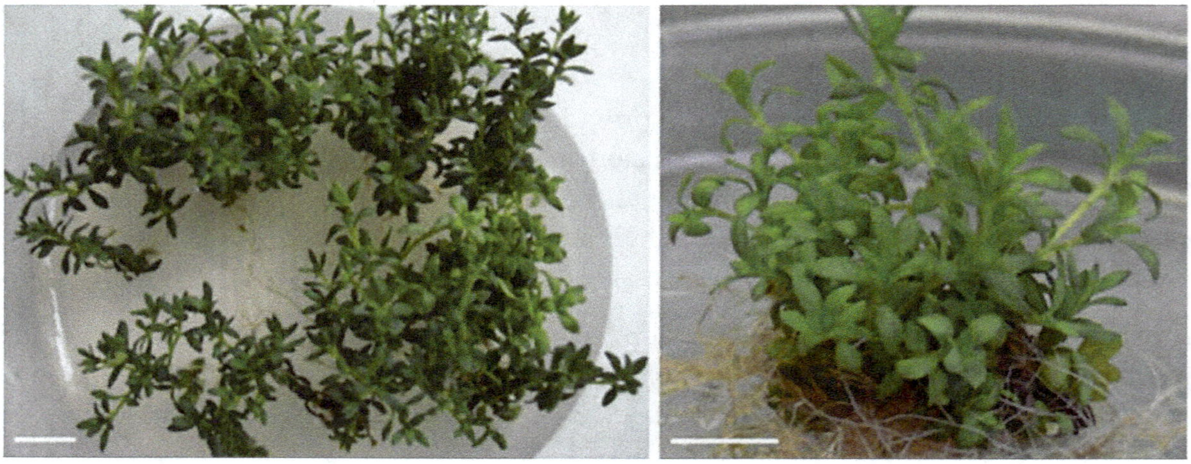

Figure 2. *Thymus caespititius* multiple shoots produced. (**A**) Outgrowth of the axillary buds maintained on MS medium with 0.4 mg L^{-1} BA and 0.1 mg L^{-1} IBA. (**B**) Detail of spontaneous root formation in shoot cultures (bars = 1 cm) [43].

Cryopreservation procedures, PVS2 vitrification, encapsulation—vitrification and droplet—and freezing methods showed to be effective to induce cryotolerance and long-term conservation of thyme shoot tips obtained from in vitro propagated plantlets [49]: Different *Thymus* species have already been studied, *Thymus moroderi* [50], *T. vulgaris* and *T. longicaulis* [2], *T. cariensis* and *T. vulgaris* [41], and *Thymus lotocephalus* [51].

4. Genetic analysis

Researchers, from different areas, use the genetic analysis of plants as the basis of their work in order to identify and to characterize plant materials in nature, to detect genetic diversity or the genetic homogeneity, and to select plants with desired compounds.

The pool of genetic variation in plants, namely, the medicinal and the aromatic ones, serves as the base for plant breeding as well as for selection. Molecular markers are very useful in breeding program allowing germplasm screening independent to the developmental stage of the plants and/or environmental factors [52].

Applications of DNA methods, with different purposes, in *Thymus* genus are few when compared with other economically important plant species. A few reports are available about genetic characterization of species of *Thymus* genus (**Table 2**), using different molecular markers, being the techniques of random amplified polymorphic DNA markers (RAPD) and inter-simple sequence repeat (ISSR) the most commonly used. Amplified fragment length polymorphisms (AFLPs) and microsatellites are also utilized for genetic analysis and genetic relationships in *Thymus* species [56, 63].

Beyond the genetic characterization of different species, the knowledge of genetic diversity within species is necessary for any improvement of cultivars and biodiversity maintenance and restoration [64]. Yousefi et al. [54] studied ecotypes grown in different parts of Iran using ISSRs and verified that the accessions were relatively grouped according to their location and conclude that ISSRs provided a powerful and reliable molecular tool for detecting genetic variation and relationships. A similar study was done by Rahimmalek et al. [55] with the purpose to assess the genetic diversity of *Thymus daenensis* Celak accessions toward the conservation of the endangered aromatic species. Solyman and Alkowni [59] studied genetic diversities of five Palestinian *Thymus* species using RAPD markers and concluded that it could be useful tools for identifying *Thymus* species in any putative breeding programs that will be carried in the country. A study, with AFLPs, in *Thymus*, section *Serpyllum* [63], demonstrated that this markers could be suitable for complex genetic relationships analysis, including frequent interspecies hybridization events. Recently Karaca et al. [56] present the first report of genomic microsatellite markers for the genus *Thymus*, used in 48 individuals representing 9 species and subspecies of *Thymus*.

The overexploitation of wild plants for commercial purposes (and consequent decreased of populations) associated to the increasing demand for secondary metabolites has intensified the application of biotechnological methods to propagate and reproduce high-yielding plants under controlled growing conditions and/or to obtain homogenous and stable genotypes. Other application of molecular markers in this genus is the analysis of the reliability of the in vitro propagation regarding the genetic homogeneity, most of times associated to the phytochemical productivity of the produced plantlets, as the experiment reported by Bakhtiar et al. [48] using RAPDs. In this work RAPD profiles confirmed the homogeneity and high-performance liquid chromatography (HPLC) confirmed the phytochemical productivity of the in vitro regenerated plants.

Mendes et al. [53], using in vitro genotypes, characterized *Thymus caespititius* terpene synthase 2 (*Tctps2*) gene and identified other terpene synthase genes responsible for the chemical polymorphism observed in *T. caespititius* essential oils.

Another genetic approach is the analysis of the chemical and the genetic relationships among species as the study described by [58] that also determinate the correlation between these two sets of data, the essential-oil composition and genetic variability of six populations of *Thymus*. RAPD markers allowed a perfect distinction between the six species, based on their distinctive genetic background: however, they did not show identical clustering with the volatile-oil profiles [58]. Contrary Echeverrigaray et al. [60], also based in RAPD profiles, observed that the cultivars (*T. vulgaris* L.) could be divided into two clusters, which coincided with results obtained by oil GS-MS analysis. Chemical and genetic differences of four *Thymus* species were studied by Pluhár et al. [61] in order to determine whether molecular characters (RAPDs) and essential oil components could be used as taxonomic markers and obtained a partial correlation between molecular and chemical assessments. In

Species	Achievements	Markers	References
Thymus caespititius	Identification of terpene synthase genes in *Lamiaceae*	TPS gene	[53]
Thymus daenensis *Thymus kotschyanus* *Thymus vulgaris*	Assessment of genetic diversity and relationships	ISSRs	[54]
Thymus daenensis subsp. *daenensis*	Assessment of genetic diversity and geographic differentiation	ISSRs	[55]
Thymus cilicicus *Thymus revolutus* *Thymus cherlerioides* *Thymus leucotrichus* *Thymus zygioides* *Thymus sipyleus* *Thymus longicaulis*	Development of 23 microsatellite primer pairs for *Thymus* genus and assessment of genetic diversity and relationships of 48 samples representing nine species and subspecies of the genus *Thymus*	Microsatellites	[56]
Thymus persicus	Confirmation of genetic homogeneity in in vitro regenerated plants	RAPDs	[48]
Thymus kotschyanus	Assessment of genetic diversity of wild populations	RAPDs	[57]
Thymus daenensis *Thymus fallax* *Thymus fedtschenkoi* *Thymus migricus* *Thymus vulgaris*	Assessment of genetic diversity and chemical polymorphism of *Thymus* species	RAPDs	[58]
Thymus syriacus *Thymus fruticosus* *Thymus incanus* *Thymus majorana* *Thymus capitatus*	Assessment of thyme genetic diversity in Palestine	RAPDs	[59]
Thymus vulgaris	Correlation between the chemical and genetic relationships among commercial *Thymus* cultivars	RAPDs	[60]
Thymus glabrescens *Thymus pannonicus* *Thymus praecox* *Thymus pulegioides*	Essential oil composition and molecular analysis	RAPDs	[61]
Thymus caramanicus	Assessment of genetic and chemical variability	ISRRs	[62]
Thymus pulegioides *Thymus glabrescens* *Thymus marschallianus* *Thymus pannonicus* *Thymus balcanus* *Thymus moesiacus* *Thymus praecox*	Assessment of genetic diversity and relationships among species of the genus *Thymus* L. (section *Serpyllum*)	AFLPs	[56]

Table 2. Employment of molecular markers in genetic characterization of *Thymus* genus plants.

Thymus caramanicus Jalas, Hadian et al. [62] assessed the genetic (using ISSRs) and chemical variability and observed a relationship between genetic and chemical variability and geographic distribution.

5. Fungal infections

Fungal infections are a serious problem of public health concern and have been increasing in recent years due to several factors given increased international travel, immigration, changing climate conditions, and the increased incidence of high-risk patients [65]. Invasive mycoses are especially problematic for immunocompromised individuals and patients in intensive care units, and some conditions can predispose as organ transplantation, the use of drugs in treatments as corticosteroids and antineoplastics, and complex surgical procedure acts [66, 67]. Other cases may be found in patients suffering from diabetes mellitus, patients with human immunodeficiency virus infection, patients with neoplasias after receiving chemotherapy, patients with transplantation surgeries, or those with prolonged antibiotherapy [68].

Oral and vulvovaginal candidiases caused by *Candida albicans* are the most common fungal diseases [69]. Invasive fungal diseases can be less frequent but much more severe. Other mycotic diseases or complications associated included asthma, bronchopulmonary and invasive aspergillosis, pneumocystosis, meningeal cryptococcosis, mucormycoses, or invasive candidiasis [70]. Deaths related with fungal infections are mostly associated with *Cryptococcus, Candida, Aspergillus,* and *Pneumocystis* [71].

Aromatic plants have been empirically used as antimicrobial compounds, but the mechanisms of action are still under study [72]. Inhibitory action of aromatic plants possibly includes cytoplasm granulation, cytoplasmic membrane lesion, and inhibition and/or inactivation of extracellular and intercellular enzymes [72, 73] and might be due to different compounds, including phenolics, terpenoids, and alkaloids. These compounds together or independently use different levels of antifungal effect ending with mycelium germination inhibition [73]. Also, it is described that plant lytic enzymes act in the fungal cell wall causing breakage of β-1,6 [72]glycan, β-1,3 glycan, and chitin polymers [74]. The antimicrobial activity of the aqueous extracts could be due to the anionic components such as chlorides, thiocyanate, nitrate, and sulfates besides other water-soluble constituents which are naturally occurring in the plant material [75].

6. Antifungal activity

Only limited numbers of new antifungal drugs were developed in recent years, and there are only small numbers of drugs available for their treatment [68]. Toxicity and drug resistance have become an increasing problem. The resistance to antifungal drugs, the high costs associated with treatment, and the fungistatic activity of most of the antifungal drugs are problems making their treatment difficult and expensive [67]. So, alternatives for treating invasive fungal infections are necessary [67].

The spread of multidrug-resistant strains of fungi is a medical problem worldwide, and the reduced number of drugs available led to a search for therapeutic substitutes, namely, among aromatic and medicinal plants and compounds isolated from them used for their antifungal [76, 77].

Numerous molecules obtained from the natural environment are investigated and described in bibliography with antimycotic activity. Several extracts are investigated for antifungal activities like crude extracts or isolated constituents as essential oils, saponins, terpenoids, alkaloids, phenolic compounds, peptides, and proteins [78, 79].

The in vitro evaluation methods of antifungal activity can be divided into diffusion methods and dilution methods. The diffusion methods yielding to inhibition diameters are used mostly for the qualitative screening. Examples are the agar overlay technique [80]. Dilution methods offer more quantitative results regarding the action of essential oils. Serial dilutions are used for detecting the minimal inhibitory concentration (MIC in mg ml^{-1}) of an essential oil in a liquid medium its antimicrobial properties and rank it among the most potent essential oils in this respect [81].

A wide range of aromatic and medicinal plants with therapeutic properties have been explored and used for the extraction of essential oils all over the world due to their antimicrobial capacity against fungal pathogens [79]. Several studies have shown that thyme oils possess antimicrobial activity [82–84].

Thymus spp., most of them possessing a large quantity of phenolic monoterpenes, revealed activity against fungi [83].

Medicinal plants have the capacity to inhibit the growth of a wide range of opportunistic or pathogenic microorganisms due to the presence of essential oils [85]. Essential oils are natural, volatile liquid, complex compounds characterized by rarely colored and a strong odor, soluble in lipid and organic solvents [85]. About 60% of essential oils show antifungal activity [84].

The essential oils and their components have been used broadly against molds [85]. The essential oil extracts from many plants have shown their considerable antifungal activity against the wide range of fungal pathogens [73].

Thyme essential oils are apparently among the greatest inhibitors of fungal microorganisms because of the presence of the phenolic compounds such as thymol as main components which might disrupt the fungal cell membrane [85]. Another component that appears to show antimicrobial activity is terpene hydrocarbons (γ-terpinene) [86]. *p*-Cymene is a compound of essential oil that does not show antibacterial efficacy when used alone which suggest a synergistic effect of the compounds [86, 87].

Thyme essential oils may in the future represent a new source of natural antiseptics with applications in industry of pharmaceutics and food [86]. The essential oils have the ability to penetrate and disrupt the fungal cell wall and cytoplasmic membranes, permeabilizing them and finally causing damage to mitochondrial membranes [88].

Variability in essential oil compounds might be linked to differences in concentration and amount recovered based on several factors, including species of plant used, method of extraction, solvents, and extraction time, which in turn may differ in their antifungal potency [68, 89]. Differences can also be attributed to raw materials used (dried or fresh), types of soils used for cultivation, the harvesting time in the year, or differences in oil extraction techniques [90].

These oils have been used in folk medicine in different communities for patients suffering from mycotic infections [91].

Differences in essential oil compounds might be related to variability in the dried or fresh materials used, to the harvesting time in the year, to types of soils used for cultivation, or to differences in oil extraction techniques. *T. vulgaris* has medicinal properties and is widely used in traditional medicine for its expectorant, antispasmodic, antibronchiolitic, antitussive, anthelmintic, carminative, and diuretic properties [92].

Many studies have shown that thyme (*T. vulgaris*) has antifungal activities and have suggested their integration into pharmaceutical preparations in the treatment of candidiasis [72, 86, 93]. Previous studies showed fungistatic activity of the essential oils of *T. vulgaris* as carvacrol, *p*-cymene, and thymol [94]. The antifungal mechanism of action by which thymol or carvacrol acts is actually not well understood, although the antifungal activity is probably because thymol is lipophilic and together with carvacrol can act in the fatty acyl chains of membrane lipid bilayers, and alters the fluidity and permeability of cell membranes [95]. Other mechanisms have been theorized as damaged of membrane and cell wall with disruption associated with morphological,

Thymus plant	Inhibited microorganisms	References
Thymus vulgaris	*Candida albicans*	[72, 86, 94, 99, 100]
Thymus vulgaris	*Aspergillus flavus*	[92]
Thymus vulgaris	*Aspergillus ochraceus*	[96]
Thymus eriocalyx *Thymus x-porlock*	*Aspergillus niger*	[98]
Thymus vulgaris	*Penicillium chrysogenum*	[96]
Thymus serpyllum	Dermatophytes	[101]
Thymus schimperi	*Penicillium chrysogenum*	[66]
Thymus schimperi	*Verticillium* sp.	[66]
Thymus schimperi	*Aspergillus tubingensis*	[66]
Thymus schimperi	*Aspergillus minutus*	[66]
Thymus schimperi	*Beauveria bassiana*	[66]
Thymus schimperi	*Microsporum gypseum*	[66]

Table 3. Effect of *Thymus* plants on the fungal microorganisms.

deformation, deterioration, collapse, and of the conidia and/or hyphae [96]. Thymol and carvacrol have a stronger antifungal capacity, indicating more susceptibility of *Aspergillus* spp. than that of *Penicillium* spp. [97]. Thyme essential oil showed its capabilities of inhibiting fungal development causing leakage of the cytoplasm of *Aspergillus flavus* and was responsible for degenerative alterations in hyphae alterations, which appeared degraded or with the complete absence of conidia [92]. A previous report showed capabilities of inhibiting aflatoxin production [92].

Thymus essential oil causes irreversible damage to cell wall, cell membrane, and cellular organelles which affects *Aspergillus niger* growth and morphology [98].

The fungal activity of *Thymus* plants has been summarized in **Table 3**.

7. Conclusions

Thymus plants have been playing, in recent years, an increasingly important role in the intense study being targeted to run through the different areas of biotechnology. So here we intend to present the latest developments involving this plant in such diverse areas as active compound analysis and their effect on antifungal activity, genetic analysis, micropropagation, and finally cryopreservation techniques, one of the most recent methodologies to plant preservation.

The utilization of new plant breeding technologies will be the future in aromatic and medicinal plant manipulation and production, in order to obtain a multitude of valuable characteristics like increased nutrient and metabolite production and resistance to different stresses. Next-generation sequencing (NGS) technology and the associated bioinformatics tools will allow general profiling of RNA expression in plant species with limited molecular genetics studies as the majority of aromatic and medicinal plants.

Author details

Fernanda Leal[1, 2*], Meriem Taghouti[3], Fernando Nunes[4], Amélia Silva[3], Ana Cláudia Coelho[5] and Manuela Matos[1, 2]

* Address all correspondence to: fleal@utad.pt

1 Genetics and Biotechnology Department, University of Trás-os-Montes and Alto Douro (UTAD), Vila Real, Portugal

2 BioISI—Biosystems & Integrative Sciences Institute, Faculty of Sciences University of Lisboa, Lisboa, Portugal

3 Centre for Research and Technology of Agro-Environmental and Biological Sciences (CITAB, UTAD), Vila Real, Portugal

4 CQ-VR Chemistry Research Center, UTAD, Vila Real, Portugal

5 Animal and Veterinary Research Centre (CECAV), UTAD, Vila Real, Portugal

References

[1] Morales, R. The history, botany and taxonomy of the genus Thymus. In: Stahl-Biskup, E. & Sáez, F. (eds). Thyme: The Genus Thymus. London: CRC Press Taylor & Francis Group; 2002. pp. 1–43. ISBN 0203216857

[2] Ozudogru, E. A., Kaya, E. & Kirdok, E. Development of protocols for short-, medium- and long-term conservation of thyme. Acta Horticulturae. 2011; 918: 43–50. DOI: 10.17660/ActaHortic.2011.918.3

[3] Stahl-Biskup, E. Thyme as a herbal drug pharmacopoeias and other product characteristics. In: Stahl-Biskup E. & Sáez F. (eds). Thyme: The Genus Thymus. London: CRC Press Taylor & Francis Group; 2002. pp. 293–316. ISBN 0203216857

[4] Huang, M. T., Ho, C. T., Wang, Z. Y., Ferraro, T., Lou, Y. R., Stauber, K., et al. Inhibition of skin tumorigenesis by rosemary and its constituents carnosol and ursolic acid. Cancer Research. 1994; 54(3): 701–708.

[5] Liu, J. Pharmacology of oleanolic acid and ursolic acid. Journal of Ethnopharmacology. 1995; 49: 57–68.

[6] Liu, J.Oleanolic acid and ursolic acid: research perspectives. Journal of Ethnopharmacology. 2005; 100: 92–94.

[7] Rey, C. & Sáez, F. Field culture, in vitro culture and selection of Thymus. In: Stahl-Biskup E. & Sáez F. (eds) Thyme, the Genus Thymus. London: Taylor & Francis; 2002. pp. 177–196.

[8] Shabnum, S. & Wagay, M. G. Micropropagation of different species of Thymus. Journal of Research & Development. 2011; 11: 71–81. ISSN 0972-5407

[9] Martins, N., Barros, L., Santos-Buelga, C., Silva, S., Henriques, M. & Ferreira, I. C. F. R. Decoction, infusion and hydroalcoholic extract of cultivated thyme: antioxidant and antibacterial activities, and phenolic characterisation. Food Chemistry. 2015; 167: 131–137.

[10] Thompson, J. D., Chalchat, J. C., Michet, A., Linhart, Y. B. & Ehlers, B. Qualitative and quantitative variation in monoterpene co-occurrence and composition in the essential oil of *Thymus vulgaris* chemotypes. Journal of Chemical Ecology. 2003; 29: 859–880.

[11] Kaloustian, J., Abou, L., Mikail, C., Amiot, M. J. & Portugal, H. Southern French thyme oils: chromatographic study of chemotypes. Journal of the Science of Food and Agriculture. 2005; 85: 2437–2444.

[12] Cosentino, S., Tuberoso, C. I. G., Pisano, B., Satta, M., Mascia, V., Arzedi, E. & Palmas, F. In-vitro antimicrobial activity and chemical composition of Sardinian Thymus essential oils. Letters in Applied Microbiology. 1999; 29: 130–135.

[13] Turner, G., Gershenzon, J., Nielson, E. E., Froehlich, J. E. & Croteau, R. Limonene synthase, the enzyme responsible for monoterpene biosynthesis in peppermint, is localized to leucoplasts of oil gland secretory cells. Plant Physiology. 1999; 120: 879–886.

[14] Degenhardt, J., Kollner, T. G. & Gershenzon, J. Monoterpene and sesquiterpene synthases and the origin of terpene skeletal diversity in plants. Phytochemistry. 2009; 70: 1621–1637.

[15] De Vincenzi, M., Stammati, A., De Vincenzi, A. & Silano, M. Constituents of aromatic plants: carvacrol. Fitoterapia. 2004; 75: 801–804.

[16] Rota, M. C., Herrera, A., Martinez, R. M., Sotomayor, J. A. & Jordan, M. J. Antimicrobial activity and chemical composition of *Thymus vulgaris, Thymus zygis* and *Thymus hyemalis* essential oils. Food Control. 2008; 19: 681–687.

[17] Bounatirou, S., Smiti, S., Miguel, M. G., Faleiro, L., Rejeb, M. N., Neffati, M., Costa, M. M., Figueiredoe, A. C., Barroso, J. G. & Pedro, L. G. Chemical composition, antioxidant and antibacterial activities of the essential oils isolated from Tunisian *Thymus capitatus* Hoff. et Link. Food Chemistry. 2007; 105: 146–155.

[18] Pina-Vaz, C., Rodrigues, A. G., Pinto, E., Costa-De-Oliveira, S., Tavares, C., Satgueiro, L., Cavaleiro, C., Goncalves, M. J. & Martinez-De-Oliveira, J. Antifungal activity of *Thymus* oils and their major compounds. Journal of the European Academy of Dermatology and Venereology. 2004; 18: 73–78.

[19] Loziene, K., Vaiciuniene, J. & Venskutonis, P. R. Chemical composition of the essential oil of different varieties of thyme (*Thymus pulegioides*) growing wild in Lithuania. Biochemical Systematics and Ecology. 2003; 31: 249–259.

[20] Lima, I. O., Pereira, F. D., De Oliveira, W. A., Lima, E. D., Menezes, E. A., Cunha, F. A. & Diniz, M. D. F. M. Antifungal activity and mode of action of carvacrol against *Candida albicans* strains. Journal of Essential Oil Research. 2013; 25: 138–142.

[21] Chavan, P. S. & Tupe, S. G. Antifungal activity and mechanism of action of carvacrol and thymol against vineyard and wine spoilage yeasts. Food Control. 2014; 46: 115–120.

[22] Nobrega, R. O., Teixeira, A. P., Oliveira, W. A., Lima, E. O. & Lima, I. O. Investigation of the antifungal activity of carvacrol against strains of *Cryptococcus neoformans*. Pharmaceutical biology. 2016; 54: 2591–2596.

[23] Hsu, C. C., Lai, W. L., Chuang, K. C., Lee, M. H. & Tsai, Y. C. The inhibitory activity of linalool against the filamentous growth and biofilm formation in *Candida albicans*. Medical Mycology. 2013; 51: 473–482.

[24] Houmani, Z., Azzoudj, S., Naxakis, G. & Skoula, M. The essential oil composition of Algerian Zaâtar: *Origanum* spp. and *Thymus* spp. Journal of Herbs Spices & Medicinal Plants. 2002; 9: 275–280.

[25] Omidbaigi, R., Sefidkon, F. & Hejazi, M. Essential oil composition of *Thymus x citriodorus* L. cultivated in Iran. Flavour and Fragrance Journal. 2005; 20: 237–238.

[26] Salgueiro, L. R., Vila, R., Tomas, X., Canigueral, S., Dacunha, A. P. & Adzet, T. Composition and variability of the essential oils of *Thymus* species from Section *Mastichina* from Portugal. Biochemical Systematics and Ecology. 1997; 25: 659–672.

[27] Elhadj Ali, I. B., Zaouali, Y., Bejaoui, A. & Boussaid, M. Variation of the chemical composition of essential oils in Tunisian populations of *Thymus algeriensis* Boiss. et Reut. (*Lamiaceae*) and implication for conservation. Chemistry and Biodiversity. 2010; 7: 1276–1289.

[28] Fatma, G., Mouna, B., Mondher, M. & Ahmed, L. In-vitro assessment of antioxidant and antimicrobial activities of methanol extracts and essential oil of *Thymus hirtus* sp. *algeriensis*. Lipids in Health and Disease. 2014; 13: 114.

[29] Koes, R. E., Quattrocchio, F. & Mol, J. N. M. The flavonoid biosynthetic-pathway in plants – function and evolution. BioEssays. 1994; 16: 123–132.

[30] Riceevans, C. A., Miller, N. J. & Paganga, G. Structure-antioxidant activity relationships of flavonoids and phenolic acids. Free Radical Biology and Medicine. 1996; 20: 933–956.

[31] Loziene, K., Venskutonis, P. R., Sipailiene, A. & Labokas, J. Radical scavenging and antibacterial properties of the extracts from different *Thymus pulegioides* L. chemotypes. Food Chemistry. 2007; 103: 546–559.

[32] Jordan, M. J., Martinez, R. M., Martinez, C., Monino, I. & Sotomayor, J. A. Polyphenolic extract and essential oil quality of *Thymus zygis ssp gracilis* shrubs cultivated under different watering levels. Industrial Crops and Products. 2009; 29: 145–153.

[33] Jabri-Karoui, I., Bettaieb, I., Msaada, K., Hammami, M. & Marzouk, B. Research on the phenolic compounds and antioxidant activities of Tunisian *Thymus capitatus*. Journal of Functional Foods. 2012; 4: 661–669.

[34] Pereira, O. R., Peres, A. M., Silva, A. M. S., Domingues, M. R. M. & Cardoso, S. M. Simultaneous characterization and quantification of phenolic compounds in *Thymus x citriodorus* using a validated HPLC-UV and ESI-MS combined method. Food Research International. 2013; 54: 1773–1780.

[35] Delgado, T., Marinero, P., Asensio-S-Manzanera, M. C., Asensio, C., Herrero, B., Pereira, J. A. & Ramalhosa, E. Antioxidant activity of twenty wild Spanish *Thymus mastichina* L. populations and its relation with their chemical composition. LWT--Food Science and Technology. 2014; 57: 412–418.

[36] Galasso, S., Pacifico, S., Kretschmer, N., Pan, S. P., Marcianci, S., Piccolella, S., Monaco, P. & Bauer, R. Influence of seasonal variation on *Thymus longicaulis* C. Presl chemical composition and its antioxidant and anti-inflammatory properties. Phytochemistry. 2014; 107: 80–90.

[37] Pereira, O. R. & Cardoso, S. M. Overview on *Mentha* and *Thymus* polyphenols. Current Analytical Chemistry. 2013; 9: 382–396.

[38] Furmanowa, M. & Olszowska, O. *Thymus vulgaris* L. propagation through tissue culture. Acta Poloniae Pharmaceutica. 1980; 37: 243–247

[39] Furmanowa, M. & Olszowska, O. Micropropagation of Thyme (*Thymus vulgaris* L.). In: Bajaj, Y. P. S. (ed) Biotechnology in Agriculture and Forestry. Vol. 19. Berlin: Springer; 1992. pp. 230–243.

[40] Mendes, M. L. & Romano, A. In vitro cloning of *Thymus mastichina* L. field-grown plants. Acta Horticulturae. 1999; 502: 303–306.

[41] Ozudogru, E. A., Kaya, E., Kirdok, E. & Issever-Ozturk, S. In vitro propagation from young and mature explants of thyme (*Thymus vulgaris* and *T. longicaulis*) resulting in genetically stable shoots. In Vitro Cellular & Developmental Biology – Plant. 2011; 47(2): 309–320. DOI: 10.1007/s11627-011-9347-6

[42] Coelho, N., Gonçalves, S., González-Benito, M. E. & Romano, A. Establishment of an in vitro propagation protocol for *Thymus lotocephalus*, a rare aromatic species of the Algarve (Portugal). Plant Growth Regulation. 2012; 66: 69–74. DOI: 10.1007/s10725-011-9630-x

[43] Mendes, M. D., Figueiredo, A. C., Oliveira, M. M. & Trindade, H. Essential oil production in shoot cultures versus field-grown plants of *Thymus caespititius*. Plant Cell, Tissue and Organ Culture (PCTOC). 2013; 113: 341–351. DOI 10.1007/s11240-012-0276-9

[44] Bakhtiar, Z., Mirjalili, M. H., Sonboli, A., Sonboli, A., Farimani, M. M. & Ayyar, M.. In vitro propagation, genetic and phytochemical assessment of Thymus persicus — a medicinally important source of pentacyclic triterpenoids. Biologia. 2014; 69(5): 594–603. DOI: 10.2478/s11756-014-0346-z

[45] Nordine, A., Tlemcani, C. R. & Meskaoui, A. Regeneration of plants through somatic embryogenesis in *Thymus hyemalis* Lange, a potential medicinal and aromatic plant. In Vitro Cellular & Developmental Biology – Plant. 2014; 50: 19–25. DOI: 10.1007/s11627-013-9577-x

[46] Bernard, F., Navab Moghadam, N. & Mirzajani, F. The effect of colloidal silver nanoparticles on the level of lignification and hyperhydricity syndrome in *Thymus daenensis* vitro shoots: a possible involvement of bonded polyamines. In Vitro Cellular & Developmental Biology – Plant. 2015; 51(5): 546–553 DOI: 10.1007/s11627-015-9700-2.

[47] Marco-Medina, A. & Casasi, J. L. In vitro multiplication and essential oil composition of *Thymus moroderi* Pau ex Martinez, an endemic Spanish plant. Plant Cell, Tissue and Organ Culture (PCTOC). 2015; 120(1): 99–108.

[48] Bakhtiar, Z., Mirjalili, M. H. & Sonboli, A. In vitro callus induction and micropropagation of Thymus persicus (*Lamiaceae*), an endangered medicinal plant. Crop Breeding and Applied Biotechnology. 2016; 16: 48–54. DOI: 10.1590/1984-70332016v16n1a8

[49] Kaya, E. Development of efficient micropropagation and cryopreservation protocols for *Thymus* germplasm. In Vitro Biology Meeting held in collaboration with the 12th IAPB Congress, 2010, P283

[50] Marco-Medina, A., Casasi, J. L., Swennen, R., Panis, B. Cryopreservation of *Thymus moroderi* by droplet vitrification. Cryoletters. 2010; 31(1): 14–23. ISSN 0143-2044

[51] Coelho, N., González-Benito, M. E., Martín, C. & Romano, A.. Cryopreservation of *Thymus lotocephalus* shoot tips and assessment of genetic stability. Cryoletters. 2014; 35(2): 119–128.

[52] Kumar, P., Gupta, V. K., Misra, A. K., Modi, D. R. & Pandey, B. K.. Potential of molecular markers in plant biotechnology. Plant Omics Journal. 2009; 2(4): 141–162. ISSN 1836-3644

[53] Mendes, M. D., Barroso, J. G., Oliveira, M. M. & Trindade, H. Identification and characterization of a second isogene encoding γ-terpinene synthase in *Thymus caespititius*. Journal of Plant Physiology. 2014; 171: 1017–1027. DOI: 10.1016/j.jplph.2014.04.001

[54] Yousefi, V., Najaphy, A., Zebarjadi, A. & Safari, H. Molecular characterization of *Thymus* species using ISSR markers. The Journal of Animal & Plant Sciences. 2015; 25(4): 1087–1094. ISSN 1018-7081

[55] Rahimmalek, M., Bahreininejad, B., Khorrami, M. & Tabatabaei, B. E. Genetic variability and geographic differentiation in *Thymus daenensis* subsp. *daenensis*, an endangered medicinal plant, as revealed by inter simple sequence repeat (ISSR). Markers. Biochemical Genetics. 2009; 47(11–12): 831–842. DOI: 10.1007/s10528-009-9281-z

[56] Karaca, M., Ince, A. G., Aydin, A., Elmasulu, S. Y. & Turgut, K. Microsatellites for genetic and taxonomic research on thyme (*Thymus* L.). Turkish Journal of Biology. 2015; 39: 147–159. DOI: 10.3906/biy-1406-20

[57] Khoshsokhan, F., Babalar, M., Fatahi, M. & Poormeidani, A.. Assessment of genetic diversity of some wild populations of *Thymus Kotschyanus* using RAPD molecular markers. Cercetări Agronomice în Moldova. 2014; 3(159): 71–81. DOI: 10.2478/cerce-2014-0028

[58] Rustaiee, A. R., Yavari, A., Nazeri, V., Shokrpour, M., Sefidkon, F. & Rasouli, M. Genetic diversity and chemical polymorphism of some *Thymus* species. Chemistry & Biodiversity. 2013; 10: 1088–1098. DOI: 10.1002/cbdv.201200020

[59] Solyman, E. & Alkowni, R. RAPD for assessment of thymes genetic diversity in Palestine. Palestine Technical University Research Journal. 2014; 2(2): 01–08.

[60] Echeverrigaray, S., Agostini, G., Atti-Serfini, L., Paroul, N., Pauletti, G. F. & Atti dos Santos, A. C. Correlation between the chemical and genetic relationships among commercial thyme cultivars. Journal of Agricultural and Food Chemistry. 2001; 49: 4220–4223. DOI: 10.1021/jf010289j

[61] Pluhár, Z., Kocsis, M., Kuczmog, A., Csete, S., Simkó, H., Sárosi, S., Molnár, P. & Horváth, G.. Essential oil composition and preliminary molecular study of four Hungarian *Thymus* species. Acta Biologica Hungarica. 2012; 63(1): 81–96. DOI: 10.1556/ABiol.63.2012.1.7

[62] Hadian, J., Bigdeloo, M., Nazeri, V. & Khadivi-Khub, A.. Assessment of genetic and chemical variability in *Thymus caramanicus*. Molecular Biology Reports. 2014; 41(5): 3201–3210. DOI: 10.1007/s11033-014-3180-z

[63] Sostaric, I., Liber, Z., Grdisa, M., Marin, P. D., Stevanovi, Z. D. & Satovic, Z.. Genetic diversity and relationships among species of the genus *Thymus* L. (section *Serpyllum*). Flora. 2012; 207: 654–661. DOI: 10.1016/j.flora.2012.06.018.

[64] Karp, A., Edwards, K. J., Bruford, M., Funk, S., Vosman, B., Morgante, M., Seberg, O., Kremer, A., Boursot, P., Arctander, P., Tautz, D. & Hewitt, G. M. Molecular technologies for biodiversity evaluation: opportunities and challenges. Nature Biotechnology. 1997; 15(7): 625–628. DOI: 10.1038/nbt0797-625

[65] Kollipara, R., Peranteau, A. J., Nawas, Z. Y., Tong, Y., Woc-Colburn, L., Yan, A. C, Lupi, O. & Tyring, S. K. Emerging infectious diseases with cutaneous manifestations: Fungal, helminthic, protozoan and ectoparasitic infections. Journal of the American Academy of Dermatology. 2016; 75(1): 19–30. DOI: 10.1016/j.jaad.2016.04.032

[66] Pagiotti, R., Angelini, P., Rubini, A., Tirillini, B., Granetti, B. & Venanzoni, R.. Identification and characterisation of human pathogenic filamentous fungi and susceptibility to *Thymus schimperi* essential oil. Mycoses. 2011; 54(5): e364–e376. DOI: 10.1111/j.1439-0507.2010.01926.x

[67] Voltan, A. R., Quindós, G., Alarcón, K. P. M., Fusco-Almeida, A. M., Mendes-Giannini, M. J. S. & Chorilli, M. Fungal diseases: could nanostructured drug delivery systems be a novel paradigm for therapy? International Journal of Nanomedicine. 2016; 11: 3715–3730. DOI: 10.2147/IJN.S93105

[68] Labib, G. S. & Aldawsari, H. Innovation of natural essential oil-loaded Orabase for local treatment of oral candidiasis. Drug Design, Development and Therapy. 2015; 9: 3349–3359. DOI: 10.2147/DDDT.S85356

[69] Dorgan, E., Denning, D. W. & McMullan, R. Burden of fungal disease – Ireland. Journal of Medical Microbiology. 2015; 64(pt 4): 423–426.

[70] Chander, J., Stchigel, A. M., Alastruey-Izquierdo, A., et al. Fungal necrotizing fasciitis, an emerging infectious disease caused by *Apophysomyces* (Mucorales). Revista Iberoamericana de Micología. 2015; 32(2): 93–98.

[71] Brown, G. D., Denning, D. W., Gow, N. A., Levitz, S. M., Netea, M. G. & White, T. C. Hidden killers: human fungal infections. Science Translational Medicine. 2012; 4: 165rv13 DOI: 10.1126/scitranslmed.3004404.

[72] Pinto, E., Pina-Vaz, C., Salgueiro, L., Gonçalves, M. J., Costa-de-Oliveira, S., Cavaleiro, C., Palmeira, A., Rodrigues, A. & Martinez-de-Oliveira, J. Antifungal activity of the essential

oil of *Thymus pulegioides* on Candida, *Aspergillus* and dermatophyte species. Journal of Medical Microbiology. 2006; 55: 1367–1373.

[73] Cowan, M. M.. Plant products as antimicrobial agents. Clinical Microbiology Reviews. 1999; 12(4): 564–582.

[74] Brull, S. & Coote, P.. Preservative agents in foods: mode of action and microbial resistance mechanisms. International Journal of Food Microbiology. 1999; 50(1–2): 1–17. ISSN 0168–1605

[75] Darout, I., Cristy, A., Skaug, N. & Egeberg, P. Identification and quantification of some potential antimicrobial anionic components in miswak extract. Indian Journal of Pharmacology. 2000; 32: 11–14.

[76] Sharma, R., Sharma, C. L. & Kapoorl, B. Antibacterial resistance: current problems and possible solutions. Indian Journal of Medical Sciences. 2005; 59(3): 120–129. ISSN 0019–5359

[77] Moghaddam, K. M., Arfan, M., Rafique, J., Rezaee, S., Fesharaki, P. J., Gohari, A. R. & Shahverdi, A. R. The antifungal activity of Sarcococca saligna ethanol extract and its combination effect with fluconazole against different resistant *Aspergillus* species. Applied Biochemistry and Biotechnology. 2010; 162(1): 127–133. ISSN 1559–0291

[78] Edeoga, H. O., Okwu, D. E. & Mbaebie, B. O. Phytochemical constituents of some Nigerian medicinal plants. African Journal of Biotechnology. 2005; 4(7): 685–688. ISSN 1684–5315

[79] Panghal, M., Kaushal, V. & Yadav, J. P. In vitro antimicrobial activity of ten medicinal plants against clinical isolates of oral cancer cases. Annals of Clinical Microbiology and Antimicrobials. 2011; 10: 21 DOI: 10.1186/1476-0711-10-21, ISSN 14760711

[80] Janssen, A. M., Chin, N. L., Scheffer, J. J. & Baerheim Svendsen, A. Screening for antimicrobial activity of some essential oils by the agar overlay technique. Pharmaceutisch Weekblad. Scientific Edition. 1986; 8(6): 289–292.

[81] Rios, J. L., Recio, M. C. & Villar, A. Screening methods for natural products with antimicrobial activity: a review of the literature. Journal of Ethnopharmacology. 1988; 23: 127–149.

[82] Bruneton, J. Partie 3. Terpeenes et steroids. In Pharmacognosie, Phytochimie, Plantes médicinales. 4ª Édition. Paris: E′ ditions Tec&Doc & Éditions Médicales Internationals; 2009, pp. 547–934.

[83] Pina-Vaz, C., Sansonetty, F., Rodrigues, A., Costa-de-Oliveira, S., Martinez-de-Oliveira, J. & Fonseca, A. F. Cytometric approach for rapid evaluation of susceptibility of Candida strains to antifungals. Clinical Microbiology and Infection. 2001; 7: 609–618.

[84] Stahl-Biskup, E. & Sáez, F. Thyme – The Genus Thymus. London: Taylor & Francis; 2002.

[85] Mohd, S., Birhanu, D. & Tanweer, A.. Antimicrobial activity of essential oils extracted from medicinal plants against the pathogenic microorganisms: a review. Issues in Biological Sciences and Pharmaceutical Research. 2014; 2(1): 001–007.

[86] Dorman, H. J. D. & Deans, S. G. Antimicrobial agents from plants: antibacterial activity of plant volatile oils. Journal of Applied Microbiology. 2000; 88(2): 308–316.

[87] Arnal-Schnebelen, B., Hadji-Minaglou, F., Peroteau, J. F., Ribeyre, F. & de Billerbeck, V. G. Essential oils in infectious gynaecological disease: a statistical study of 658 cases. International Journal of Aromatherapy. 2004; 14(4): 192–197.

[88] Villanueva Bermejo, D., Angelov, I., Vicente, G., Stateva, R. P., Rodriguez García-Risco, M., Reglero, G., Ibañez, E. & Fornari, T. Extraction of thymol from different varieties of thyme plants using green solvents. Journal of the Science of Food and Agriculture. 2015; 95(14): 2901–2907.

[89] Wohlmuth, H., Smith, M. K., Brooks, L. O., Myers, S. P. & Leach, D. N. Essential oil composition of diploid and tetraploid clones of ginger (*Zingiber officinale* Roscoe) grown in Australia. Journal of Agricultural and Food Chemistry. 2006; 54: 1414–1419.

[90] Kalemba, D. & Kunicka, A. Antibacterial and antifungal properties of essential oils. Current Medicinal Chemistry. 2003; 10(10): 813–829.

[91] Kohiyama, C. Y., Yamamoto Ribeiro, M. M., Mossini, S. A., Bando, E., Bomfim Nda, S., Nerilo, S. B., Rocha, G. H., Grespan, R., Mikcha, J. M. & Machinski, M. Jr. Antifungal properties and inhibitory effects upon aflatoxin production of *Thymus vulgaris* L. by *Aspergillus flavus* link. Food Chemistry. 2015; 15(173): 1006–1010. DOI: 10.1016/j.foodchem.2014.10.135. Epub 2014 Nov 3.

[92] Manou, I., Bouillard, L., Devleeschouwer, M. J. & Barel, A. O.. Evaluation of the preservative properties of *Thymus vulgaris* essential oil in topically applied formulations under a challenge test. Journal of Applied Microbiology. 1998; 84(3): 368–376.

[93] Tampieri, M. P., Galuppi, R., Macchioni, F., Carelle, M. S., Falcioni, L., Cioni, P. L. & Morelli, I.. The inhibition of *Candida albicans* by selected essential oils and their major components. Mycopathologia. 2005; 159: 339–345. DOI: 10.1007/s11046-003-4790-5

[94] Ahmad, A., Khan, A., Akhtar, F., Yousuf, S., Xess, I., Khan, L. A. & Manzoor, N.. Fungicidal activity of thymol and carvacrol by disrupting ergosterol biosynthesis and membrane integrity against Candida. European Journal of Clinical Microbiology and Infectious Diseases. 2011; 30: 41–50. DOI: 10.1007/s10096-010-1050-8

[95] Sharifzadeh, A., Javan, A. J., Shokri, H., Abbaszadeh, S. & Keykhosravy, K. Evaluation of antioxidant and antifungal properties of the traditional plants against foodborne fungal pathogens. Journal of Medical Mycology. 2016; 26(1): e11–e17. DOI: 10.1016/j.mycmed.2015.11.002

[96] Markovic, T., Chatzopoulou, P., Siljegovic, J., Nikolic, M., Glamoclija, J. & Ciric, A. Chemical analysis and antimicrobial activities of the essential oils of *Satureja thymbra* L. and *Thymbra spicata* L. and their main components. Archives of Biological Sciences. 2011; 63: 457–464.

[97] Rasooli, I., Rezaei, M. B. & Allameh, A. Growth inhibition and morphological alterations of *Aspergillus niger* by essential oils from *Thymus eriocalyx* and Thymus x-porlock. Food Control. 2006; 17: 359–364.

[98] Mandras, N., Nostro, A., Roana, J., Scalas, D., Banche, G., Ghisetti, V., Del Re, S., Fucale, G., Cuffini, A. M. & Tullio, V. Liquid and vapour-phase antifungal activities of essential oils against *Candida albicans* and non-albicans Candida. BMC Complementary and Alternative Medicine. 2016; 16(1): 330. DOI: 10.1186/s12906-016-1316-5

[99] Leal, F., Matos, M., Coelho, A. C. & Pinto-Carnide, O. *In vitro* multiplication of aromatic and medicinal plants and fungicide activity. In: Dhanasekaran D., Thajuddin, N. & Panneerselvam, A. (eds). Fungicides for Plant and Animal Diseases. Croacia: Intech Open Access Publisher; 2011. pp. 119–138. ISBN 978-953-307-804-5

[100] Nardoni, S., Giovanelli, S., Pistelli, L., Mugnaini, L., Profili, G., Pisseri, F. & Mancianti, F. In vitro activity of twenty commercially available, plant-derived essential oils against selected dermatophyte species. Natural Product Communications. 2015; 10(8): 1473–1478.

[101] Lima, O. I., Oliveira, R. A. G., Lima, E. O., Porto Farias, N. M. & Souza, E. L. Antifungal activity from essential oils on Candida species. Revista Brasileira de Farmacognosia. 2006; 16: 197–201.

12

Vanillin and its Detection in Air

Saaya Minematsu and Xing-Zheng Wu

Abstract

Vanillin (4-hydroxy-3-methoxybenzaldehyde) is an important flavor and aroma molecule, which has been widely used in not only foods and beverages such as chocolate and dairy products, but also masking unpleasant tastes in medicines or livestock fodder. Its chemical properties, manufacturing methods, novel applications, and developments in fast detections in air are discussed in detail.

Keywords: vanillin, properties, detection, capillary electrophoresis

1. Introduction

Vanillin (4-hydroxy-3-methoxybenzaldehyde) is an important flavor and aroma molecule but is also of interest because of its biogenetic relationship to the phenylpropanoid pathway and to other molecules of physiological significance, notably salicylate [1]. Vanillin is the most important ingredient of the well-known vanilla, which is a complex blend of flavor and fragrance ingredients extracted from the seed pods of the vanilla orchid. As a flavorings agent, vanillin is used in not only foods and beverages such as chocolate and dairy products, but also masking unpleasant tastes in medicines or livestock fodder [2].

Here, its properties, manufacturing methods, and novel applications are discussed. Furthermore, its detection in air is introduced.

2. Molecular structure and properties of vanillin

Vanillin is the common name for 3-methoxy-4-hydroxybenzaldehyde, and its molecular structure is shown in **Figure 1**.

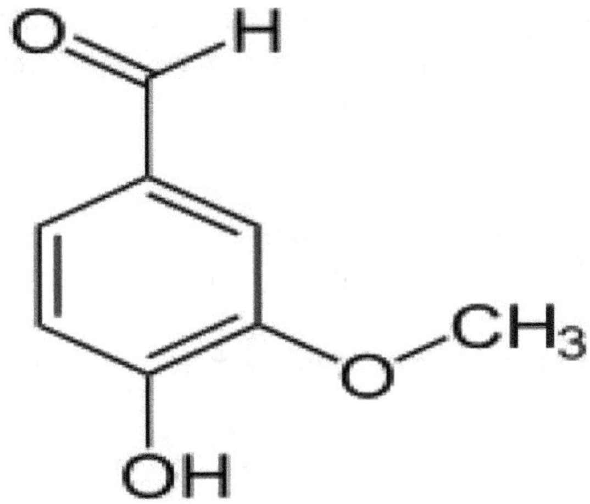

Figure 1. Molecular structure of vanillin.

2.1. Toxicity about vanillin

Toxicity about vanillin was studied as early as 1940 [3]. Generally, vanillin does not give human skin irritation and produce no sensitization reactions. Vanillin is considered to be a secondary allergen because sensitivity was found only in patients sensitive to vanilla, isoeugenol, and coniferyl benzoate. Animal studies showed that vanillin was not carcinogenic.

2.2. Antioxidant, antifungal or antimicrobial, and antimutagenic properties of vanillin and vanillin derivatives

Vanillin and vanillin derivatives have antioxidant and antimutagenic properties. Antifungal activities of vanillin and 33 vanillin derivatives against the human fungal pathogen Cryptococcus neoformans, which was the main pathogen of cryptococcal meningitis in immunocompromised patients, have been studied [4]. Functional groups in the vanillin derivatives seemed to affect antifungal activity. The hydroxyl or alkoxy group seemed to be more effective than the halogenated or nitrated group in benzaldehyde in antifungal ability. O-vanillin and o-ethyl vanillin were with the highest antifungal activity against *C. neoformans* in the vanillin derivatives. O-Vanillin was further found to be able to cause mitochondrial dysfunction and trigger oxidative stress. These antifungal mechanisms of o-vanillin were experimentally confirmed by the significantly reduced growth of the mutants lacking the genes involved in mitochondrial functions and oxidative stress response.

Evaluation in which structural elements of the vanillin molecule are responsible for its antifungal activity was also investigated [5]. Minimum inhibitory concentrations (MICs) of vanillin, its six direct structural analogs, and several other related compounds were determined in yeast extract peptone dextrose broth against a total of 18 different food spoilage molds and yeasts. Experimental results showed that the antifungal order of isomers of hydroxybenzaldehyde and anisaldehyde was 2- > 3- > 4- and 3- > 2- > 4-, respectively. The aldehyde moiety of vanillin seems to play a key role in its antifungal activity, but side-group position on the benzene ring also influences this activity.

Antimicrobial activities and the MICs of solutions containing vanillin and vanillic acid against *Staphylococcus aureus, Staphylococcus epidermidis, Bacillus cereus, Enterobacter aerogenes, Escherichia coli,* and *Yersinia enterocolitica* were experimental studied by the agar well-diffusion method [6]. The experimental results showed that the vanillin and vanillic acid was with inhibitory activity against all of the bacteria. Moreover, the MIC of the vanillin and vanillic acid decreased with the vanillic acid concentration. It suggested that thermal treatment of vanillin-containing food may lead to products with higher antioxidant and antimicrobial properties.

2.3. Protection human keratinocyte stem cells against ultraviolet-B irradiation

Ultraviolet-B (UVB) irradiation is one of major factors, which induce cellular damages in the epidermis. Protective effects and mechanisms of vanillin against UVB-induced cellular damages in keratinocyte stem cells (KSC) have been investigated recently [7]. Experimental results indicated that vanillin significantly decreased the UVB irradiation-induced cytotoxicity. Also, vanillin seemed to be able to induce production of pro-inflammatory cytokines. It was explained that vanillin could significantly reduce phosphorylation of ataxia telangiectasia mutated (ATM), tumor suppressor protein 53 (p53), serine threonine kinase checkpoint kinase 2 (Chk2), c-Jun N-terminal kinase/stress-activated protein kinase (JNK), S6 ribosomal protein (S6RP), p38/mitogen-activated protein kinase (p38), and histone 2A family member X (H2A.X) generated by the UVB. Vanillin also could inhibit UVB-induced activation of p53 luciferase reporter. The results suggested that vanillin protects KSC from UVB irradiation. Vanillin may play its role through the suppression of downstream step of MDM2 in UVB irradiation-induced p53 activation.

3. Manufacturing methods of vanillin

A simple laboratory synthesis is illustrated in **Figure 2** to make a small amount of vanillin. This synthesis scheme involves electrophilic bromination of 4-hydroxybenzaldehyde, followed by copper-catalyzed methoxylation.

For large-scale industrial syntheses, a classic early method starts from eugenol, which occurs naturally in cloves, nutmeg, and cinnamon. This isomerizes to isoeugenol in alkaline solution, and this in turn can be oxidized (by nitrobenzene) to vanillin (**Figure 3**).

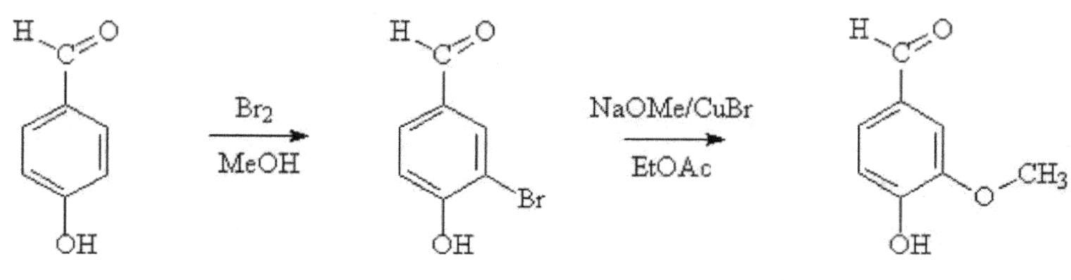

Figure 2. Laboratory synthesis scheme of vanillin.

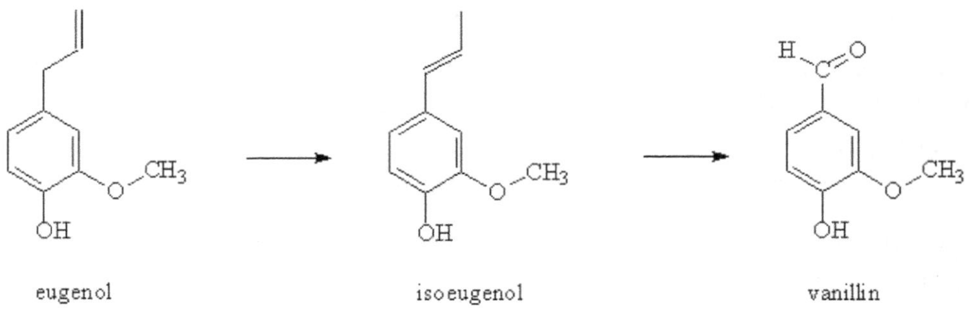

Figure 3. Industrial synthesis scheme of vanillin.

Lignin was known to be a source of vanillin as early as at the beginning of the twentieth century. Lignin is a well-known polymer, which plays strengthening role in woods and in the cell walls of plants. Since the 1920s, much of the world's vanillin was extracted from lignin waste from the cellulose industry [8].

Recently, potential of industrial Eucalyptus globulus sulfite liquor and kraft liquors was evaluated for the production of syringaldehyde and vanillin by oxidation with O_2 in alkaline medium [9]. The Eucalyptus globulus sulfite liquor and kraft liquors were collected at different stages of processing before the recovery boiler. Under controlled temperature and pressure, the oxidations were performed in a jacketed reactor by two methods. One was the direct oxidation of pulping liquors, and the other was the one of kraft lignins isolated from liquors. Products profiles were established, as well as the yields, temperature and O_2 uptake during the reaction. Results showed that sulfite liquor was the best raw material leading to the highest yield by direct oxidation. Thin kraft liquor (KL) was with the second high yield. Proportion of by-products such as syringic and vanillic acids was low.

Natural vanillin was obtained by plant tissue culture early. Molecular biology and microbial biotransformation techniques can also be used to produce natural vanillin [10]. These techniques rely on natural vanillin precursor molecules (eugenol, isoeugenol, curcumin, or ferulic acid), and their enzymatic reaction pathways are very different. Among them, microbial biotransformation method seems to be the most promising for large amount of natural vanillin production with high efficiency and high quality.

Screening of bacteria to produce vanillin and/or vanillic acid from isoeugenol was carried out [11]. *Achromobacter, Aeromonas, Agrobacerium, Alcaligenes, Arthrobacter, Bacillus, Micrococcus, Pseudomonas, Rhodobacter*, and *Rhodococcus* were found to be able to produce vanillin and/or vanillic acid, in addition of isoeugenol to the culture medium [11]. In particular, a soil isolate strain IE27 showed the highest vanillin-producing activity, and it was identified as *Pseudomonas putida*. Under the optimized culture conditions, *P. putida* IE27 cells produced 16.1 g/l vanillin from 150 mM isoeugenol. The molar conversion yield from isoeugenol to vanillin was as high as 71% at 20°C after a 24-h incubation. Therefore, it is expectable to produce natural vanillin with high efficiency.

Production of vanillin from vanillic acid and *O*-benzylvanillic acid was investigated by using whole cells and enzyme preparations of *Nocardia* sp. strain NRRL 5646 [12]. With growing cultures of the whole cells, 69 and 11% of vanillic acid were found to be decarboxylated to guaiacol and reduced to vanillyl alcohol, respectively. On the other hand, no decarboxylation of 4-*O*-benzylvanillic acid was found in conversion to the corresponding alcohol product. Purified *Nocardia* carboxylic acid reductase, an ATP and NADPH-dependent enzyme, was found to be able to reduce vanillic acid to vanillin quantitatively.

In addition to make use of the microbial biotransformation, enzymatic synthesis of natural vanillin was studied [13]. Flavoprotein vanillyl alcohol oxidase (VAO) could convert both creosol and vanillylamine to vanillin with high production yield. This conversion of creosol was realized via a two-step process. The first step was to convert creosol to vanillyl alcohol, and then, the second step was the oxidation of the vanillyl alcohol to vanillin. In the second step, the conversion of vanillyl alcohol to vanillin was inhibited by the competitive binding of creosol. The VAO-catalyzed conversion yield of vanillylamine to vanillin was high at alkaline solutions. Furthermore, mechanism study showed that vanillylamine was firstly converted to a vanillylimine intermediate product. The intermediate product was then hydrolyzed to vanillin nonenzymatically.

4. Novel applications of vanillin

4.1. Preparation of benzoxazine resin and reactive monomeric surfactant containing oxazine ring

Vanillin is used to synthesize polybenzoxazine with the expected desirable benzoxazine properties as well as a high char yield of 55.3% [14]. The synthesized monomer provides an unused aldehyde group from vanillin. The aldehyde can be further reacted with other materials to enhance properties. As a model, the unused aldehyde is reacted with amine terminated poly (ethylene oxide) to form a surfactant, which retains 1,3-benzoxazine's reactivity. The chemical structure of the synthesized monomers, surfactant, and polymers is characterized by Fourier transform infrared spectroscopy (FT-IR) and proton nuclear magnetic resonance spectroscopy (^{1}H NMR). Thermal properties are also characterized by differential scanning calorimetry (DSC) and thermogravimetric analysis (TGA). Miniemulsions with stability up to 2 weeks are created with the newly synthesized surfactant and polystyrene. Dynamic light scattering (DLS) indicates 627 nm as the average diameter of the emulsion droplets.

4.2. Renewable polymers prepared from vanillin and its derivatives

Methacrylated derivatives of vanillin and vanillyl alcohol are synthesized and used as two monomers, respectively. The two monomers were further polymerized by a free-radical process [15]. Rheokinetics of their polymerization were studied to determine the cure behaviors. Thermomechanical properties of the resulting polymers affected by the structure and functionalities of the monomers were discussed. In comparison with methacrylated vanillin monomer, the methacrylated vanillyl alcohol gave a higher cross-linking density of the polymers, which in turn resulted a higher storage modulus and glass transition temperature, a better thermal resistance. Methacrylated vanillyl alcohol monomer was also with low viscosity at room temperature. Therefore, methacrylated vanillyl alcohol monomer is an expectable bio-based reactive diluent for unsaturated polyester resins and vinyl esters.

5. Detection and analysis of vanillin and vanillin-type aromatic compounds

Vanillin and other purely olfactory odorants such as coumarin, octanoic acid, and phenylethyl alcohol cannot be identified when presented oral cavity only (OCO), because the oral cavity trigeminal system is fully unresponsive to these odorants in vapor phase [16]. Therefore, modern analytical methods are usually required for detection and analysis of vanillin and its derivatives.

5.1. Detection of real natural vanilla from synthetic one

Because of the extremely different in price of natural real vanilla from synthetic one, detection of fake vanilla is required. Basically, gas or liquid chromatography can tell the real natural from synthetic vanilla because some impurities such as 4-hydroxybenzaldehyde present in natural vanilla essence could be detected. Another way is to investigate amount of radioactive carbon-14. Natural plant-sourced vanillin contains a certain level of carbon-14, whose half-life is 5730 years. On the other hand, vanillin derived from crude oil has no radiocarbon since it has decayed away over the millions of years; the oil was trapped underground. Ratio of the natural isotopes, carbon-13 to carbon-12, also can be used for identify the real natural vanilla from the synthetic ones, because the vanilla orchid uses a different biosynthetic pathway to other plants. Orchid-derived vanillin has a greater ratio of carbon-13 to carbon-12 than synthetic vanillin [17].

A solid phase micro-extraction (SPME)-GC-MS method seems to be able to distinguish the natural real vanilla extracts from the synthetic one too [18]. The fiber material in SPME, sampling time, desorption time, and other experimental conditions were optimized. Under the optimized conditions, a relative standard deviation (RSD) of 2.5–6.4% indicated good reproducibility of the method. Because GC profile of the natural extracts was different from synthetic ones, it is easily to determine whether the sample is natural or synthetic. The method is also applicable to identify the type of vanilla extract/flavoring used in flavor foods.

5.2. Analysis of vanillin

The presence of vanillin in orange, tangerine, lemon, lime, and grapefruit juices could be easily identified and confirmed using GC-MS [19]. Vanillin concentrations in the orange, tangerine, lemon, lime, and grapefruit juices were determined to be 0.20, 0.35, 0.41, 0.35, and 0.60 ppm, respectively.

A headspace-solid phase micro-extraction (HS-SPME) GC-MS method was also proposed to determine of vanillin in vanilla products [20]. Detection limits were reported to be 1.33–13.2 ppb. Furthermore, LC-ESI-MS determinations of the vanillin were carried out at the same time, and the results were compared. Totally, 24 commercially available vanilla products were analyzed with the two methods. Vanillin was detected in all of the 24 products. Also, 18 other flavor related compounds were detected in the samples.

As illustrated in **Figure 4**, the sampling system allowed real-time and continuously sampling of the aroma volatiles from model liquid foods [21]. The sample samples could be kept at a certain temperature (e.g., at 37°C), and aroma volatiles released into the headspace. A carrier gas was flowed into the headspace and further into a quadrupole MS via a jet separator. The MS analysis could monitor and identify the volatile molecular weight. Also, this sampling system can examine the dynamic flavor releasing process of liquid samples.

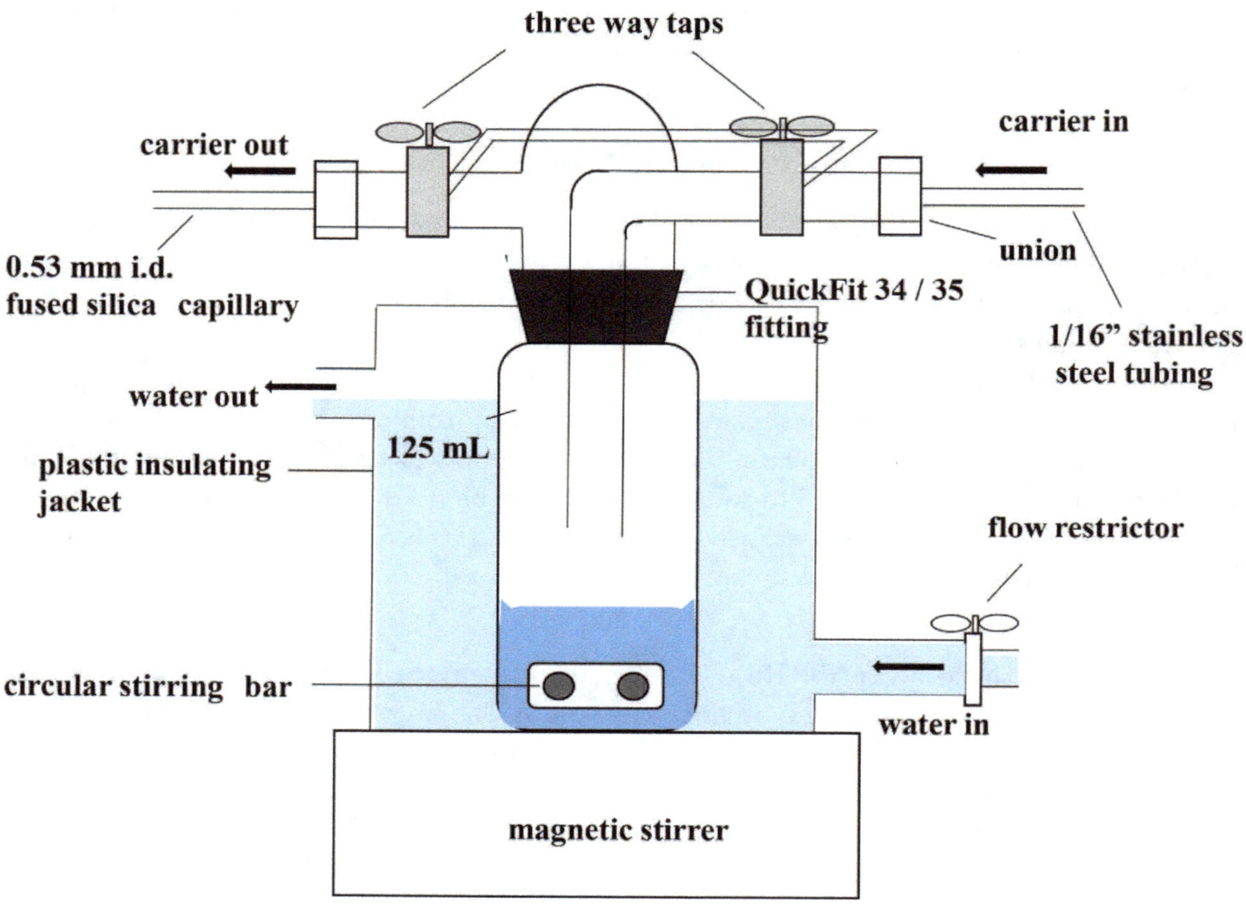

Figure 4. Illustration of a sampling system for the measurement of dynamic flavor release.

Recently, odor imaging sensing with multi-probe film is reported [22]. Odor substances are determined by fluorescent quenching with imaging film and a cooled CCD camera. The system could detect gaseous odor flow and visualize shape, spread, and concentration distribution of odor. A multi-film and FRET probes consisted of a certain combination of fluorescence dyes such as tryptophan and vanillin have been used for high sensitive and selective detection of odor. This approach is expectable in near future for more sensitivity and selectivity.

There are a lots of other analytical methods for the analysis of vanillin, based on spectrophotometric [23, 24], FIA [25], ion selective electrodes [26], flourimetric [27], thin layer chromatography [28], GC-MS [20, 29], HPLC [30, 31], and capillary electrophoresis (CE) [32–35]. Because CE is not only fast (usually shorter than 10 min), but also with nano-liter amount of injection volume for samples, it is particularly noticeable. Recently, direct sampling method for CE determination of vanillin in indoor air has been developed [36]. Here, the CE determination of vanillin is discussed in detail.

5.3. CE detection of vanillin in indoor air

Generally, a fused silica capillary is used in CE. When running buffer solution is filled into the capillary, silanol groups (**Figure 5A**) in the surface of capillary dissociate, and inner surface of the capillary is charged negatively (**Figure 5B**). Cations in the running buffer solution are pulled toward the inner surface. As a result, an electric double layer is formed (**Figure 5C**). When an electric voltage is applied across the two ends of the capillary, an electroosmotic flow (EOF) toward cathode arises.

$$\mathrm{EOF}= (\varepsilon Z/(4\pi\rho))E \tag{1}$$

where ε, Z, ρ, and E are the dielectric constant, zeta potential, solution viscosity, and electric field, respectively.

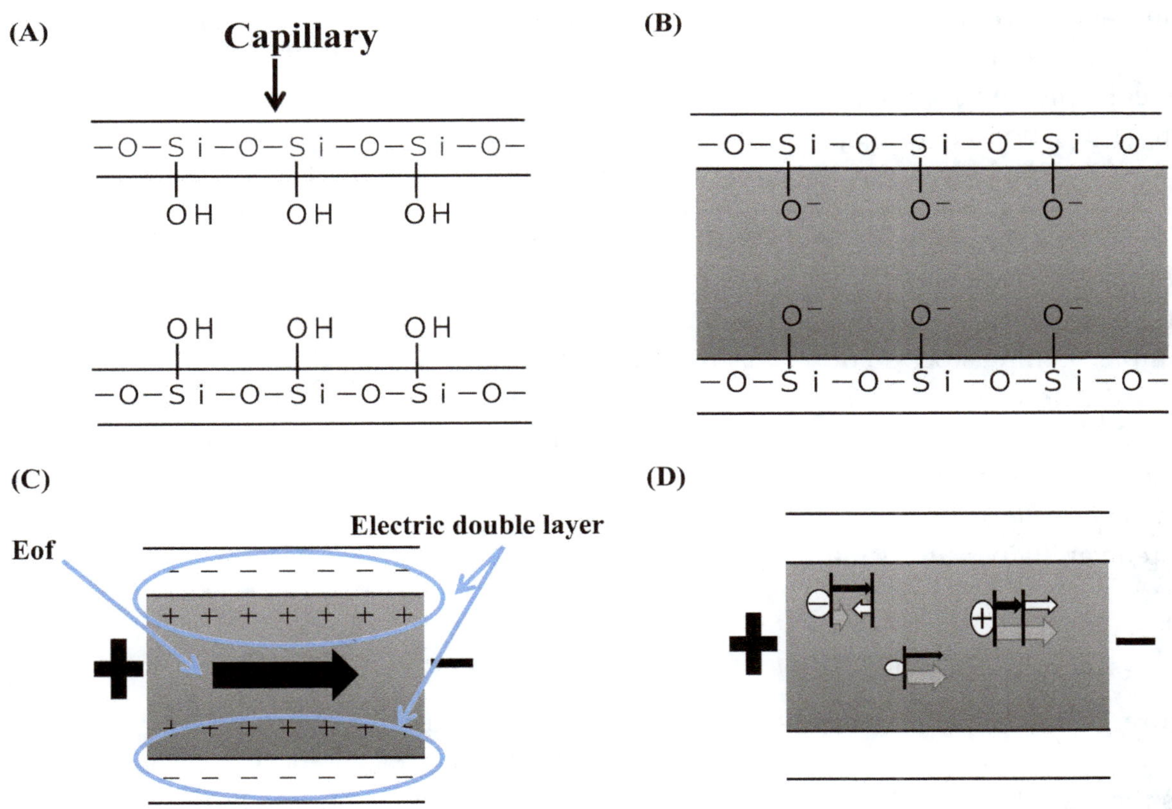

Figure 5. Illustration of molecular structure of the capillary inner surface and principle of CE separation. (A) molecular structure of inner surface of capillary; (B) dissociation of silanol group; (C) formation of electric double layer; (D) electromigration of analytes in CE.

On the other hand, electrophoretic velocity (Vep) of an ion toward the electrode of opposite charge is:

$$Vep = (q/(6\pi\rho r))E \tag{2}$$

where q and r are the electric charge and radius of the ion, respectively. Usually, EOF is larger than Vep for most of ions, and detector is usually close to the cathode end of the capillary. Electromigration velocity of a cation will be (EOF + Vep) while that of an anion (EOF–Vep). Neutral molecule will move with the electroosmotic flow (EOF). Then, cations, anions, and neutral molecules are separated (**Figure 5D**). Because different ions are with different q/r, their Vep is different. Thus, ions can be separated from each other by CE.

CE instrument is relatively simple. Basically, it consists of an electric power supply, a capillary, and a detector. **Figure 6** illustrates a typical laboratory-built CE apparatus [35]. It was consisted of a 30 kV high-voltage power supply and an UV-absorbance detector. Wavelength of the UV-absorbance detector could be set at 254 nm for detection of aromatic compounds. A capillary (inner diameter of 50–100 μm, out diameter of 364 μm) could be used. Its total length and the effective length (length from the anode end to the detector) could be about 30–70 and 20–60 cm, respectively. The capillary was usually cleaned thoroughly by subsequently flushing 1 mol/L NaOH, distilled-deionized water, and finally running buffer. Sample injection could be performed with either an electrophoretic method (e.g., injection voltage 1 kV, injecting time 30 s) or a hydrodynamic flow method with a height difference (e.g., 1 cm) between the two ends of the capillary.

Buffer solutions such as phosphate buffers or boric buffers with certain pH and concentration can be used in CE. Samples are usually dissolved or diluted with the buffers. For example, vanillin stock solution was prepared by dissolving a certain amount of vanillin into distilled-deionized water directly [35]. Its concentration was 10^{-3} mol/L. This stock solution was diluted to required concentrations with the running buffer when used. Vanilla perfume was also diluted with the buffer solutions to concentrations of 1 and 10%. For vanillin spiked vanilla perfume sample, a certain amount of the vanillin standard solution was added into the diluted vanilla perfume sample.

5.3.1. CE of vanillin standard solution [35]

Figure 7 showed the CE results of vanillin at running buffers with different pH. It is well known that the higher the pH of the running buffer, the faster the EOF. Therefore, EOF was the fastest in running buffer of pH 11.5, while slowest in running buffer of pH 7.2. On the other hand, vanillin is a weak acid, and its acid dissociation constant Ka is about $10^{-9.25}$. At pH 11.5, almost all of vanillin molecules behavior as anions, while at pH 7.2 most of them as neutral molecules. At pH 9.3, about half vanillin molecules dissociated to anions.

Therefore, Vep of vanillin was the largest at pH 11.5, slowest at pH 7.2. As a result of V = EOF-Vep, the vanillin was detected at about 500, 450, and 600 s at pH of 11.5, 9.3, and 7.2, respectively.

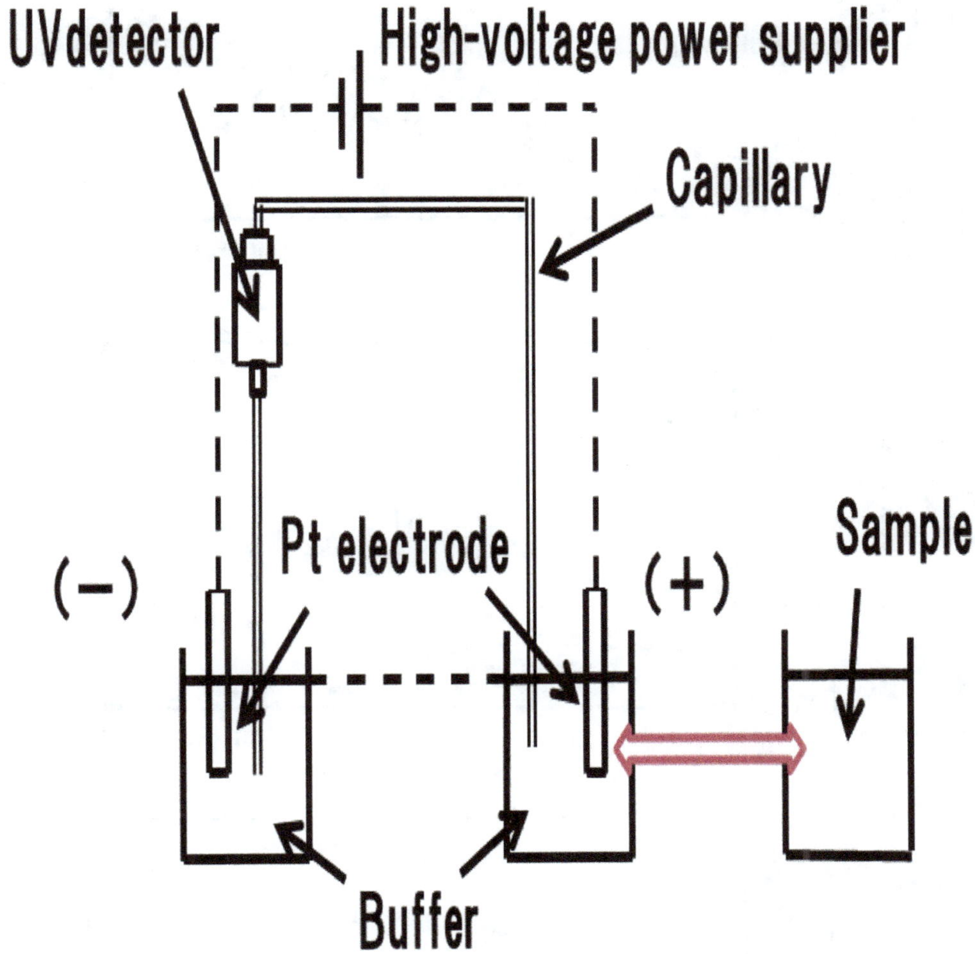

Figure 6. Illustration of a laboratory-built CE instrument.

Figure 8 showed the calibration curve of vanillin at the running buffer of pH 9.3. It can be seen that the peak area is proportional to the vanillin concentration in the range of 10^{-6}–10^{-2} mol/L. The detection limit was about 10^{-6} mol/L.

5.3.2. CE of vanilla perfume [35]

Figure 9 showed electropherogram of 10% vanilla perfume sample solution (A) and 10% vanilla perfume sample solution spiked with 10^{-3} mol/L vanillin standard solution (B). In **Figure 9A**, three peaks were detected. In order to confirm which peak was vanillin, the vanilla perfume sample was spiked with vanillin standard solution. **Figure 9B** showed that only the third peak became large in the spiked sample. Therefore, the third peak was confirmed to be vanillin in the vanilla perfume. Vanillin concentration in the 10% vanilla perfume sample was determined to be about 3×10^{-3} mol/L by a standard addition method. The first and second peaks have not been identified.

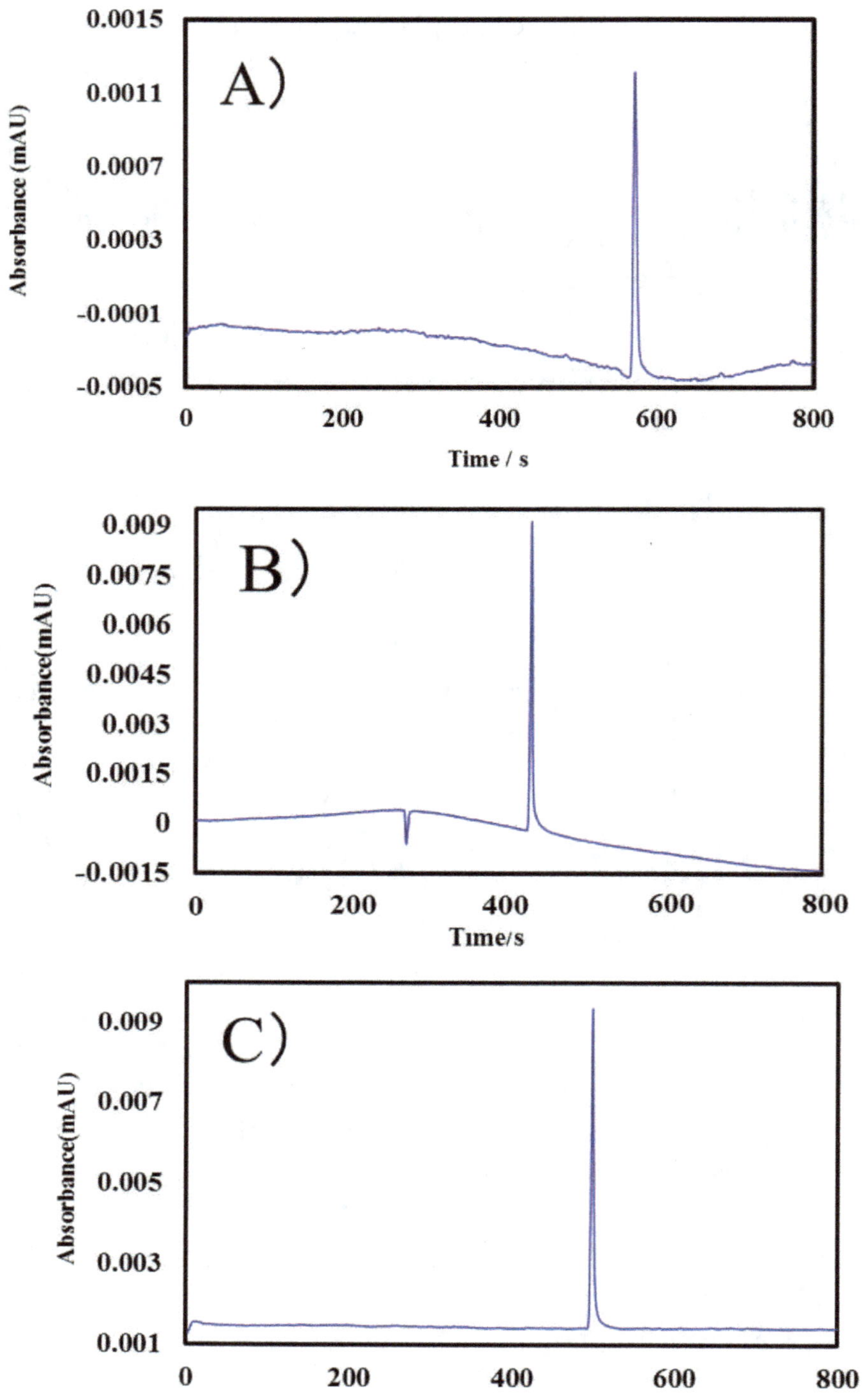

Figure 7. Electropherograms of vanillin standard solution (10^{-4} mol/L) in running buffers of pH 7.2 (A), 9.3 (B), and 11.5 (C).

5.3.3. Detection of vanillin in indoor air by offline combination of CE with absorption and desorption of vanillin with active carbon [35]

In order to detect vanillin in indoor air with CE, about 0.02 g active carbon was spread on a glass slide for adsorption of vanillin in air. The glass slide was placed in a room of about 80 m^2, where a vanilla perfume of 5 ml was placed too for a certain period of time. Then, the active carbon on the glass slide was collected into a vial, and 0.5 ml ethanol or mixture of ethanol/pH 11.5 running buffer with a mixing ratio of 1:1 was added for desorption of vanillin adsorpted on the active carbon. The vial was centrifuged for 5 min at a centrifugation speed of 3000 rpm. The supernatant was directly injected into the capillary, and CE was carried out. **Figure 11** showed CE results.

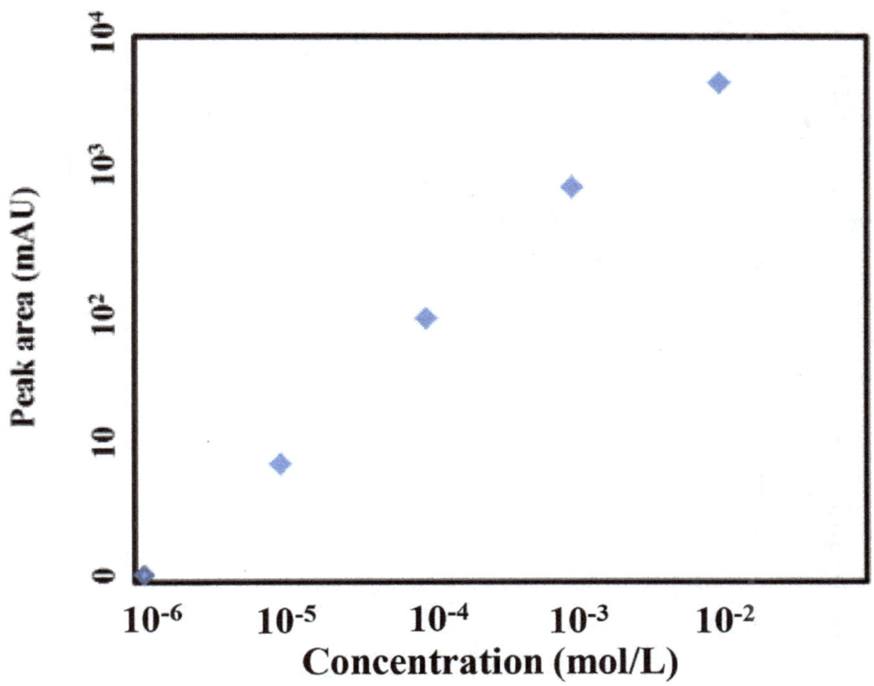

Figure 8. Vanillin calibration curves in running buffers of pH 9.3.

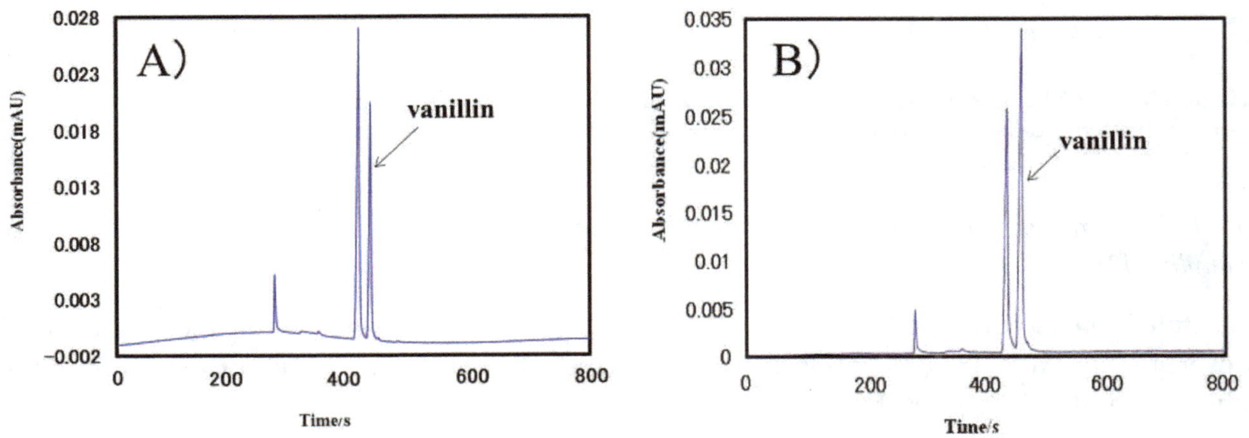

Figure 9. Electropherograms of 10% vanilla perfume sample (A) and the 10% vanilla perfume spiked with 10^{-3} (mol/L) vanillin (B) in the pH 9.3 phosphate buffer.

When the active carbon placed in the room for 2 days, the peak of vanillin was not detectable (top figure in **Figure 10**). When the active carbon placed in the room for 4 days, the vanillin peak was clearly detected (bottom figure in **Figure 10**). This meant that the CE method could be used for detection of vanillin in air by combination with the active carbon adsorption.

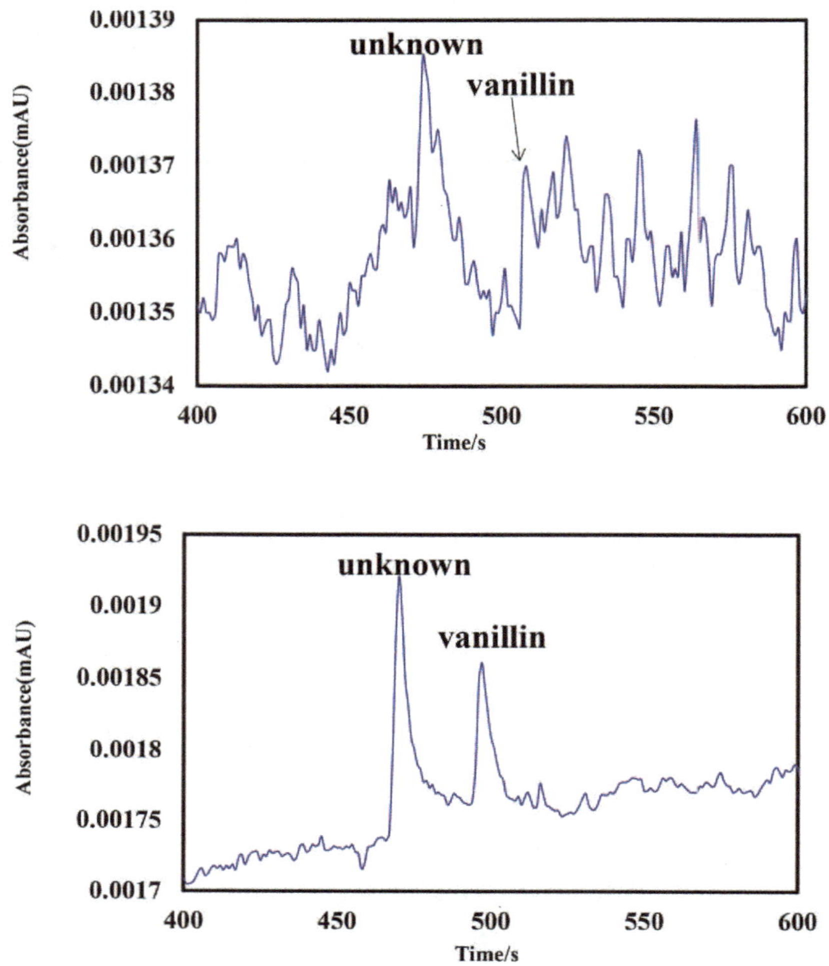

Figure 10. Electropherograms of supernatant of the ethanol/pH 11.5 running buffer after desorption from the active carbons. The active carbons adsorption time was 2 (top) and 4 (bottom) days, respectively.

5.3.4. Fast detection for trace vanillin and vanillin-type aromatic compounds in air by direct sampling [36]

As stated above, CE could detect vanillin in air by offline combining with the adsorption/desorption method. However, it is usually time- and labor-consuming. Recently, a direct sampling of vanillin in the air of CE was demonstrated [36].

As shown in **Figure 11**, the inlet end of a fused silica capillary filled with a pH 7.2 phosphate buffer was directly placed in the air, while the outlet end was immersed into a buffer vial at the low electric potential side. Then, gaseous or volatile components such as vanillin and its derivatives would absorb at the air/buffer interface of the capillary inlet end. That meant a direct sampling of the vanillin in air at capillary inlet end for CE. After a certain period of sampling time, the inlet end was immersed into another buffer vial at the high electric potential side; CE was carried out by applying a high electric voltage of 20 kV. Evaporated vanillin in indoor air was detected fast.

It was found that the CE peak area increased with the direct sampling time. This was easily understood because the longer the sampling time, the more the vanillin absorbed at the running /air/buffer interface, the larger the peak area. Also, the peak area in the direct sampling-CE was considered to be proportional to the vanillin concentrations in air.

Figure 12 showed results of a conventional CE of 10% vanilla perfume sample (A) and direct sampling-CE in indoor air with a sampling time of 5 min (B), respectively. A conventional CE usually gave two peaks for vanilla perfume sample. The detection time of the two peaks was about 420–600 s. In particular, the second peak was identified to be vanillin [35].

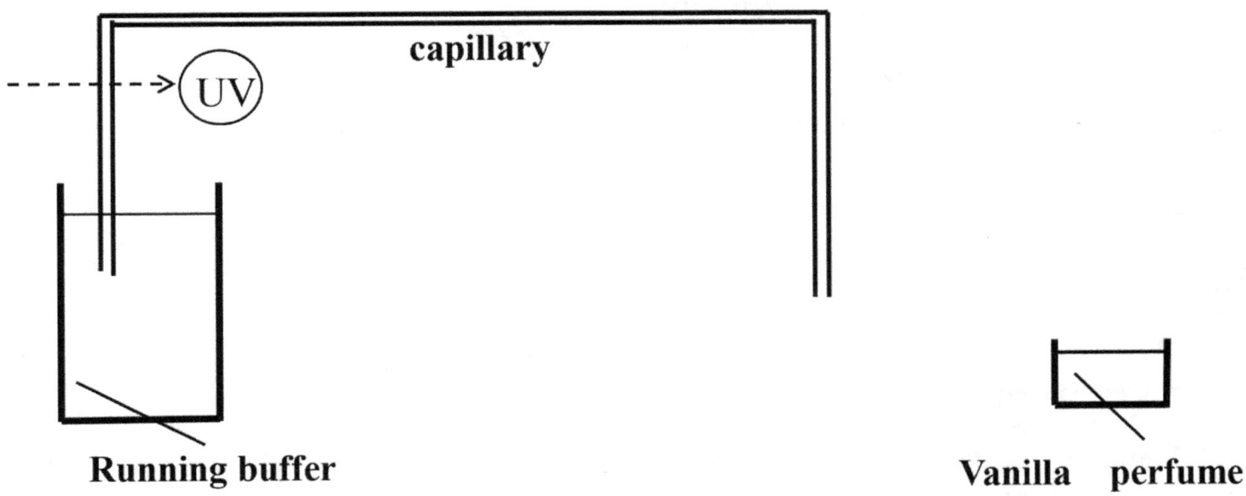

Figure 11. Illustration of the direct sampling of CE in air for vanillin in indoor air.

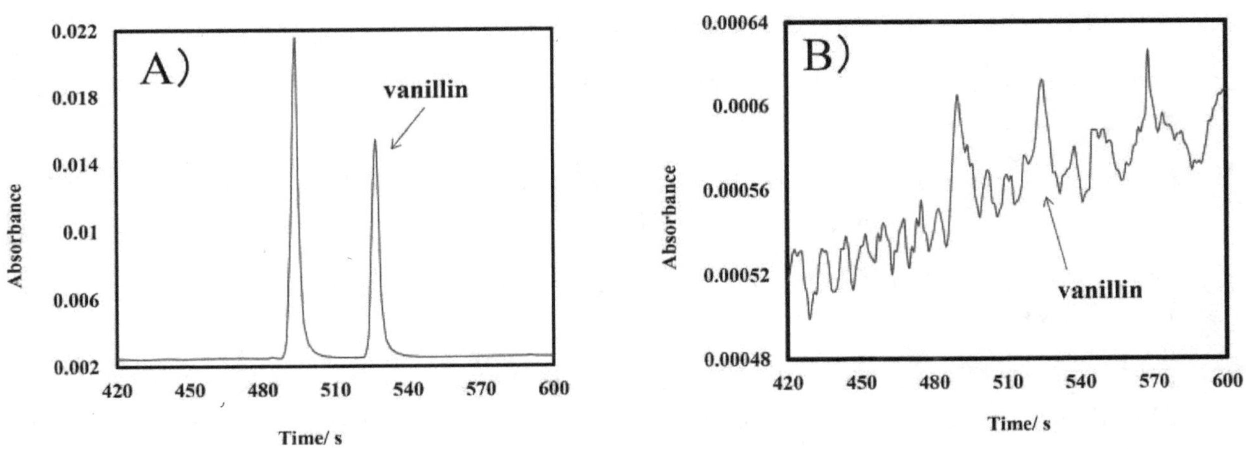

Figure 12. Results of a conventional CE of 10% vanilla perfume solution (A) and direct sampling-CE in indoor air with a sampling time of 5 min (B), respectively.

As shown in **Figure 12B**, there were also two peaks detected in the direct sampling-CE in air, and they were from vanilla perfume. Moreover, they were detected even with a sampling time as short as 5 min. This sampling time was extremely short in comparison with the offline active carbon adsorption/desorption-CE determinations [35]. In the offline active carbon adsorption/desorption-CE, it took more than 2 days to detect vanillin in indoor air [35]. Therefore, the direct sampling-CE is much faster and simpler than the offline active carbon adsorption/desorption-CE. The direct sampling-CE is promising and expectable in fast gas analysis.

Author details

Saaya Minematsu[1] and Xing-Zheng Wu[2*]

*Address all correspondence to: wu@fit.ac.jp

1 Environmental Chemistry, Fukuoka Technical High School Fukuoka, Japan

2 Department of Life, Environment and Materials Science, Fukuoka Institute of Technology Fukuoka, Japan

References

[1] Walton N.J., Mayer M.J., Narbad A.: Phytochemistry. 2003; **63**: 505–515. doi: 10.1002/jps.3030291001

[2] Vanillin: PubChem Open Chemistry Database [Internet] 2004. Available from: https://pubchem.ncbi.nlm.nih.gov/compound/vanillin

[3] Deichmann W., Kitzmiller K.V.: J Am Pharm Assoc (Scientific ed.). 1940; **29**(10): 425–428. doi: 10.1002/jps.3030291001

[4] Kim J.H., et al.: PLoS One. 2014; **9**(2): e89122. doi: 10.1371/journal.pone.0089122

[5] Fitzgerald D.J., Gasson M.J., Narbad A.: J Agric Food Chem. 2005; **53**: 1769–1775. doi: 10.1021/jf048575t

[6] Mourtzinos I., Kalogeropoulos N., Karathanos V.T., Konteles S.: Food Chem. 2009; **114**: 791–797. doi: 10.1016/f.foodchem.2008.10.014

[7] Lee J., Lee K.-W., Song J.-Y., Cho J.Y., et al.: Food Chem Toxicol. 2014; **63** :30–37. doi: 10.1016/j.fct.2013.10.031

[8] Fahlbusch K.-G., et al: Flavors and Fragrances. Ullmann's Encyclopedia of Industrial Chemistry, 7th ed. (1999–2015) New York, NY: John Wiley & Sons. Online Posting Date: January 15, 2003.

[9] Pinto P.C.R., Costa C.E., Rodrigues A.E.: Ind Eng Chem Res. 2013; **52**: 4421–4428. doi: 10.1021/ie303349j

[10] Burdock G.A. (ed.): Fenaroli's Handbook of Flavor Ingredients. 6th ed. CRC Press, Taylor & Francis Group, Boca Raton, FL 2010. 2001 p.

[11] Yamada M., Okada Y., Yoshida T., Nagasawa T.: Appl Microbiol Biotechnol. 2007; **73**: 1025–1030. doi: 10.1007/s00253-006-0569-1

[12] Li T., Rosazza J.P.N.: Appl Environ Microbiol. 2000; **66**: 684–687. doi: 10.1128/AEM.66.2.684-687.2000

[13] Robert H. H. van den Heuvel, Marco W. Fraaije, Colja Laane, and Willem J. H. van Berkel: J Agric Food Chem. 2001;**49**: 2954–2958. doi:10.1021/jf010093j

[14] Van A., Chiou K., Ishida H.: Polymer. 2014; **55**: 1443–1451. doi: 10.1016/j.polymer.2014.01.041

[15] Zhang C., Kessler M.R., Madbouly S.A.: Macromol Chem Phys. 2015; **216**: 1816–1822. doi: 10.1002/macp.201500194

[16] Stephensin D., Halpern B.P.: Chem Senses. 2009; **34**: 121–126. doi: 10.1093/chemse/bjn063

[17] Vanillin. Toxicology Data Nerwork [Internet] 1983. Available from http://www.rsc.org/chemistryworld/podcast/CIIEcompounds/transcripts/vanillin.asp

[18] Sostaric T., Boyce M.C., Spickett E.E.: J Agric Food Chem. 2000; **12**: 5802–5807. doi: 10.1021/jf000515+

[19] Goodner K.L., Jella P, Rouseff R.L.: J Agric Food Chem. 2000; **48**: 2882–2886. doi: 10.1021/jf990561d

[20] de Jager L.S., Perfetti G.A., Diachenko G.W.: Food Chem. 2008; **107**: 1701–1709. doi: 10.1016/j.foodchem.2007.09.070

[21] Elmore J.S., Langley K.R.: J Agric Food Chem. 1996; **44**: 3560–3563. doi: 10.1021/jf950687k

[22] Frusawa Y., Yokoyama R., Liu C., Hayashi K.: Inst Electr Eng Japan. 2013; **133**: 199–205. doi: 10.1541/ieejsmas.133.199

[23] Rind F.M.A., Mughal U.R., Memon A.H. et al.: Asian J Chem. 2009; **21**: 2849–2856.

[24] Longares-Patron A., Canizares-Macias M.P.: Talanta. 2006; **69**: 882–887. doi: 10.1016/j.talanta.2005.11.030

[25] Linares P., Luque de Castro M.D., Valcarcel M.: Microchem. J. 1987; **35**: 120–124. doi: 10.1016/0026-265x(87)90206-2

[26] Chan W.H., Lee W.M., Foo C.L., Tang W.K.: Analyst. 1987; **112**: 845–848. doi: 10.1039/AN9871200845

[27] Katayama M., Mukai Y., Taniguchi H.: Anal Sci. 1987; **3**: 369–372. doi: 10.2116/analsci.3.369

[28] Belay M.T., Poole C.F.: Chromatographia. 1993; **37**: 365–373. doi: 10.1007/BF02272250

[29] Gassenmeier K.: Lebensm Wiss Technol. 2003; **36**: 99–103. doi: 10.1016/S0023-6438(02)00183-4

[30] Sinha A.N., Verma S.C., Sharma U.K.: J Separation Sci. 2007; **30**: 15–20. doi: 10.1002/jssc.200600193

[31] Guenther L.: Food Chem. 2009; **114**: 1130–1134. doi: 10.1016/j.foodchem.2008.10.071

[32] Masataka O., Hisako O., Misako H., et al.: J Chromatogr A. 2007; **1138**: 262–267. doi: 10.1016/j.chroma.2006.10.031

[33] Toshiro W., Akira Y., Shiro N., et al.: J Chromatogr A. 1998; **793**: 409–413. doi: 10.1016/S0021-9673(97)00931-X

[34] Jozef L.B.: J Chem Educ. 2005; **82**: 604–606. doi: 10.1021/ed082p604

[35] Minematsu S., Xuan G.S., Wu X.-Z.: J Environ Sci. 2013; **25**: 8–14. doi: 10.1016/S1001-0742(14)60617-3

[36] Minematsu S., Wu X.-Z.: Anal. Sci. 2013; **29**: 373–375. doi: 10.2116/analsci.29.373

13

Medicinal Plants of the Indigenous Tribes in Peninsular Malaysia: Current and Future Perspectives

Pozi Milow, Sorayya Malek and
Raznan Mohd. Ramli

Abstract

The main aim of this paper is to compile information on plant that is known to be medicinal to the indigenous tribes in Peninsular Malaysia. Information is compiled from various sources. Current trends on studies of medicinal plants of the indigenous tribes and threats to the sustainability of the plants are also discussed. Focus of future studies on medicinal plants utilized by the indigenous tribes will also be discussed.

Keywords: Jah Hut, medicinal, Negrito, Semai, Semang, Temuan, proto-Malay

1. Introduction

The indigenous tribes in Peninsular Malaysia are collectively known as the Orang Asli. The Orang Asli consists of 18 subethnic groups or tribes which anthropologists and administrators grouped into the Semang (Negrito), Senoi, and aboriginal Malay (proto-Malay). Documentation on the plant resources, particularly medicinal plants, utilized by the people is still far from complete as most of the villages of the tribes have not been studied. Documentation on traditional uses of medicinal plants is important because it helps to preserve traditional culture of indigenous tribes, provide leads to the discovery medicinal compounds, and find ways to conserve the medicinal plants.

The main aims of this paper are to compile information on medicinal plants of the indigenous tribes in Peninsular Malaysia based on previous studies and to provide direction for future studies on the medicinal plants of the indigenous tribes.

2. List of medicinal plants of the indigenous tribes in Peninsular Malaysia

Two hundred and thirteen species of plants (**Table 1**) have been reported as medicinal to the indigenous tribes in Peninsular Malaysia. The medicinal plants were based on uses by the tribes Jah Hut, Semai, Semang and Temuan. Information on the plants is compiled from Refs. [1–8]. Leaves and roots are the most common parts that have medicinal uses. Destructive harvest, i.e., those that involve the removal of barks, roots, or whole plants, is among the most susceptible to overharvest because of destruction of the entire plants [9].

3. Current approaches of research on medicinal plants of indigenous tribes in Peninsular Malaysia

The most common approach to illicit information on the medicinal plants of the indigenous tribes is through semistructure interviews with traditional medicine practitioners known as *batin*. Two issues that have not been adequately addressed in previous studies are the veracity of information obtained from such approach and the extent of use or usage of medicinal by the indigenous tribes.

The veracity of information on medicinal properties plants utilized by the indigenous tribes in Peninsular Malaysia can be verified by laboratory analysis of bioactive compounds extracted from the plants. Several such studies have already been carried on some of the species that are listed in **Table 1**. Mohd Zin et al. [10] had carried out antioxidative activity of extracts from *Morinda citrifolia* L. and had concluded that active compounds in root of the plant might be both polar and nonpolar in nature, whereas compounds that contribute to antioxidative activity of both its leaf and fruit are probably nonpolar in nature. Hakimi Wan Salleh et al. [11] studied the chemical compositions and antioxidant and antimicrobial activities of essential oils of *Piper caninum* Blume. Safrole, β-caryophyllene, β-pinene, and germacrene D were the main components from the leave and stem oil of the plant. They noted that the highest activity was observed for inhibition of lipid peroxidation in the β-carotene/linoleic acid system by the stem oil and the essential oil showed strong antimicrobial activity.

by examining the effects of *E. longifolia* Jack on sexual qualities in middle-aged male rats. They demonstrated that *E. longifolia* Jack enhanced the sexual qualities of the middle-aged male rats. Bhat and Karim [13] reviewed the ethnobotany and pharmacological importance and *E. longifolia* Jack and noted that the plant possesses adequate therapeutic potential and could be explored further for commercial purposes and could be designated as a "wonder drug plant."

Information on usages of medicinal plants by the indigenous tribes was very limited in previous reports, thus making the assessment of this aspect of traditional culture practice difficult. Persistent usage of the medicinal plants by the tribes is important to ensure that the knowledge on the medicinal uses of plants is conserved and subsequently should contribute to the conservation of the plants. This is of concern because as modernization moves toward the

No.	Species	Indigenous tribe(s) [plant part(s) used]	Sources of information
1.	*Abutilon indicum* L.	Semang [leaves]	[3]
2.	*Acorus calamus* L.	Semai [rhizomes]	[6]
3.	*Acrotrema costatum* Jack	Semang [roots and leaves]	[7]
4.	*Agelaea macrophylla* (Zoll.) Leenh.	Semang [leaves]	[3]
5.	*Aglaia odorata* Lour.	Semang [flowers]	[3]
6.	*Aglaia yzermannii* Boerl. & Koord.	Semang [leaves]	[1]
7.	*Albizia myriophylla* Benth.	Jah Hut [roots]	[5]
8.	*Aloe barbadensis* Mill.	Jah Hut [leaves], Temuan [leaves]	[4, 5]
9.	*Alpinia galanga* (L.) Willd.	Temuan [rhizomes]	[4]
10.	*Alstonia angustiloba* (L.) Miq.	Jah Hut [leaves]	[2]
11.	*Ancistrocladus extensus* Wall. ex Planch	Jah Hut [roots]	[5]
12.	*Ancistrocladus tectorius* (Lour.) Merr.	Semang [roots]	[7]
13.	*Annona muricata* L.	Semang [leaves]	[3]
14.	*Apama tomentosa* Engl.	Temuan [roots]	[4]
15.	*Aquilaria malaccensis* Lamk.	Jah Hut [stems and leaves], Semai [barks]	[5, 6]
16.	*Archidendron ellipticum* Blume	Semang [leaves]	[3]
17.	*Archidendron jiringa* Niels.	Temuan [barks, leaves, and roots]	[4]
18.	*Ardisia colorata* Roxb.	Semang [leaves]	[3]
19.	*Ardisia crenata* Sims.	Jah Hut [leaves], Semang [whole plants]	[3, 5]
20.	*Ardisia crispa* (Thunb.) DC	Semang [whole plants]	[7]
21.	*Ardisia sanguinolenta* Bl.	Jah Hut [roots]	[5]
22.	*Areca catechu* L.	Semang [fruits]	[7]
23.	*Argostemma pictum* Wall.	Semang [whole plants]	[7]
24.	*Artemisia argyi* Levi. et Vant.	Semang [leaves]	[3]
25.	*Arthrophyllum diversifolium* Blume	Semang [roots]	[3]
26.	*Averrhoa bilimbi* L.	Semang [leaves]	[3]
27.	*Averrhoa carambola* L.	Temuan [barks, leaves, and roots]	[4]
28.	*Azadirachta indica* Juss.	Temuan [leaves]	[4]
29.	*Barringtonia acutangula* (L.) Gaertn.	Semang [stems]	[7]
30.	*Baccaurea motleyana* (Muell. Arg.) Muell. Arg.	Temuan [fruits]	[4]
31.	*Baccaurea ramiflora* Lour.	Jah Hut [roots]	[5]
32.	*Barleria lupulina* Lindl.	Semang [leaves]	[3]
33.	*Barleria prionitis* L.	Semang [leaves]	[3]
34.	*Bauhinia semibifida* Roxb.	Semang [roots]	[3]

No.	Species	Indigenous tribe(s) [plant part(s) used]	Sources of information
35.	*Bixa orellana* L.	Semai [seeds]	[6]
36.	*Blechnum orientale* L.	Semai [leaves]	[6]
37.	*Bombax ceiba* L.	Semang [leaves]	[3]
38.	*Bonnaya veronicaefolia* Spreng.	Temuan [leaves]	[4]
39.	*Bulbophyllum mutabile* (Bl.) Lindl.	Semang [leaves]	[3]
40.	*Caesalpinia crista* L.	Semang [seeds]	[3]
41.	*Calamus ornatus* Bl.	Semai [stem saps]	[6]
42.	*Cassytha filiformis* L.	Semang [whole plants]	[3]
43.	*Catharanthus roseus* (L.) Don	Temuan [whole plants]	[4]
44.	*Centella asiatica* (Linn.) Urban	Semang [whole plants], Semang [leaves] Temuan [whole plants]	[3, 4, 7]
45.	*Champereia manillana* (Bl.) Merr.	Semang [roots]	[7]
46.	*Chassalia chartacea* Craib	Semang [roots]	[7]
47.	*Chroesthes longifolia* (Wight) Hansen	Jah Hut [roots]	[5]
48.	*Cinnamomum aureofulvum* Gamb.	Jah Hut [roots]	[5]
49.	*Cinnamomum iners* Reinw. ex Blume	Semang [roots]	[7]
50.	*Cinnamomum javanicum* Bl.	Temuan [leaves]	[4]
51.	*Citrus medica* L.	Jah Hut [fruits]	[5]
52.	*Cnestis platantha* Griff.	Semang [leaves]	[3]
53.	*Cnestis ramiflora* Griff.	Semang [roots]	[7]
54.	*Cocos nucifera* L.	Temuan [fruits]	[5]
55.	*Connarus grandis* Jack	Jah Hut [roots]	[5]
56.	*Coptosapelta tomentosa* (L.) (Blume) Valeton ex K. Heyne	Jah Hut [roots]	[2]
57.	*Costus speciosus* (Koenig.) Smith	Semang [stems], Jah Hut [leaves], Semai [leaves]	[5–7]
58.	*Crinum asiaticum* L.	Temuan [leaves]	[4]
59.	*Croton caudatus* Geisel	Semang [roots]	[3]
60.	*Curcuma longa* L.	Temuan [rhizomes]	[4]
61.	*Curcuma petiolata* Roxb.	Semang [rhizomes]	[3]
62.	*Curcuma xanthorrhiza* Roxb.	Semang [rhizomes]	[7]
63.	*Cyclea laxiflora* Miers	Semai [whole plants]	[6]
64.	*Cymbopogon citratus* (DC.) Stapf.	Jah Hut [leaves]	[5]
65.	*Cymbopogon nardus* (L.) Rendle	Jah Hut [leaves], Temuan [leaves]	[4, 5]
66.	*Cyrtandra pendula* Bl.	Jah Hut [roots]	[5]

No.	Species	Indigenous tribe(s) [plant part(s) used]	Sources of information
67.	*Daemonorops didymorphyllus* Becc.	Semang [saps]	[1, 7]
68.	*Dendrophoetoe constricta* Dans.	Semang [leaves]	[3]
69.	*Desmos chinensis* Lour.	Jah Hut [roots]	[5]
70.	*Dianella ensifolia* Red.	Semai [roots]	[6]
71.	*Dicranopteris linearis* (Burm.) Underw.	Semai [leaves]	[6]
72.	*Dioscorea hispida* Dennst.	Temuan [tubers]	[4]
73.	*Dipteracanthus repens* (L.) Hassk.	Semang [leaves]	[3]
74.	*Durio zibethinus* Murray	Semang [leaves]	[1, 2, 7]
75.	*Dysoxylum alliaceum* (Bl.) Bl.	Semang [roots]	[7]
76.	*Elephantopus scaber* L.	Temuan [leaves]	[4]
77.	*Elephantopus tomentosus* L.	Temuan [leaves]	[4]
78.	*Etlingera elatior* (Jack) Smith	Semang [leaves]	[7]
79.	*Eleiodoxa conferta* (Griff.) Burret	Semang [stems]	[8]
80.	*Epiprinus malayanus* Griff.	Jah Hut [roots]	[5]
81.	*Eranthemum borneense* Hook f.	Semang [leaves]	[3]
82.	*Eugenia urceolata* King.	Jah Hut [roots]	[5]
83.	*Eupatorium odoratum* L.	Semang [leaves]	[3, 7]
84.	*Euphorbia hirta* L.	Jah Hut [latex]	[5]
85.	*Euphorbia tirucalli* L.	Semang [latex]	[3]
86.	*Eurycoma apiculata* Benn.	Semai [leaves]	[6]
87.	*Eurycoma longifolia* Jack	Semang [roots], Jah Hut [roots], Temuan [leaves, roots], Semang [roots]	[2–5, 7]
88.	*Fibraurea chloroleuca* Miers	Semang [roots]	[7]
89.	*Ficus aurantiaca* Griff.	Jah Hut [stems and roots], Temuan [stems]	[4, 5]
90.	*Freycinetia javanica* Bl.	Semang [roots]	[7]
91.	*Garcinia mangostana* L.	Semang [fruits]	[3]
92.	*Garcinia scortechinii* King.	Jah Hut [roots]	[4]
93.	*Gnetum leptostachyum* Blume	Semang [whole plants]	[3]
94.	*Gomphandra lanceolata* King.	Temuan [roots]	[4]
95.	*Goniothalamus macrophyllus* (Bl.) Miq.	Jah Hut [roots], Semai [barks]	[5, 6]
96.	*Guioa pubescens* (Zoll. & Mor.) Radlk.	Semang [roots and leaves]	[7]
97.	*Gynura procumbens* (Lour.) Merr.	Semang [leaves]	[3]
98.	*Hedyotis capitellata* (L.) Wall. ex G. Don	Jah Hut [roots], Semai [roots]	[2, 5]
99.	*Hevea brasiliensis* Muell. Arg.	Jah Hut [stems]	[5]

No.	Species	Indigenous tribe(s) [plant part(s) used]	Sources of information
100.	*Hedychium longicornutum* Baker	Semang [roots]	[7]
101.	*Helminthostachys zeylanica* (L.) Hook.	Semang [whole plants], Jah Hut [roots]	[5, 7]
102.	*Hibiscus rosa-sinensis* L.	Temuan [leaves], Semang [roots and barks]	[3, 4]
103.	*Hibiscus tiliaceus* L.	Semang [barks]	[3]
104.	*Hippocratea indica* Willd.	Jah Hut [roots]	[5]
105	*Homalanthus populneus* (L.) (Geisel.) Pax	Jah Hut [leaves]	[2]
106.	*Homalomena griffithii* Hk.f.	Semai [stems]	[6]
107.	*Homalomena rostrata* Griff.	Jah Hut [roots]	[5]
108.	*Hoya coronaria* Blume	Semang [leaves]	[3]
109.	*Iguanura geonomiformis* Mart.	Semai [leaves]	[6]
110.	*Imperata cylindrica* (L.) Beauv.	Semang [whole plants]	[3]
111.	*Jasminum sambac* (L.) Ait.	Semang [leaves]	[3]
112.	*Jatropha curcas* L.	Semai [saps], Semang [leaves]	[3, 6]
113.	*Justicia betonica* L.	Jah Hut [leaves]	[5]
114.	*Kaempferia galanga* L.	Semang [rhizomes]	[3]
115.	*Kalanchoe pinnata* (Lam.) Pers.	Semang [leaves]	[7]
116.	*Labisia pothoina* Lindl.	Jah Hut [roots and stems], Semai [roots]	[5, 6]
117.	*Labisia pumila* (Blume) Mez	Semang [roots]	[7]
118.	*Languas conchigera* Burkill	Semang [rhizomes]	[3]
119.	*Lantana camara* L.	Semang [leaves]	[3]
120.	*Lasia spinosa* Thwaites	Semang [tubers], Jah Hut [leaves]	[5, 7]
121.	*Lasianthus oblongus* King & Gamble	Jah Hut [roots]	[5]
122.	*Lasianthus villosus* Ridl.	Semai [leaves]	[6]
123.	*Lawsonia inermis* (L.) Pers.	Semang [leaves]	[7]
124.	*Leea indica* (Burm. f.) Merr.	Semang [leaves]	[7]
125.	*Lepidagathis incurva* Buch.-Ham.	Jah Hut [leaves]	[5]
126.	*Leptaspis urceolata* R. Br.	Jah Hut [roots]	[5]
127.	*Licuala spinosa* Wurm	Jah Hut [meristems]	[5]
128.	*Limacia oblonga* (Miers.) Hk.f. et. Thoms.	Temuan [stems]	[4]
129.	*Lindera lucida* (Bl.) Boerl.	Semai [leaves]	[6]
130.	*Lindera pipericarpa* (Miq.) Boerl.	Jah Hut [roots]	[5]
131.	*Lophatherum gracile* Brongn.	Semang [roots], Semai [roots]	[7]
132.	*Loranthus cochinchinensis* Lour.	Semang [whole plants]	[7]

No.	Species	Indigenous tribe(s) [plant part(s) used]	Sources of information
133.	*Luvunga scandens* Buch.-Ham.	Semai [leaves]	[5]
134.	*Lycopodiella cernua* (L.) Pic. Serm.	Jah Hut [leaves]	[2]
135.	*Lygodium circinnatum* (Burm.) Sw.	Semang [leaves]	[3, 7]
136.	*Lygodium flexuosum* (L.) Sw.	Jah Hut [leaves]	[2]
137.	*Lygodium microphyllum* (Cav.) R.Br.	Semai [leaves]	[6]
138.	*Maranta arundinacea* L.	Jah Hut [roots]	[2]
139.	*Marumia nemorosa* Bl.	Semai [leaves]	[6]
140.	*Melastoma malabathricum* L.	Jah Hut [roots]	[2]
141.	*Mikania micrantha* Kunth ex H.B.K.	Semang [whole plants]	[7]
142.	*Millettia sericea* Benth.	Semai [stems]	[6]
143.	*Mitragyna speciosa* Korth	Semang [leaves]	[7]
144.	*Morinda citrifolia* L.	Semang [fruits], Jah Hut [leaves and fruits]	[2, 3]
145.	*Musa sapientum* L.	Semang [fruits]	[7]
146.	*Neodissochaeta gracilis* (Jack) Bakh.	Semang [leaves]	[7]
147.	*Nephelium lappaceum* L.	Semang [leaves]	[7]
148.	*Oldenlandia diffusa* (Willd.) Roxb.	Semang [leaves]	[3]
149.	*Orchidantha longiflora* Ridl.	Semai [leaves]	[6]
150.	*Oroxylum indicum* (L.) Kurz	Semang [barks]	[7]
151.	*Oryza sativa* L.	Semai [seeds]	[6]
152.	*Parameria barbata* (Blume) K.Schum.	Semang [roots]	[7]
153.	*Parkia speciosa* Hassk.	Semai [roots], Temuan [roots], Semang [seeds]	[3, 4, 6]
154.	*Peliosanthes lurida* Ridl.	Semang [roots]	[7]
155.	*Peliosanthes violacea* Wall.	Semang [roots], Jah Hut [roots], Semai [leaves]	[5–7]
156.	*Pellacalyx saccardianus* Scort.	Semai [leaves]	[6]
157.	*Peltophorum pterocarpum* (DC.) K. Heyne	Semang [barks]	[3]
158.	*Peristrophe acuminata* Nees	Jah Hut [leaves]	[5]
159.	*Peucedanum japonica* Thunb.	Temuan [roots]	[4]
160.	*Phyllagathis rotundifolia* (Jack) Bl.	Jah Hut [roots]	[5]
161.	*Phyllanthus niruri* L.	Semang [whole plants]	[3]
162.	*Phyllanthus oxyphyllus* Miq.	Temuan [whole plants]	[4]
163.	*Phyllanthus pulcher* Wall. ex Muell. Arg.	Jah Hut [roots]	[5]
164.	*Phyllanthus urinaria* L.	Semai [whole plants]	[6]
165.	*Physalis minima* L.	Jah Hut [leaves]	[2]

No.	Species	Indigenous tribe(s) [plant part(s) used]	Sources of information
166.	*Pinanga polymorpha* Becc.	Jah Hut [leaves]	[5]
167.	*Piper betle* L.	Temuan [leaves]	[4]
168.	*Piper caninum* Blume	Semang [fruits and barks]	[7]
169.	*Piper muricatum* Bl.	Semai [leaves]	[6]
170.	*Planchonella obovata* (R. Br.) Pierre	Semang [leaves]	[3]
171.	*Platycerium bifurcatum* (Cav.) C. Chr.	Semang [tubers]	[7]
172.	*Plumeria obtusa* L.	Semai [flowers]	[6]
173.	*Polyalthia bullata* King.	Jah Hut [roots]	[5]
174.	*Pongamia pinnata* L.	Semang [leaves and seeds]	[3]
175.	*Pseuderanthemum crenulatum* (L.) Lindl.	Jah Hut [leaves]	[2]
176.	*Pseuderanthemum piloselloides* (L.) M.G. Price	Jah Hut [leaves]	[2]
177.	*Psidium guajava* L.	Jah Hut [leaves], Temuan [leaves]	[4, 5]
178.	*Psychotria montana* Bl.	Jah Hut [roots]	[5]
179.	*Rafflesia cantleyi* Solms.-Laub.	Semai [flowers]	[6]
180.	*Rennellia speciosa* (Wall. ex Kurz) Hk.f.	Jah Hut [roots]	[5]
181.	*Rourea concolor* Bl.	Temuan [roots]	[4]
182.	*Salacca affinis* Griff.	Jah Hut [leaves]	[5]
183.	*Sambucus javanica* Reinw. ex Blume	Semang [leaves]	[3]
184.	*Sansevieria trifasciata* Prain	Semang [leaves]	[3]
185.	*Smilax calophylla* Wall.	Semang [roots], Temuan [whole plants]	[4, 7]
186.	*Smilax lanceifolia* (L.) Roxb.	Jah Hut [leaves]	[2]
187.	*Smilax myosotiflora* L.	Jah Hut [bulbs]	[2]
188.	*Solanum nigrum* L.	Semang [fruits and leaves]	[3]
189.	*Spilanthes paniculata* Wall. ex DC.	Semang [flowers]	[7]
190.	*Stachyphrynium jagoranum* Schum.	Jah Hut [roots]	[5]
191.	*Stachytarpheta jamaicensis* (L.) Vahl.	Semang [whole plants]	[3]
192.	*Striga asiatica* (L.) Kuntze	Jah Hut [whole plants], Temuan [whole plants]	[4, 5]
193.	*Strobilanthes crispus* Blume	Semang [leaves]	[3]
194.	*Styrax benzoin* Dryand	Jah Hut [resin], Semai [resin]	[5, 6]
195.	*Syzygium cerina* Hend.	Semang [roots]	[3]
196.	*Syzygium samarangenese* Blume	Semang [leaves]	[3]
197.	*Tagetes patula* L.	Semai [flowers]	[6]
198.	*Talinum triangulare* (Jacq.) Willd.	Semang [flowers]	[3]

No.	Species	Indigenous tribe(s) [plant part(s) used]	Sources of information
199.	*Tectaria angulata* (Willd.) Copel	Semang [roots]	[7]
200.	*Tetracera macrophylla* Wall. ex Hk.f. & Thoms	Jah Hut [leaves], Temuan [leaves]	[4, 5]
201.	*Timonius wallichianus* (Korth.) Val.	Semang [roots], Jah Hut [whole plants]	[5, 7]
202.	*Tinospora crispa* (L.) Miers. ex Hk.f. and Thoms.	Temuan [stems], Semang [stems]	[3, 4]
203.	*Trema orientalis* (L.) Bl.	Temuan [leaves and shoots]	[4]
204.	*Trichilia trijuga* Roxb.	Semang [barks]	[3]
205.	*Urena lobata* L.	Semai [stems]	[6]
206.	*Uvaria sorsogonensis* C.Presl.	Semang [leaves]	[3]
207.	*Vernonia arborea* Buch.-Ham.	Jah Hut [roots]	[5]
208.	*Vernonia cinerea* (L.) Less.	Jah Hut [leaves and roots]	[2]
209.	*Zingiber griffithii* Baker	Semai [rhizomes]	[6]
210.	*Zingiber officinale* Rosc.	Temuan [rhizomes]	[4]
211.	*Zingiber ottensii* Valeton	Semang [rhizomes]	[3]
212.	*Zingiber spectabile* Griff.	Jah Hut [leaves], Semai [leaves]	[5, 6]
213.	*Zingiber zerumbet* (L.) Roscoe ex Sm.	Semang [latex]	[7]

Table 1. Annotated medicinal plant species list of the indigenous tribes in Peninsular Malaysia.

doorstep of the indigenous tribes, knowledge and usage of biodiversity decrease and eventually become adulterated or lost to humanity [4].

4. Future studies on medicinal plants of indigenous tribes in Peninsular Malaysia

Future studies on medicinal plants should be extended to more villages of the indigenous tribes in Peninsular Malaysia. The studies should include aspects that have not been adequately addressed in the previous studies. Other aspects that can be included in future studies are the use of geographical information system to analyze the spatial trend on medicinal plants of the indigenous tribes and also the development of automated identification system for medicinal plant species.

Geographic information systems (GIS) have not been used in any studies on the medicinal plants in Peninsular Malaysia, although the use of GIS for conserving medicinal and herbal plants elsewhere has been reported [14–17]. GIS application together with remote sensing data could be used for comprehensive vegetation mapping and analysis of data attained from ground surveys. In terms of mapping medicinal plants, remote sensing data can be useful to obtain information on land usage or coverage, vegetation, terrain attributes, distribution, and accessibility to area. Besides this, GIS could be used to produce map layers and to develop comprehensive databases on physical, biological, and environmental parameters which govern the spatial distribution and abundance of medicinal plants.

Serious consideration should be given to the use of machine learning for rapid identification of medicinal plants, especially those utilized by the indigenous tribes in Peninsular Malaysia. As medicinal plants utilized by most of the indigenous tribes have not been studied, these techniques will facilitate urgent documentation of the plants which are needed for their conservation. Machine learning methods such as artificial neural networks (ANN) and support vector machine (SVM) have been used to develop automated plant species identification despite the claims that leaf morphology is not a reliable indicator in identifying tree species. ANN is a mathematical model composed of many processing units that communicate by interconnected variables. It is trained using data for which the classes are known, followed by being used for class prediction of unidentified data. Multilayer structure of ANN enables learning from complex input image features and generates single output. Support vector machine (SVM) is a supervised learning method proposed by Cortes and Vapnik [18], generating hyperplanes for classification, based on statistical learning theory and structural risk minimization. The boundary of hyperplanes separates the sample data mapped in space, clearly dividing them into categories. New data will be predicted to belong to a category by the hyperplanes.

Studies conducted by Clark et al. [19] applied ANN to extract features from species of the genus *Tilia* and achieved 44% accuracy rate. Kumar et al. [20] developed a "Leafsnap," a computerized system that searches on database for species matching and retrieval. Hearn [21] used a combination of Fourier analysis and Procrustes analysis (a simple shape registration method, based on rotation, translation, and scaling) to perform species identification using a large database of 2420 leaves from 151 different species.

5. Conclusion

Two hundred and thirteen species of plants have been reported as medicinal to the indigenous tribes in Peninsular Malaysia. Leaves and roots are the two most common medicinal plant parts used by the indigenous tribes in Peninsular Malaysia. Medicinal use of roots requires destructive harvesting which may lead to overharvesting of the plant species. Future studies on medicinal plants of the indigenous tribes in Peninsular Malaysia should extend to more tribes as information that is available up to now is only to the Jah Hut, Semai, Semang, and Temuan tribes. Aspects of the medicinal plants of the indigenous tribes have been overlooked in previous studies; such veracity of information and usage need to be emphasized in future studies. To facilitate spatial analysis and identification of the medicinal plants, geographical information system and machine learning techniques can also be employed in future studies.

Acknowledgements

We would like to thank the Department of Orang Asli Development for granting us permission to carry out study at Kampung Lubuk Legong. We are thankful to the University of Malaya for providing the research grants (PS018/2011A and RG044/09SUS) to carry out this study.

Author details

Pozi Milow*, Sorayya Malek and Raznan Mohd. Ramli

*Address all correspondence to: pozimilow@um.edu.my

Institute of Biological Sciences, University of Malaya, Kuala Lumpur, Malaysia

References

[1] Burkill IH. A Dictionary of the Economic Products of the Malay Peninsula. 4th edition. Dept. of Agriculture, Kuala Lumpur, Malaysia. 2002.

[2] Lin KW. Ethnobotanical Study of Medicinal Plants Used by the Jah-Hut Peoples in Malaysia. Indian Journal of Medical Sciences. 2005; 59(4): 156–158.

[3] Samuel AJSJ, Kalusalingam A, Chellappan DK, Gopinath R, Radhamani S, Husain HA, et al. Ethnomedical Survey of Plants Used by the Orang Asli in Kampung Bawong, Perak, West Malaysia. Journal of Ethnobiology and Ethnomedicine. 2010; 6: http://www.ethnobiomed.com/content/6/1/5

[4] Ong HC, Ahmad N, Milow P. Traditional Medicinal Plants Used by the Temuan Villagers in Kampung Tering, Negeri Sembilan, Malaysia. Ethno Medicine. 2011; 5(3): 169–173.

[5] Ong HC, Faezah AW, Milow P. Medicinal Plants Used by the Jah Hut Orang Asli at Kampung Pos Penderas, Pahang, Malaysia. Ethno Medicine. 2012; 6(1): 11–15.

[6] Ong HC, Lina E, Milow P. Traditional Knowledge and Usage of Medicinal Plants among the Semai Orang Asli at Kampung Batu 16, Tapah, Perak, Malaysia. Ethno Medicine. 2012; 6(3): 207–211.

[7] Mohammad NS, Milow P, Ong HC. Traditional Medicinal Plants Used by the Kensiu Tribe of Lubuk Ulu Legong, Kedah, Malaysia. Ethno Medicine. 2012; 6(3): 149–153.

[8] Lim TK. Edible Medicinal and Non-Medicinal Plants. Volume 1, Fruits. Springer, Dordrecht, Heidelberg, London, New York. 2012; pp. 396–398.

[9] Schippman U, Leaman DJ, Cunningham AB. Impact of Cultivation and Gathering of Medicinal Plants on Biodiversity: Global Trends and Issue. Paper published in Biodiversity and the Ecosystem Approach in Agriculture, Forestry and Fisheries in Rome, October 12–13. 2002.

[10] Mohd Zin Z, Abdul-Hamid A, Osman A. Antioxidative Activity of Extracts from Mengkudu (*Morinda citrifolia* L.) Root, Fruit and Leaf. Food Chemistry. 2002; 78: 227–231.

[11] Hakimi Wan Salleh WMN, Ahmad F, Yen KH, Mohd Sirat H. Chemical Compositions, Antioxidant and Antimicrobial Activities of Essential Oils of *Piper caninum* Blume. International Journal of Molecular Sciences. 2011; 12: 7720–7731. DOI: 10.3390/ijms12117720

[12] Ang HH, Ngai TH, Tan TH. Effects of *Eurycoma longifolia* Jack on Sexual Qualities in Middle Aged Male Rats. Phytomedicine. 2003; 10: 590–593.

[13] Bhat R, Karim AA. Tongkat Ali (*Eurycoma longifolia* Jack): A Review on Its Ethnobotany and Pharmacological Importance. Fitoterapia. 2010; 81: 669–679.

[14] Porwal MC, Sharma L, Roy PS. Stratification and Mapping of *Ephedra gerardiana* Wall in Poh (Lahul and Spiti) Using Remote Sensing and GIS. Current Science. 2003; 84: 208–212.

[15] Anderson DM, Salick J, Moseley RK, Xiaokun O. Conserving the Sacred Medicine Mountains: A Vegetation Analysis of Tibetan Sacred Sites in Northwest Yunnan. Biodiversity and Conservation. 2005; 14: 3065–3091.

[16] Roy PS, Behera MD. Assessment of Biological Richness in Different Altitudinal Zones in the Eastern Himalayas, Arunachal Pradesh, India. Current Science. 2005; 88: 250–257.

[17] Yang X, Skidmore AK, Melick DR, Zhou Z, Xu J. Mapping Non-wood Forest Product (Matsutake Mushrooms) Using Logistic Regression and a GIS Expert System. Ecological Modeling. 2006; 198: 208–218.

[18] Cortes C, Vapnik V. Support-vector Networks. Machine Learning. 1995; 20(3): 273–297.

[19] Clark JY, Corney DP, Tang H. Automated Plant Identification Using Artificial Neural Networks. 2012 IEEE Symposium on Computational Intelligence in Bioinformatics and Computational Biology (CIBCB). San Diego, CA: IEEE. 2012; pp. 343–348. DOI: 10.1109/CIBCB.2012.6217250

[20] Kumar N, Belhumeur PN, Biswas A, Jacobs DW, Kress WJ, Lopez I, Soares JV. Leafsnap: A Computer Vision System for Automatic Plant Species Identification. 12th European Conference on Computer Vision (ECCV). Berlin: Springer-Verlag Heidelberg. 2012; pp. 502–516.

[21] Hearn DJ. Shape Analysis for the Automated Identification of Plants from Images of Leaves. TAXON. 2009; 58(3): 934–954.

14

Comparative Proteomic Analysis of *Panax ginseng* C. A. Meyer × *Panax quinquefolius* L. Leaves and Parental Lines

Xiujuan Lei, Zhiqing Wang, Juan Song, Shao Liang,

Lina Yao, Zhifang Hou and Yingping Wang

Abstract

Heterosis refers to the superior performance of heterozygous F1 hybrid plants with respect to those of their genetically distinct parents. Despite its wide use in crops, heterosis is seldom applied in the Panax genus, and its molecular basis remains unclear. Thus, this study is aimed to obtain hybrid F1s and identify the proteins associated with heterosis. Hybrid F1 plants and parental inbred lines were obtained using the embryo rescue technique, and the proteomes of their leaves were analyzed using two-dimensional gel electrophoresis. A total of 236 differentially expressed proteins were found, among which 84 nonadditive proteins indicated a heterosis pattern in the hybrid. Gene Ontology (GO) and Kyoto Encyclopedia of Genes and Genomes analysis revealed that photosynthesis, carbohydrate metabolism, and protein and amino acid synthesis were the most abundant classes of nonadditive proteins. Of the proteins in these categories, 10, 6, and 4 proteins, respectively, showed above high parent expression in the hybrid leaves. These results imply that the increment in photosynthetic capacity, carbohydrate decomposition, and nitrogen fixation might be related to the heterosis of the hybrid biomass and ginsenoside production in the hybrid leaves. This study could provide a basis for hybrid breeding of the Panax genus.

Keywords: hybridization, heterosis, proteomic analysis, morphological traits, ginsenoside, Panax genus

1. Introduction

Hybridization is a commonly used breeding method for plants because it allows gene transfer and optimization of the best plant features [1]. Wheat, maize, and soybean hybrids have been produced from conventional hybrid breeding, and these hybrids tend to exhibit better traits than those of their parents [2–4]. This phenomenon is called heterosis. *Panax ginseng* C. A. Meyer (Asian ginseng) and *Panax quinquefolius* L. (American ginseng) are two medicinal plants of the Araliaceae ginseng species widely used in Asia because of their purported therapeutic effects on cancer, diabetes, and Parkinson's disease [5–7]. The ability to enhance the hybridization of Panax plants may improve yield and quality, which is an essential goal of the ginseng industry. However, research into the hybrid breeding of each species, especially the molecular basis of heterosis, remains to be clarified, although several hypotheses and models have been proposed, such as locus-specific overdominant effects and genome dominance complementation [8, 9]. Recently, several studies on maize, rice, and Arabidopsis analyzed heterosis at the genome, transcriptome, and proteome levels by applying a variety of molecular tools [10–13].

Protein profiling plays an important role in comparative proteomic analysis, thereby enabling the comparison of proteins across different genotypes, organs, or treatments. Two-dimensional electrophoresis (2-DE) combined with mass spectrometry (MS) is commonly used to appoint correlations among the polymorphism of individual protein amounts, indications, and hybrid vigor for agronomic traits [14–17]. However, to date, no report is available on the differences in the proteomic profiling of the leaves of the Panax hybrid and its parents. In this study, we report research into the differences in leaf proteome profiles between the hybrid F1 and its parental inbred lines at the seedling stage. The proteomic analysis in this work reveals that the proteins involved in photosynthesis, carbohydrate metabolism, and protein and amino acid synthesis may be responsible for heterosis in Panax. The molecular insights provided by this study might help in improving understanding of the possible molecular networks involved in Panax heterosis.

2. Materials and methods

2.1. Plant materials and hybridization

All plant materials were collected from Fusong, Jilin province, China, in 2012. Among them, "FX01" (*Panax ginseng*, female parental inbred line) is a landrace with high yield and ginsenoside content, and "ZNYS01" (*Panax quinquefolius*, male parental inbred line) was introduced from America in 1975. Samples were cultivated in an experimental greenhouse of Special Wild Economic Animals and Plants Institute of Chinese Academy of Agricultural Sciences, Changchun, China. To ensure matching flowering periods, seeding stage was regulated for four years for "ZNYS01" and "FX01" on 5 April and 1 May, respectively. When flowering, pollen was collected from "ZNYS01," dried with silica gel, and kept at 4°C until use. Interspecific hybridization was accomplished by selecting the unopened but fully developed flowers of "FX01" emasculating and pollinating them with dried pollen of "ZNYS01," and bagging the pollinated flowers immediately to prevent contamination from other pollen sources. Abortive seeds were removed 21 days after pollination and stored at 4°C.

2.2. Embryo rescue and plant regeneration

Embryo rescues were performed according to Suputtitada et al. [18] with modifications. Three weeks after pollination, abortive fruits were collected and surfaces were washed with running water for 2 h, and then, seeds were removed and sterilized with 75% ethanol for 1 min, followed by 0.1% $HgCl_2$ treatment for 10 min, and five washes in sterilized water. Ovules were excised from seeds and cultured in Erlenmeyer flasks containing solid embryo induction medium (Murashige and Skoog basal medium supplement with 1.0 mg/L 6-benzyladenine, 2.0 mg/L gibberellin, 0.5% lactalbumin hydrolysate, 3.0% sucrose, and 6.0% agar), with 3–4 ovules/flask [19]. Cultures were kept in the dark at 25 ± 2°C. After 3–4 weeks of culture, developed embryos were excised from ovules and then transferred to White's basal medium [20], containing 1.0 mg/L 6-benzyladenine, 0.2 mg/L α-naphthalene acetic acid, 3.0% sucrose, and 6.0% agar for plant regeneration, and cultured under a 15-/9-h photoperiod with a light intensity of 40 μE/s/min provided by cool white fluorescent light (25 ± 2°C). pH of media was adjusted to 5.8 before autoclaving. Subculture was performed every two months. Samples were collected from the middle leaf of cultured plantlets (palmate compound leaves) after 30 days from the third subculture. For each experiment, 30 plantlets were propagated from one embryo to ensure genetic background consistency.

2.3. Molecular identification

Leaves of the F1 hybrid and parental inbred lines were frozen in liquid nitrogen and ground into fine powders. Genomic DNA was isolated with the cetyltriethylammonium bromide method. DNA was separated on agarose gel and quantified with a DNA/Protein analyzer. PCR amplification of ribosomal external transcribed spacer regions was performed on plant DNA samples. Oligonucleotide primers (**Table 1**) were designed according to Wang et al. [21] and the 20 μL PCR reaction mixture consisted of 10 ng of template DNA, 0.5 μM of each primer, 1 UE × Taq, 2 μL 10 × PCR buffer, and dNTP 0.2 mM. PCR amplification was performed using 1 predenaturation cycle of 4 min at 94°C, 39 cycles of 94°C for 30 s, 60°C for 30 s, and 72°C for 30 s, and a final extension at 72°C for 5 min. PCR products were analyzed on a 1.0% agarose gel stained with ethidium bromide.

2.4. Morphological traits measurement

Plants were carefully harvested and dried in an oven at 60°C for 96 h, for dry weight determination. Six plant traits were characterized including plant height (PH), total leaf number (TLN), leaf area (LA), leaf thickness (LT), leaf fresh weight (LFW), and leaf dry weight (LDW). Statistical analysis of the five traits was performed using F-test.

2.5. Ginsenoside analysis

For ginsenoside analysis, 250 mg of leaf samples (dry weight) was soaked in 50 mL methanol for 1 day and filtered. Filtrate was removed to a 100-mL volumetric flask, and residue was re-extracted twice. Extracts were concentrated with methanol and diluted to 100 mL. Then, 2 μL samples were analyzed with a Waters XEVE-TQ ultra-high performance liquid chromatography-tandem mass spectrometry system. Separation was achieved using a BEH C18 column (1.7 μm, 50 mm × 2.1 mm). MS/MS analyses were carried out under positive and negative ion modes. Gradient elution and ion source parameters were set as Wang et al. reported [22]. Ginsenosides were detected under negative multiple reaction monitoring mode.

2.6. Protein extraction and separation

Total protein extraction and separation were performed according to Lei et al. [23]. Leaves of hybrid F1 and two parents were removed, and each ~0.5 g was ground to powder under liquid nitrogen and homogenized in 3.0 mL of ice-cold acetone containing 10% (w/v) trichloroacetic acid and 0.07% β-mercaptoethanol. After incubation at -20°C overnight, the mixture was centrifuged at 15,000×*g* at 4°C for 15 min. The upper fraction was removed, and precipitate was collected and washed three times with 3 mL of ice-cold acetone containing 0.07% β-mercaptoethanol. Each washing was followed by centrifugation as described above. All obtained precipitates were air-dried at 4°C and dissolved in sample rehydration buffer containing 7 M urea, 2 M thiourea, 2% 3-[(3-cholamidopropyl) dimethylammonio] propanesulfonic acid, 1% phenylmethanesulfonyl fluoride, and 1% protein inhibitors. After dissolution, sample protein solutions were vortexed at 38°C for 30 min and centrifuged at 15,000×*g* at 15°C for 10 min. Protein concentration was measured with a Bradford assay [24].

Before the first dimension [isoelectric focusing (IEF)], 1.5 mg of sample protein (350 μL) was loaded on an immobilized pH gradient dry strip (17 cm, pH 4–7, linear; Bio-Rad) and rehydrated for 15 h. IEF was then performed under the following conditions: 200 V for 1.5 h, 500 V for 1.5 h, 1000 V for 3 h, and 10,000 V for 7 h. IEF was terminated after reaching 70,000 Vh. Gel strips were subsequently equilibrated for 15 min in 5 mL equilibration buffer [75 mM Tris-HCl (pH 8.8), 6 M urea, 2 M thiourea, 30% glycerol, 2% sodium dodecyl sulfate, 0.002% bromophenol blue, and 1% (w/v) dithiothreitol (DTT)] and then soaked again for an additional 15 min with the same buffer but replacing DTT with 2.5% (w/v) iodoacetamide. For the second dimension, the equilibrated strips were then separated with 12.5% sodium dodecyl sulfate polyacrylamide gel electrophoresis (SDS-PAGE) sealed with 0.5% (w/v) low temperature agarose. Gels were stained with Coomassie brilliant blue R-250 and destained with a solution containing 10% ethanol and 10% acetic acid. Three biological replicates were carried out for all samples to obtain statistically reliable results. Then, the 2-DE gels were scanned using Image Scanner 6.0 (Amersham Biosciences, location) with a resolution of 300 dpi and analyzed on the PDQuestTM 2-DE analysis Software Version 8.01 (Bio-Rad). Protein expression was estimated by the spot percent volume (vol.%), a value normalized as a percent of the total volume of all gel spots present. Percent volumes can be used to correct the variability caused by sample loading, gel staining, and destaining. Fold-changes in protein expression were calculated according to spot percent volumes, and only spots with more than twofold quantitative variation (increase/decrease) in three replicates and statistically significant when calculated by ANOVA ($p < 0.05$) were considered significantly differentially expressed proteins.

2.7. Protein MS analysis and classification

Gel digestion was performed according to Deng et al. [25] with modifications. Protein spots with significant differences in abundance were manually excised from gels. Peptide MS and MS/MS analyses were carried out on an ABI–5800 MALDI-TOF/TOF Plus mass spectrometer (Applied Biosystems, location). General MS parameters were as follows: laser, 200 Hz (UV, 355 nm); acceleration voltage, 2 kV; scans per laser spot, 2500–3000 times; mass range from 800 to 4000 kDa; eight most intense peaks were selected on each mass spectrum for further MS/MS analysis.

Data were acquired in a positive MS reflector by using a CalMix5 standard to calibrate the instrument (ABI–5800 Calibration Mixture). The following parameters were used as follows: one allowed missed cleavage site; fixed modifications of carbamidomethyl; variable modifications of oxidization; 100 ppm for precursor ion tolerance and 0.3 Da for fragment tolerance. Both MS and MS/MS data were integrated and processed by using GPS Explorer V3.6 software (Applied Biosystems) with default parameters.

Protein identification was performed by searching Viridiplantae sequences in the nonredundant National Center for Biotechnology Information (NCBI) database and ginseng Expressed Sequence Tags database using the GPS-Mascot V 2.4 search engine (www.matrixscience.com Matrix Science Ltd., London, UK). Only proteins with Mascot scores >75 based on 95% or greater confidence intervals were considered identified. Protein functions were classified using Gene Ontology (GO) annotation according to their biological processes and molecular functions (http://geneontology.org/). When no GO annotation was available, protein classification was based on literature retrieval and closely related homologous sequences.

3. Results

3.1. Plant regeneration and molecular identification

One major difficulty in interspecific hybridization is the embryogenic abortion of hybrids [26]. To overcome this problem, the embryo rescue technique was used as depicted in the "Methods," and the embryo germination rate was influenced by basal medium, hormones, and the embryonic developmental stages. **Figure 1a–d** shows "FX01 × ZNYS01" and the parent plants regenerated from immature embryos; both growth and reproduction of the hybrid plants showed the highest speed and stability. Although "FX01 × ZNYS01" displayed significant differences in trait with their parents, identification at the molecular level was considered essential. Thus, single-nucleotide polymorphism molecular markers in the ribosomal external transcribed spacer region were adopted to identify such differences. Two primers P1 and P2 were specific to *P. quinquefolius* and *P. ginseng*, respectively. Another primer P3 was used as the corresponding reverse primer of P1 and P2 (**Table 1**). The combination of three primers generated different fragment patterns for the hybrid F1s and their parents (**Figure 2**). "FX01" produced specific 388-bp bands, whereas "ZNYS01" yielded specific 501-bp bands. Two bands were detected when the DNA of "FX01 × ZNYS01" was used.

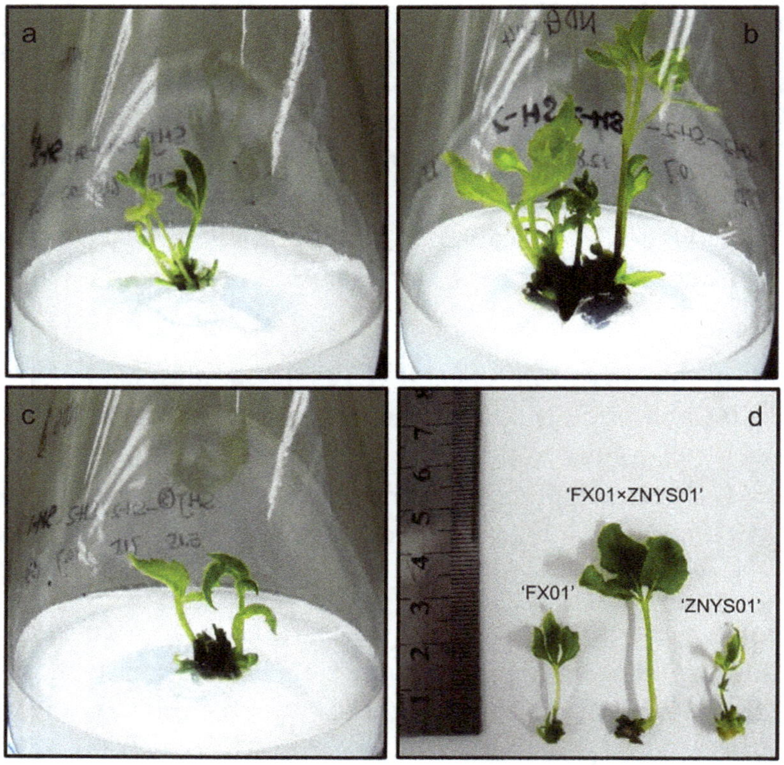

Figure 1. Hybrid F1 plants and parental inbred lines differentiated from embryos and morphology. Cultured (a) "FX01," (b) "FX01 × ZNYS01," and (c) "ZNYS01." (d) The leaf trait of plant height and leaf area in "FX01 × ZNYS01" was significantly different from that in the parents.

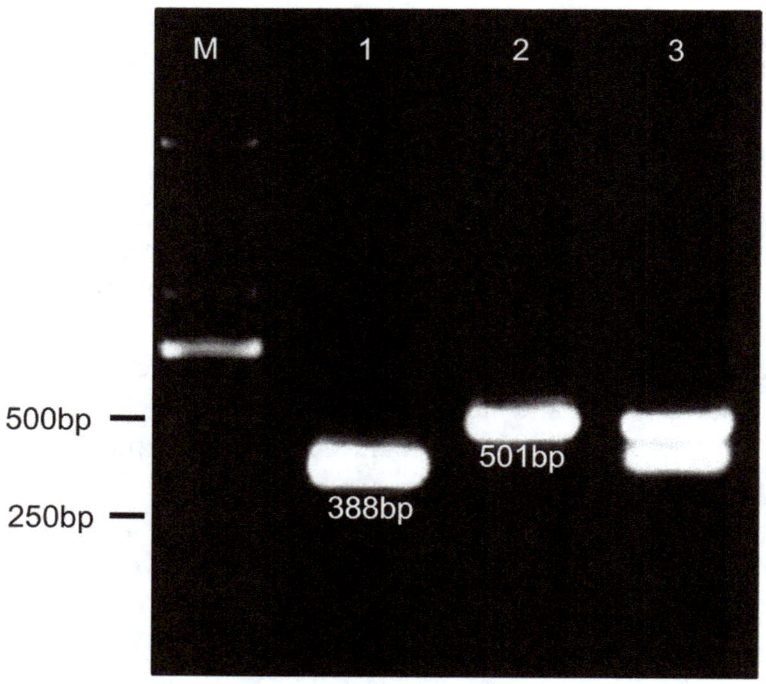

Figure 2. Multiplex allele-specific PCR products using the DNA extracted from the leaves of the hybrid and its parental inbred lines. Lane M: 2000 bp DNA marker; Lane 1: "FX01"; Lane 2: "ZNYS01"; and Lane 3: "FX01 × ZNYS01".

Primer name	Nucleotide sequence (5′–3′)
P1	GTGTTGGCATAGTGTACGTTA
P2	AGAGCAGTAAGCCTTGGAAAAT
P3	AGACAAGCATATGACTACTGGCAGG

Table 1. Oligonucleotide sequences of the primers used.

3.2. Morphological traits and ginsenoside measurement

Hybrid plants often perform better than their parents; this is a phenomenon called heterosis. This better performance manifests as increased growth speed, yield, or vigor of hybrid F1 plants compared with the average levels of traits in their parents. In this study, six plant traits, namely, PH, TLN, LA, LT, LFW, and LDW, were measured. Statistical analysis revealed the significant differences in morphological traits between the hybrid and parental inbred lines (**Table 2**). Ginsenoside is the major effective component of Panax; thus, ginsenoside production was measured as another important heterosis factor. The quantified ginsenosides and related data are listed in **Table 3**. The results on both the total ginsenosides and 20(S)-Rg2 indicate that "FX01 × ZNYS01" F1 exhibited the highest yield and showed a strong transgressive inheritance. The other seven ginsenosides also displayed increased mid-parent advantage.

SV[a]	DF[b]	PH (cm)	TLN	LT (mm)	LA (cm^2)	LFW (mg)	LDW (mg)
Genotype	2	8.04**	102.4**	3.89×10^{-2} NS[c]	1.41**	22.58**	0.66**
Error	15	0.28	4.82	3.67×10^{-2}	0.18	2.3	0.05

[a] SV, source of variance.

[b] DF, degree of freedom.

[c] NS, nonsignificant at the 0.05 probability level.

** Significant at the 0.01 probability level.

Table 2. Mean squares of variance analysis for the different characteristics of the hybrid and its parental inbred lines.

3.3. 2-DE separation of the leaf proteins of the hybrid and its parental inbred lines

The protein expression profiles of the leaves from the hybrid F1 and parental inbred lines were obtained by 2-DE. Means of 679 ± 21, 869 ± 32, and 987 ± 16 (mean ± standard deviation; $n = 3$) spots per gels were detected in "FX01," "FX01 × ZNYS01," and "ZNYS01," respectively (**Figure 3**). The spot intensities on each replicate gel were normalized with PDQuest software to compensate for the non-expression-related variations in spot intensity. The 2-DE map of the leaf proteins of the hybrid F1 was used as a reference map for comparison with the proteins of the parental inbred lines. After normalization, the average protein spot intensities of the three replicate gels per genotype were compared between "FX01 × ZNYS01" and the parental inbred lines. A total of 236 protein spots were present in significantly different quantities across the three genotypes.

Ginsenoside	"FX01" (mg/g)	"FX01 × ZNYS01" (mg/g)	"ZNYS01" (mg/g)
Rg1[&]	$22.62^{a} \pm 1.65$	$2.98^{b} \pm 0.21$	$0.61^{c} \pm 0.07$
Re[&]	$56.69^{a} \pm 1.13$	$51.41^{b} \pm 2.36$	$26.78^{c} \pm 2.28$
20(S)-Rg2[&]	$1.16^{c} \pm 0.09$	$7.38^{a} \pm 0.63$	$2.98^{b} \pm 0.13$
Rb1[&]	$5.43^{a} \pm 0.32$	$5.49^{a} \pm 0.45$	$1.12^{b} \pm 0.02$
Rb2[&]	$3.47^{c} \pm 0.49$	$6.88^{b} \pm 0.71$	$8.97^{a} \pm 0.57$
Rb3[&]	$0.41^{c} \pm 0.07$	$16.52^{b} \pm 0.39$	$30.39^{a} \pm 1.29$
Rc[&]	$3.52^{b} \pm 0.41$	$4.66^{a} \pm 0.22$	$4.01^{a} \pm 0.19$
Rd[&]	$10.21^{c} \pm 0.83$	$39.22^{b} \pm 1.28$	$40.58^{a} \pm 3.02$
Total yield[#] (mg/g DW)	$103.51^{c} \pm 2.61$	$134.54^{a} \pm 1.52$	$115.44^{b} \pm 0.98$

[&]Means with the different letters in a single line are significantly different according to Tukey's honestly significant difference multiple comparisons with (family error 0.05).
[#]Total yield = (Rg1 + Re + 20(S)-Rg2 + Rb1 + Rb2 + Rb3 + Rc + Rd).

Table 3. Ginsenoside analysis of the hybrid and its parental inbred lines.

3.4. Identification of nonadditively accumulated proteins in hybrid

The target of this study was to identify proteins in the leaf proteome of hybrid "FX01 × ZNYS01" that accumulated significantly different traits from those of the mid-parent level of the parental inbred lines. Only these so-called nonadditive proteins might be associated with heterosis in the leaf of Panax genus. Among the 236 differentially expressed protein spots, 84 (36%) displayed significant heterosis patterns and were identified. The nonadditive proteins are shown in **Figure 3**. These nonadditively accumulated proteins were then categorized on the basis of the system suggested by Stupar and Springer [27] (**Figure 4**). The proteins with significantly higher expression in the hybrid than in the better performing parental line were classified as "above high parent" (++). The proteins with significantly lower expression in the hybrid than in the less performing parent line were named "below low parent" (--). The hybrid proteins that exhibited a significantly higher expression than that of the less performing parent but with no significant difference with that of the better performing parent were classified as "high parent" (+). The hybrid proteins with significantly lower expression than in the better performing parent but with no significant difference in expression with the less performing parent were designated as "low parent" (-). Moreover, the hybrid proteins with significantly higher expression than that in the less performing parent and significantly lower expression than that in the better performing parent were classified as "partial dominance" (±). Among the different heterotic classes, 25 proteins (30% of the nonadditive expressed protein) displayed "above high parent" expression, and 2 proteins (2%) showed "below low parent" expression. Moreover, 14 proteins (17%) revealed "high parent" expression, 12 proteins (14%) demonstrated "low parent" expression, and 31 (37%) of the nonadditive proteins exhibited "partial dominance." Results showed that the class with "partial dominance" expression exhibited the highest degree of expression among the different expression patterns, followed by the "above high parent" class.

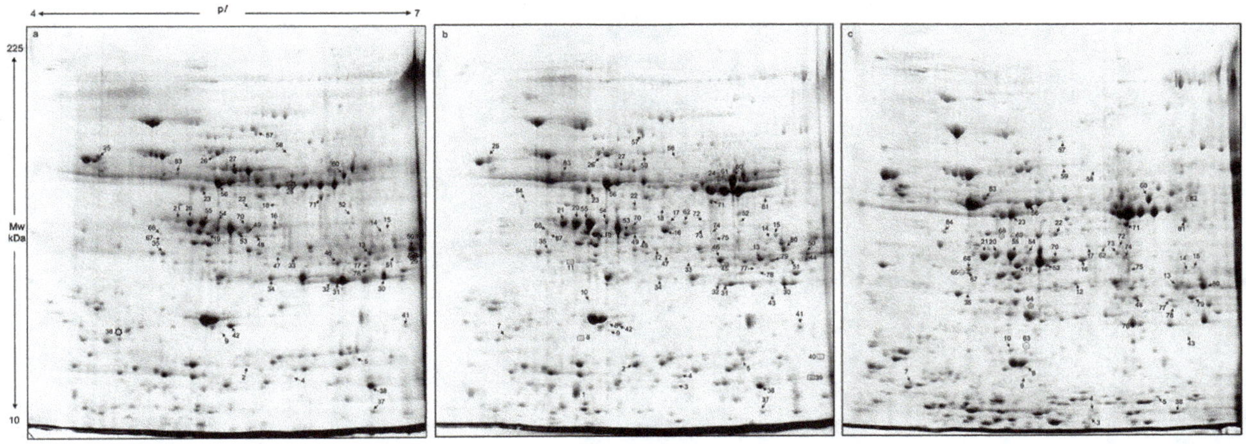

Figure 3. 2-DE profile of proteins extracted from the leaves of the hybrid and its parental inbred lines. (a) "FX01," (b) "FX01 × ZNYS01," and (c) "ZNYS01." The nonadditive accumulation proteins were marked with symbols in gel images. The spots only found in "FX01," "FX01 × ZNYS01," and "ZNYS01" are marked with stars, squares, and circles, respectively.

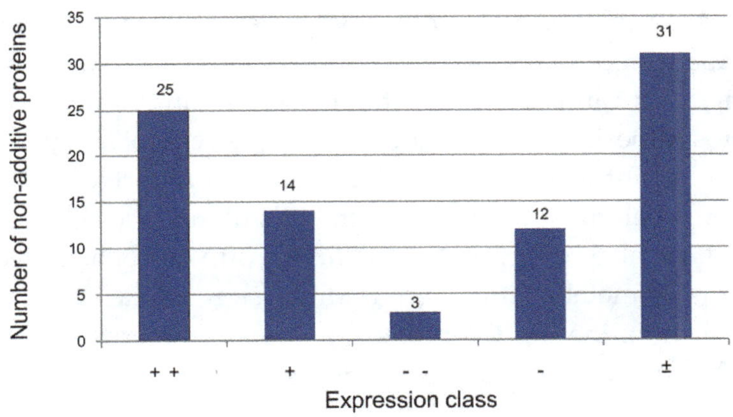

Figure 4. Classification of the nonadditive proteins expressed in the hybrid leaves and its parental inbred lines. "Above high parent expression" (++); "high parent expression" (+); "below low parent expression" (--); "low parent expression" (-); and "partial dominance" (±).

3.5. Biological functional classification

Molecular annotation and GO of these proteins were obtained using blast2GO (http://www.blast2go.com/b2ghome) and NCBI annotation (**Figure 5**). Photosynthesis, carbohydrate metabolism, and protein metabolism were the top three functional categories of the nonadditive expression proteins.

4. Discussion

P. ginseng and *P. quinquefolius* have been traditionally used as precious herbal medicines in Asia for many years. Despite its commercial importance, interspecific hybrid breeding, especially the molecular basis of heterosis, is poorly understood. In this study, comparative

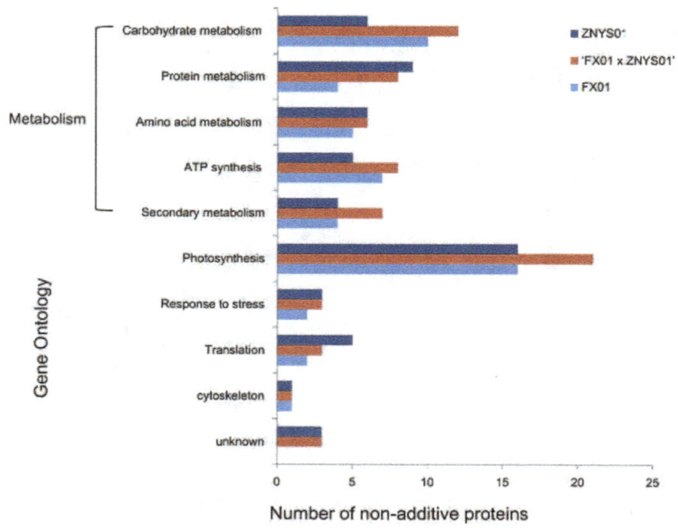

Figure 5. Functional classification of the nonadditive proteins.

proteomic analysis was employed to uncover the proteins related to heterosis in the hybrid plants. Among the 236 differentially expressed proteins, 84 exhibited a nonadditive pattern (**Figure 3**). According to GO annotation, most of these proteins were involved in the metabolism (60%) and photosynthesis (25%) categories. Mohayeji et al. [28] studied the nonadditive protein accumulation in sunflower leaves of hybrid F1 and reported that the main categories of nonadditive proteins belonged to energy metabolism and photosynthesis. Hoecker et al. [29] and Marcon et al. [4] also reported that the first group of nonadditive proteins in maize roots was classified under metabolism. These findings suggest the importance of metabolism and photosynthesis in illuminating the molecular basis of heterosis. In this light, the most important proteins that showed nonadditive patterns are discussed on the basis of their functional categories.

4.1. Photosynthesis-related proteins

Photosynthesis is a highly important biological process in plant growth. A total of 21 nonadditive proteins belonged to photosynthesis, and 10 of these proteins showed a "above high parent" pattern. Ribulose-1,5-bisphosphate carboxylase/oxygenase (Rubisco; spots 24 and 60) is a major Calvin cycle enzyme composed of eight large and eight small subunits. The high expression of these proteins indicates that the hybrid F1 could fix more CO_2 in the Calvin cycle [30, 31]. Ribulose bisphosphate carboxylase/oxygenase activase (RCA; spots 20, 54, and 55) regulates the activity of Rubisco in a light-dependent manner [32]. In most species, RCA is found in two forms (RCAI and RCAII), both of which can activate Rubisco. Studies showed that RCA physically interacts with Rubisco, thereby catalyzing ATP and facilitating the release of ribulose-1,5-bisphosphate and other tight-binding sugar phosphates from the active site of Rubisco [33, 34]. RCA expression increased, thereby suggesting increased Rubisco activation in the hybrid F1. The light-harvesting chlorophyll a/b binding protein (spot 6) was upregulated, suggesting a greater degree of light harvesting in the hybrid leaves than in the parent leaves. Carbonic anhydrase (CA; spots 2 and 39), which catalyzes the reversible interconversion of HCO_3^- and CO_2, participates in many biochemical pathways [35]. In photosynthesis, CA supports the CO_2 production for the Rubisco reaction [35]. CA was upregulated in the hybrids, thereby suggesting increased CO_2 delivery in photosynthesis. These results suggest that the enhancement of the proteins involved in photosynthesis may increase the photosynthetic capacity and efficiency of the hybrid F1 and consequently increase biomass production.

4.2. Carbohydrate metabolism-related proteins

Among the several processes involved in metabolism, carbohydrate metabolism is a critical plant process [36]. Glycolysis, the citric acid cycle, and the pentose phosphate pathway (PPP) are chief metabolic pathways for carbohydrate breakdown, which can provide not only energy but also intermediates for various activities [12]. Our results showed that most of the nonadditive proteins involved in carbohydrate metabolic pathways were expressed with "high parent" and "partial dominance" patterns. However, fructose-bisphosphate aldolase 1 (FBA1; spot 13), fructose-bisphosphate aldolase 3 (FBAIII; spot 46), and malate dehydrogenase (MDH; spots 44, 45, and 51) were expressed with an "above high parent" pattern in the "FX01 × ZNYS01" F1. In glycolysis, FBA reversibly catalyzes fructose 1,6-bisphosphate (F1,6BP) into triose phosphates dihydroxyacetone phosphate and glyceraldehyde 3-phosphate (GA3-P) [37]. The increased abundance of various isoforms of FBA indicates the enhancement of the glycolytic pathway in the hybrids. MDH reversibly catalyzes the oxidation of malate to oxaloacetate as part of multiple metabolic pathways, including secondary metabolism [38]. However, decreased or no expression of enzymes, such as enolase (spot 28), 6-phosphogluconate dehydrogenase (6-PGDH; spot 81), and some MDHs (spots 29 and 32), occurred in the hybrids. Enolase is an essential phosphopyruvate hydratase in glycolytic catabolism [39], and 6-PGDH is needed for the PPP pathway. The enzyme 6-PGDH catalyzes the reversible oxidative decarboxylation of 6-phosphogluconate to ribulose-5-phosphate and CO_2 [40]. The lower expression of proteins in the hybrid F1 is likely due to the inherence of the parent line traits. In particular, the parents naturally express such traits in lower amounts.

4.3. Protein and amino acid synthesis-related proteins

Protein and amino acid metabolism is crucial for plant growth. High accumulation of amino acid synthesis-related enzymes (spots 1 and 53) in the hybrid is evidence of the higher amino acid production. Ribonuclease-like storage protein (spot 4) and elongation factor Tu (spot 62) also showed an "above high parent" expression pattern. Elongation factor Tu is a protein that promotes the GTP-dependent binding of aminoacyl–tRNA to the A site of ribosomes during biosynthesis in mitochondria [41]. These results reveal that the amino acid synthesis capacity and protein biosynthesis are higher in the hybrid than in its parental inbred lines.

4.4. Two ginsenoside synthesis-related proteins identified in "FX01 × ZNYS01"

Two ginsenoside synthesis-related proteins, namely, 1-hydroxy-2-methyl-2-(E)-butenyl 4-diphosphate reductase (IspH; spot 61) and uridine diphosphate–glucosyltransferase (UGT;

spot 14), were identified, although 2-DE is limited for the study of low-abundance proteins. IspH is involved in the final step of the methylerythritol phosphate pathway, generating two pathway products isopentyl pyrophosphate and dimethylallyl pyrophosphate, which are needed for ginsenoside synthesis [42]. UGT is assumed to play an important role in producing different ginsenosides by adding monosaccharides to triterpene aglycones [43, 44]. The difference in UGT expression between the F1 hybrid and parents might be an important reason for the difference in ginsenoside monomers produced by the plants.

5. Conclusion

In this study, we demonstrated that "FX01 × ZNYS01" F1 exhibited heterosis in morphology and ginsenoside yield. At the proteome level, 236 differentially expressed proteins were found, among which 36% (84/236) accumulated in a nonadditive pattern. Eighty-four nonadditive proteins were identified, among which 60% (50/84) and 25% (21/84) were involved in the metabolism and photosynthesis categories, respectively. These results indicate that the greater biomass production in the hybrids than in the parental inbred lines is related to the increased carbon fixation, protein synthesis, and carbohydrate metabolism in the former. Enhanced protein and carbohydrate metabolism is important for producing additional organic compounds. Moreover, the increased release of energy for plant growth and photosynthesis

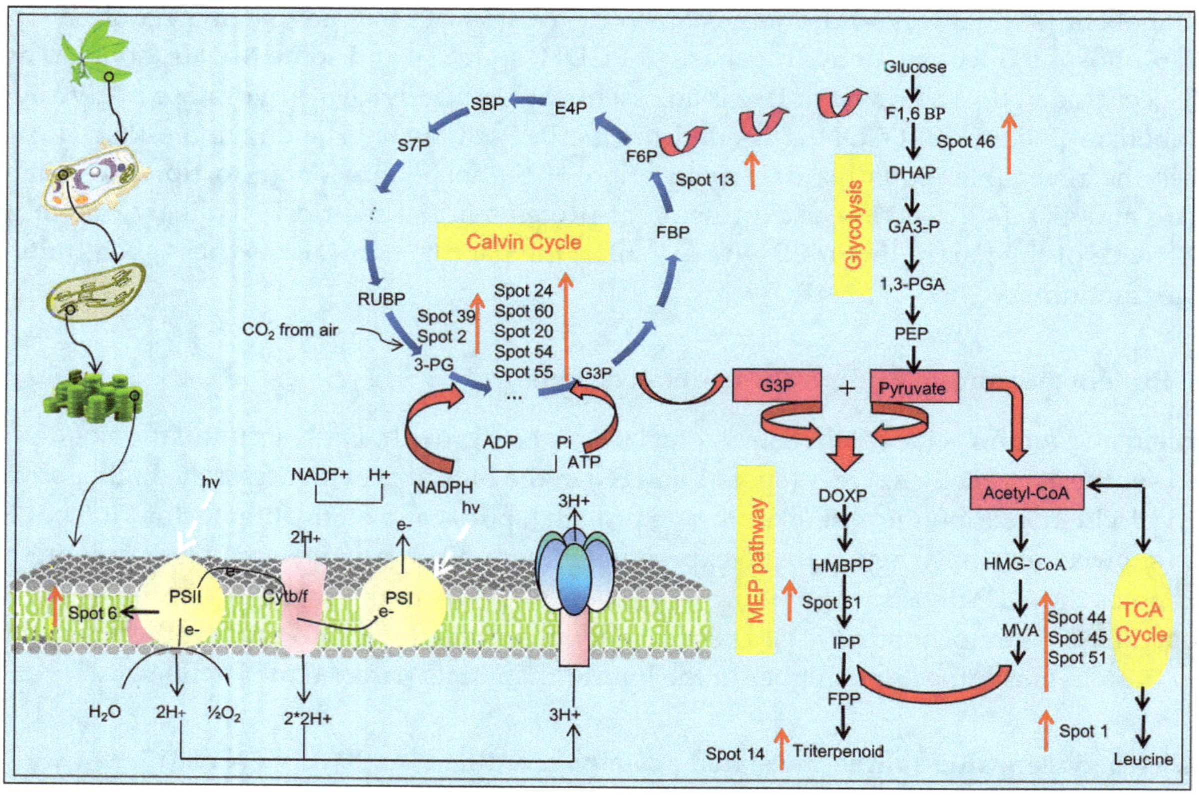

Figure 6. Schematic of heterosis in the hybrid ("FX01 × ZNYS01") from the Kyoto Encyclopedia of Genes and Genomes and UniProt database. The proteins and metabolites are indicated by spot number and red arrows (above high parent).

as the only source of assimilation plays an important role in biomass production. Leaves are the sites of ginsenoside synthesis, and a higher leaf yield implies greater ginsenoside production in the hybrid F1. Furthermore, the enhanced photosynthesis can offer a higher amount of intermediate products for plant secondary metabolism, which then improves ginsenoside yield (**Figure 6**). These data offer a foundation to better understand heterosis in the Panax genus and provide a basis for hybrid breeding.

Acknowledgements

The authors would like to thank Young People Fund of Jilin Science and Technology Department (No20140520165JH) for their finance support.

Author details

Xiujuan Lei, Zhiqing Wang, Juan Song, Shao Liang, Lina Yao, Zhifang Hou and Yingping Wang*

*Address all correspondence to: yingpingw@126.com

Institute of Special Wild Economic Animal and Plant Science of Chinese Academy of Agricultural Sciences, Changchun, P. R. China

References

[1] Xia G, Chen H. Plant regeneration from intergeneric somatic hybridization between *Triticum aestivum* L. and *Leymus chinensis* (Trin.) Tzvel. Plant Science.1996; **120**:197–203.

[2] Goff SA, Zhang Q. Heterosis in elite hybrid rice: speculation on the genetic and biochemical mechanisms. Current Opinion in Plant biology. 2013; **16**(2):221–7.

[3] Jiang Q, Chen H, Pan X, Pan Q, Shi Y, Li X, et al. Proteomic analysis of wheat (*Triticum aestivum* L.) hybrid necrosis. Plant Science. 2008; **175**(3):394–401.

[4] Marcon C, Lamkemeyer T, Malik WA, Ungrue D, Piepho HP, Hochholdinger F. Heterosis-associated proteome analyses of maize (*Zea mays* L.) seminal roots by quantitative label-free LC-MS. Journal of Proteomics. 2013; **93**:295–302.

[5] Aziz F, Wang X, Liu J, Yan Q. Ginsenoside Rg3 induces FUT4-mediated apoptosis in H. pylori CagA-treated gastric cancer cells by regulating SP1 and HSF1 expressions. Toxicology in vitro: An International Journal published in association with BIBRA. 2016; **31**:158–66.

[6] Liu YW, Zhu X, Li W, Lu Q, Wang JY, Wei YQ, et al. Ginsenoside Re attenuates diabetes-associated cognitive deficits in rats. Pharmacology, Biochemistry, and Behavior. 2012; **101(1)**:93–8.

[7] Van Kampen JM, Baranowski DB, Shaw CA, Kay DG. *Panax ginseng* is neuroprotective in a novel progressive model of Parkinson's disease. Experimental Gerontology. 2014; **50**:95–105.

[8] Birchler JA, Auger DL, Riddle NC. In search of the molecular basis of heterosis. The Plant Cell. 2003; **15**:2236–2239.

[9] Springer NM, Stupar RM. Allele-specific expression patterns reveal biases and embryo-specific parent-of-origin effects in hybrid maize. The Plant Cell. 2007; **17**:264–275.

[10] Andorf S, Selbig J, Altmann T, Poos K, Witucka-Wall H, Repsilber D. Enriched partial correlations in genome-wide gene expression profiles of hybrids (*A. thaliana*): a systems biological approach towards the molecular basis of heterosis. Theoretical and Applied Genetics (Theoretische und angewandte Genetik). 2010; **120**(2):249–59.

[11] Fu H, Dooner HK. Intraspecific violation of genetic colinearity and its implications in maize. Proceedings of the National Academy of Sciences. 2002; **99**(14):9573–78.

[12] HofiusD, Bornke Fredirik AJ. Photosynthesis, carbohydrate metabolism and source-sink relations. 1st ed. Netherlands: Elsevier; 2007. 257–285 p.

[13] Yao Y, Ni Z, Zhang Y, Chen Y, Ding Y, Han Z, et al. Identification of differentially expressed genes in leaf and root between wheat hybrid and its parental inbreds using PCR-based cDNA subtraction. Plant Molecular Biology. 2005; **58**(3):367–84.

[14] Adalatzadeh-Aghdam S, Toorchi M, Shakiba MR. Heterosis investigation of sunflower (*Helianthus annuus* L.) by two-dimensional electrophoresis. International Journal of Biosciences (IJB). 2014; **4**(10):70–79.

[15] Dahal D, Mooney BP, Newton KJ. Specific changes in total and mitochondrial proteomes are associated with higher levels of heterosis in maize hybrids. The Plant Journal: For Cell and Molecular Biology. 2012; **72**(1):70–83.

[16] Guo B, Chen Y, Zhang G, Xing J, Hu Z, Feng W, et al. Comparative proteomic analysis of embryos between a maize hybrid and its parental lines during early stages of seed germination. PloS One. 2013; **8**(6):e65867.

[17] Xiang X, Ning S, Wei D. Proteomic profiling of rice roots from a super-hybrid rice cultivar and its parental lines. Plant Omics. 2013; **6**(5):318–324.

[18] Suputtitada S, Adachi T, Pongtongkam P, Peyachoknagul S, Apisitwanich S Thongpradistha J. Breeding barriers in the interspecific cross of *Oryza sativa* L. and *Oryza minuta* Presl. Breeding Science. 2000; **50**:29–35.

[19] Murashige T, Skoong F. A revised medium for rapid growth and bio assays with tobacco tissue cultures. Physiologia Plantarum. 1962; **15**:473–497.

[20] White P. The cultivation of animal and plant cells. Ronald, New York; 1963. pp. 123–127.

[21] Wang H, Kim MK, Kwon WS, Jin H, Liang Z, Yang DC. Molecular authentication of *Panax ginseng* and ginseng products using robust SNP markers in ribosomal external

transcribed spacer region. Journal of Pharmaceutical and Biomedical Analysis. 2011; **55**(5):972–976.

[22] Wang J, Zheng P, Zheng S, Wang Y, Zhu Y, Zhou H, et al. Profiling and identification of the metabolites of ginsenoside Ro in rat faeces and urine after oral administration. European Food Research and Technology. 2016; **242**(2):199-210.

[23] Lei X, Wang Y, Li C, Zhang C, Song J, Liu L, et al. Protein expression changes in anther callus of ginseng during low-temperature acclimation. Crop Science. 2013; **53**(4):1571–1578.

[24] Bradford MM. A rapid and sensitive method for the quantitation of microgram quantities of protein utilizing the principle of protein-dyebinding. Analytical Biochemistry. 1976; **72**:248–254.

[25] Deng G, Liu LJ, Zhong XY, Lao CY, Wang HY, Wang B, et al. Comparative proteome analysis of the response of ramie under N, P and K deficiency. Planta. 2014; **239**(6):1175–1186.

[26] Karim MM, Siddika A, Tonu NN, Hossain DM, Meah MB, Kawanabe T, et al. Production of high yield short duration *Brassica napus* by interspecific hybridization between *B. oleracea* and *B. rapa*. Breeding Science. 2014; **63**(5):495–502.

[27] Stupar RM, Springer NM. Cis-transcriptional variation in maize inbred lines B73 and Mo17 leads to additive expression patterns in the F1 hybrid. Genetics.2006; **173**(4):2199–2210.

[28] Mohayeji M, Capriotti AL, Cavaliere C, Piovesana S, Samperi R, Stampachiacchiere S, et al. Heterosis profile of sunflower leaves: a label free proteomics approach. Journal of Proteomics. 2014; **99**:101–110.

[29] Hoecker N, Keller B, Muthreich N, Chollet D, Descombes P, Piepho HP et al. Comparison of maize (*Zea mays* L.) F1-hybrid and parental inbred line primary root transcriptomes suggests organ-specific patterns of non-additive gene expression and conserved expression trends. Genetics. 2008; **179**:1275–1283.

[30] Sghaier-Hammami B, Redondo-Lopez I, Valero-Galvan J, Jorrin-Novo JV. Protein profile of cotyledon, tegument, and embryonic axis of mature acorns from a non-orthodox plant species: *Quercus ilex*. Planta. 2016; **243**:369-396.

[31] Walker RP, Battistelli A, Moscatello S, Chen ZH, Leegood RC, Famiani F. Metabolism of the seed and endocarp of cherry (*Prunus avium* L.) during development. Plant Physiology and Biochemistry: PPB/Societe Francaise de Physiologie Vegetale. 2011; **49**(8):923–930.

[32] Salvucci ME, Portis AR, Ogren WL. A soluble chloroplast protein catalyzes ribulose bis-phosphate carboxylase/oxygenase activation in vivo. Photosynthesis Research.1985; **7**:193–201.

[33] Houtz RL, Portis AR. The life of ribulose 1,5-bisphosphate carboxylase/oxygenase—posttranslational facts and mysteries. Archives of Biochemistry and Biophysics. 2003; **414**(2):150–158.

[34] Salvucci ME, Ogren WL. The mechanism of rubisco activase: insights from studies of the properties and structure of the enzyme. Photosynthesis Research. 1996; **47**(1):1–11.

[35] Wei-Hong S, Yan-You W, Zhen-Zhen S, Qiu-Xia W, Xin-Yu W. Enzymatic characteristics of higher plant carbonic anhydrase and its role in photosynthesis. Journal of Plant Studies. 2014; **3**(2):39–44.

[36] Beruter J. Carbohydrate metabolism in two apple genotypes that differ in malate accumulation. Journal of Plant Physiology. 2004; **161**(9):1011–1129.

[37] Li S, Bian M, Wang X, Chen X, Xie Z, Sun H, et al. Molecular and biochemical characterizations of three fructose-1,6-bisphosphate aldolases from *Clonorchis sinensis*. Molecular and Biochemical Parasitology. 2014; **194**(1–2):36–43.

[38] Xing J, Sun Q, Ni Z. Proteomic patterns associated with heterosis. Biochimica et Biophysica Acta. 2016; **1864**(8):908-915.

[39] Polle JW, Neofotis P, Huang A, Chang W, Sury K, Wiech EM. Carbon partitioning in green algae (Chlorophyta) and the enolase enzyme. Metabolites. 2014; **4**:612–628.

[40] Ruuska SA, Andrews TJ, Badger MR, Price GD, Caemmerer SV. The role of chloroplast electron transport and metabolites in modulating rubisco activity in tobacco. Insights from transgenic plants with reduced amounts of cytochrome complex or glyceraldehyde 3-phosphate dehydrogenase1. Plant Physiology. 2000; **122**:491–504.

[41] Inaba K, Fujiwara T, Hayashi H, Chino M, Komeda Y, Naito S. Isolation of an *Arabidopsis thaliana* mutant, mto1, that over accumulates soluble methionine (temporal and spatial patterns of soluble methionine accumulation). Plant Physiology. 1994; **104**:881–887.

[42] Lee MH, Jeong JH, Seo JW, Shin CG, Kim YS, In JG, et al. Enhanced triterpene and phytosterol biosynthesis in *Panax ginseng* overexpressing squalene synthase gene. Plant & Cell Physiology. 2004; **45**(8):976–984.

[43] Khorolragchaa A, Kim YJ, Rahimi S, Sukweenadhi J, Jang MJ, Yang DC. Grouping and characterization of putative glycosyl transferase genes from *Panax ginseng* Meyer. Gene. 2014; **536**:186–192.

[44] Kim YJ, Zhang D, Yang DC. Biosynthesis and biotechnological production of ginsenosides. Biotechnology Advances. 2015; **33**(6 Pt 1):717–735.

15

Chemical Structure, Quality Indices and Bioactivity of Essential Oil Constituents

Nashwa Fathy Sayed Morsy

Abstract

Essential oil (EO) is a mixture of low molecular weight constituents that are responsible for its characteristic aroma. These constituents include terpenoid and non-terpenoid hydrocarbons and their oxygenated derivatives. This chapter focuses on the heterogeneous composition of the essential oils. It discusses the usage of essential oil constituents as a key marker of the oil quality, freshness and unique characteristics. It describes the biological activity and synergistic effect of the essential oil constituents as antioxidant, antibacterial, antifungal and anticancer agents.

Keywords: chemical structure, quality characteristics, bioactivity, antioxidant, antimicrobial, antitumor

1. Introduction

Essential oil (EO) is defined as odorous product, of complex composition, obtained from part of plant or whole plants through various methods. It has the characteristic taste and odor of the plant from which it was derived [1, 2]. This variation in composition could be due to a variety of plants [3], geographical locations [3, 4], harvesting seasons [5–7], drying methods [8] and extraction methods [9, 10].

The quality, freshness and uniqueness of an essential oil are major considerations pertaining to its value [11]. Essential oils are highly sensitive to heat, moisture and oxygen [12]. Formation of oxygenated terpenes, chemical transformations, or polymerization are features of aging processes that led to quality loss. Therefore, quality control of essential oils needs to be monitored by producers, traders, or essential oil manufacturers [13, 14].

Essential oils have wide variety of bioactivities and play an important role as ideal natural sources of antimicrobial, antioxidant and chemopreventive agents [15–17]. They have potential therapeutic applications in the prevention of cancer [18].

2. Chemical composition of essential oil

Essential oils (EOs) are volatile constituents obtained from aromatic plant material, including leaves, rhizomes, flowers, roots, bark, seeds, peel, fruits, wood and whole plants [19]. A few of the essential oils are found in animal sources, for example, musk and sperm whale, or are produced by microorganisms [20]. In plants, essential oils occur in oil cells, secretory ducts or cavities, or in glandular hairs. Essential oils can be isolated by steam distillation from an aromatic plant because of their volatility [21]. Different constituents in EOs exhibit varying smell or flavor [9]. The perception of individual volatile compounds depends on their threshold [22].

Essential oils are a complex mixture of polar and non-polar compounds [23]. The essential oil composition depends on the species of the extracted plant, the geographic location of this plant, harvest time and extraction technique [24].

EOs can be classified into the four main groups: [25, 26]

1. Terpenes, related to isoprene
2. Straight-chain compounds not containing any side chain
3. Phenylpropanoids (benzene derivatives)
4. Miscellaneous group having varied structures not included in first three groups (sulfur- or nitrogen-containing compounds)

2.1. Terpenes, related to isoprene or isopentene

Essential oils constituents can be divided into two major groups: terpene hydrocarbons and oxygenated compounds [27].

2.1.1. Terpene hydrocarbons

Terpenes are the most common class of chemical compounds found in essential oils [28]. Terpenes are synthesized in the cytoplasm of plant cells, through the mevalonic acid pathway [19]. Terpenes have been regarded as polymers of isoprene (C_5H_8) joined in a repetitive head-to-tail manner [29] as shown in **Figure 1**.

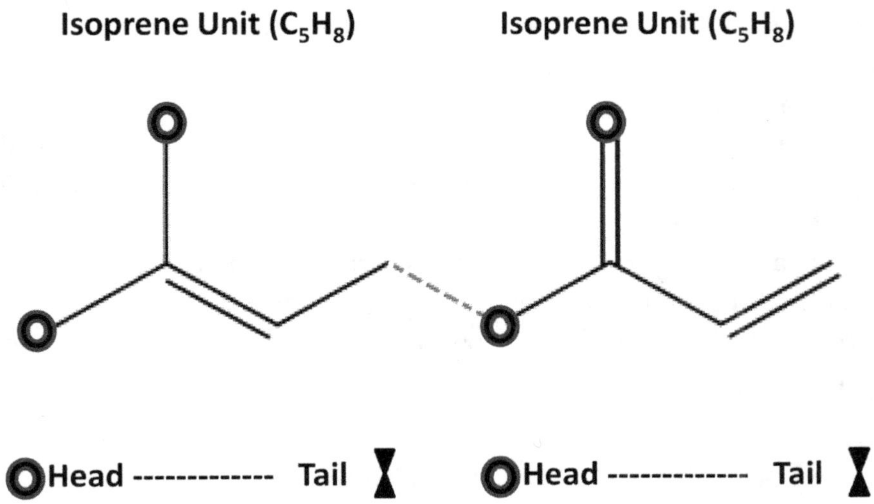

Figure 1. Link of isoprene molecules.

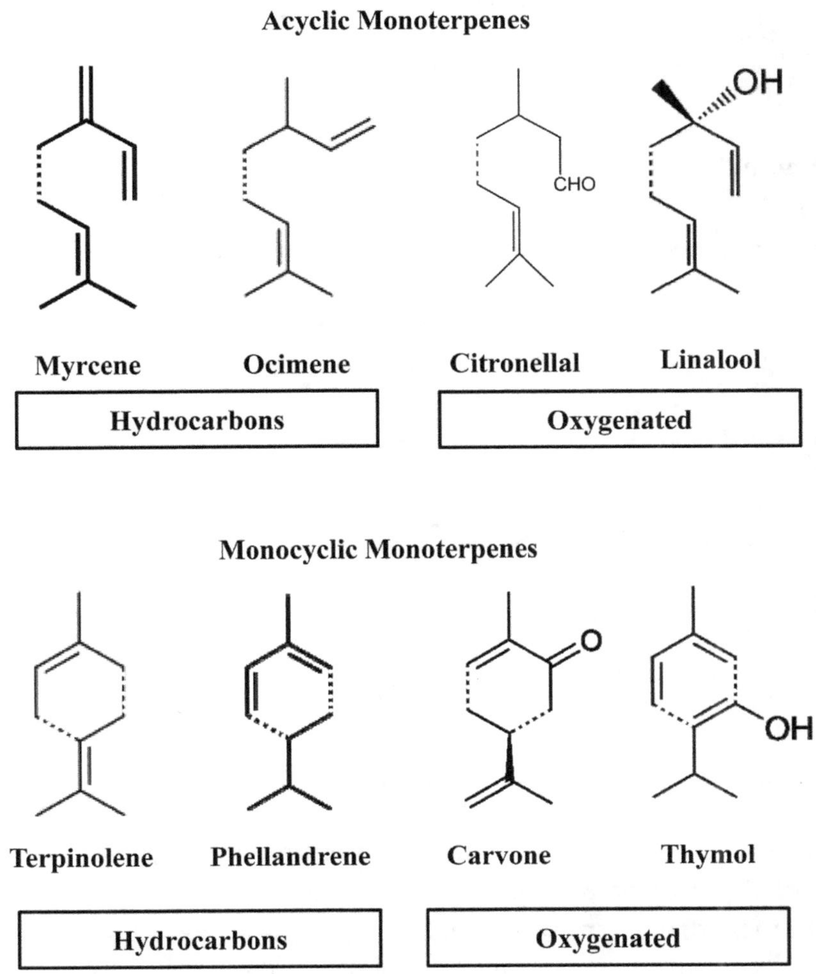

Figure 2. Chemical structures of acyclic and monocyclic monoterpenes.

They could be classified according to the fusion of the isoprene units or to the number of the rings [28]. Terpenes can be classified into hemiterpenes (1 unit), monoterpenes (2 units), sesquiterpenes (3 units), diterpenes (4 units), sesterterpenes (5 units), triterpenes (6 units) and polyterpenes (many units) [30]. The combinations of two isoprene units are called a "terpene unit." Monoterpenes ($C_{10}H_{16}$) are formed by the attachment of two isoprene units (at least one double bond). These terpenes have a hydrocarbon skeleton which can be rearranged into acyclic, cyclic, or aromatic (**Figure 2**). Cyclic monoterpenes can be classified according to their ring size such as monocyclic monoterpenes, bicyclic monoterpenes and tricyclic monoterpenes [31] **Figure 3**. These compounds oxidize easily because of their rapid reaction to air and heat sources [32].

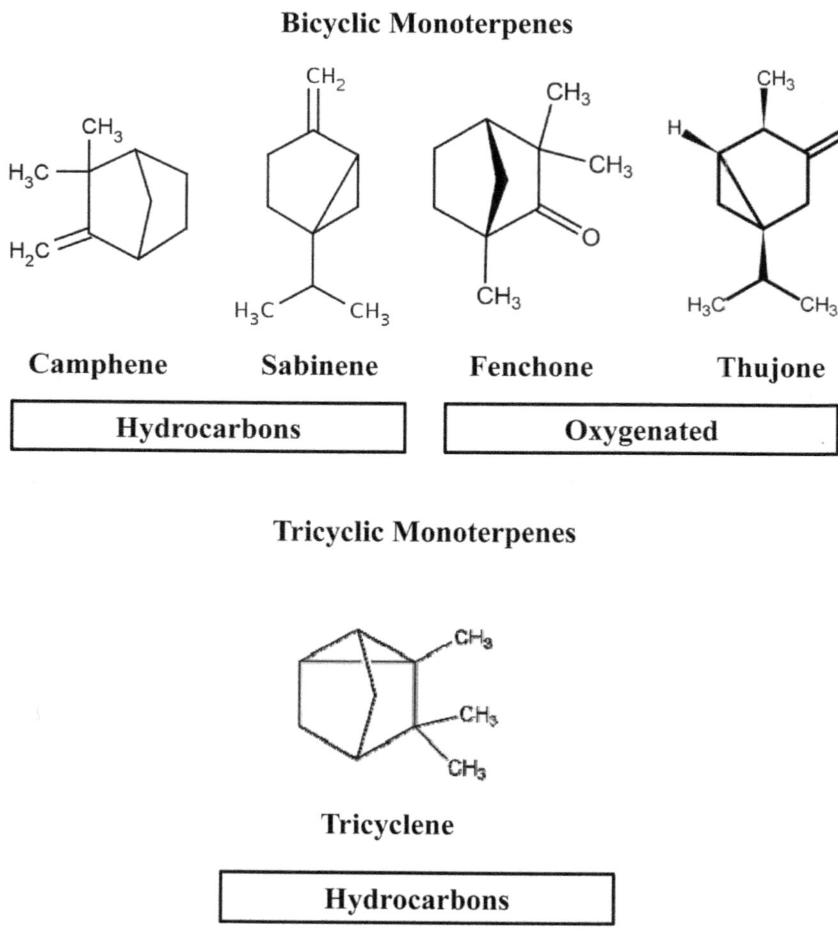

Figure 3. Chemical structures of bicyclic and tricyclic monoterpenes.

Sesquiterpenes ($C_{15}H_{24}$) are the second to the dominant monoterpenes. They are formed from the combination of three isoprene units [29]. Sesquiterpenes are unsaturated compounds. There are linear, branched, or cyclic sesquiterpenes (**Figure 4**). Sesquiterpenes are unsaturated compounds. Cyclic sesquiterpenes can be classified into monocyclic, bicyclic, or tricyclic [31] (**Figure 5**). Diterpenes are formed by the head-to-tail combinations of four isoprene units followed by rearrangement and/or substitutions (**Figure 6**).

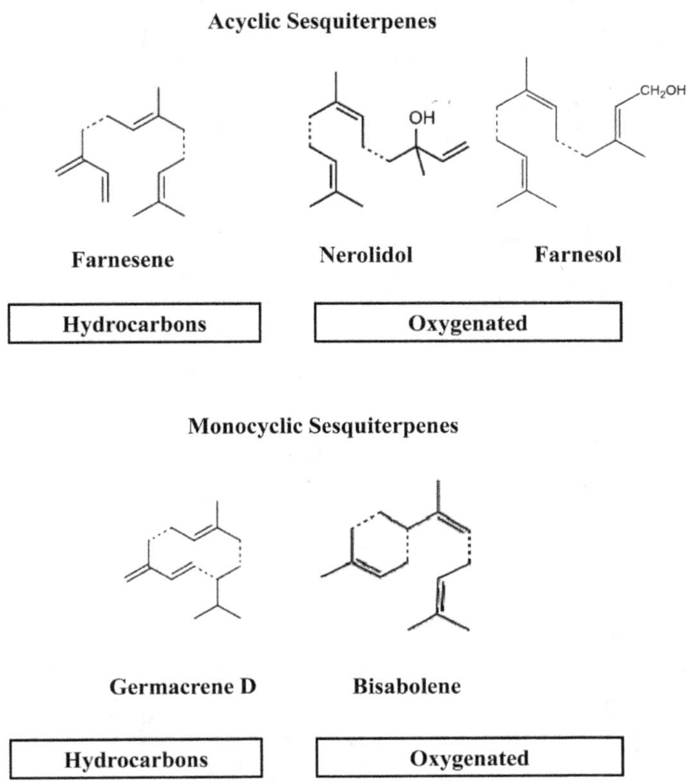

Figure 4. Chemical structures of acyclic and monocyclic sesquiterpenes.

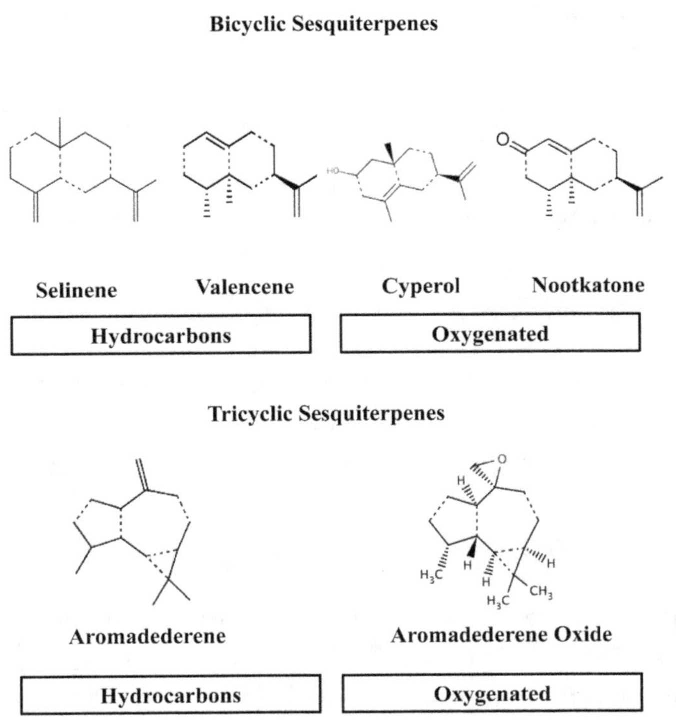

Figure 5. Chemical structures of bicyclic and tricyclic sesquiterpenes.

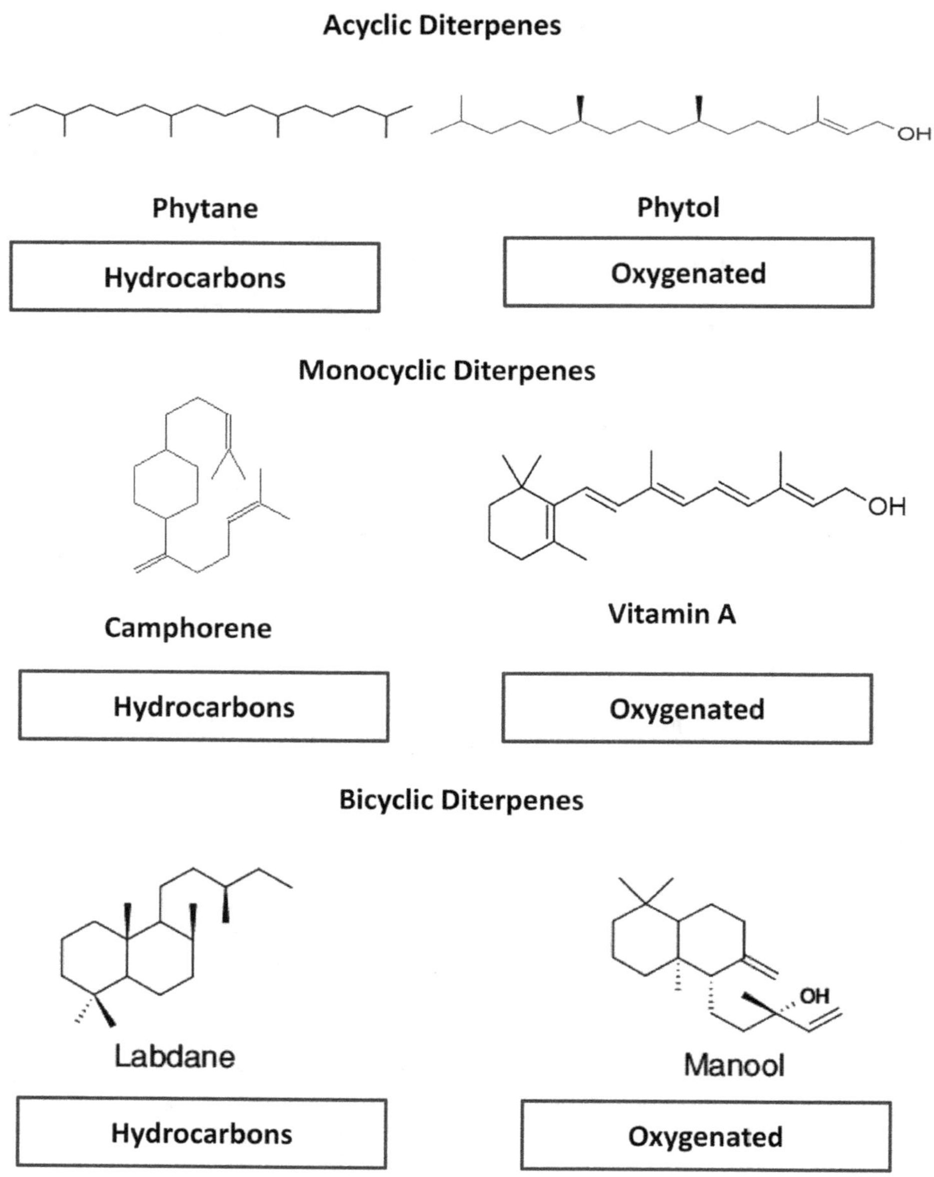

Figure 6. Chemical structures of acyclic, monocyclic and bicyclic diterpenes.

They are important components of plant resins [33]. Diterpenes, triterpenes and tetraterpenes are present at a very low concentration in essential oils [27, 34]. Their recovery increases with increasing steam distillation times [35] and influenced by the extraction method.

2.1.2. *Oxygenated compounds (terpenoids)*

The oxygenated compounds are highly odoriferous [36]. Terpenoids are volatile secondary metabolites which give plants their fragrance [37]. Terpenoids can be subdivided into aldehydes, ethers, alcohols, esters, ketones, phenols and epoxides [19]. Examples: (+)-Borneol occurs in camphor, rosemary and lavender oils. It has a camphor-like odor, with a slightly peppery note [38]. Carvacrol is found in oregano and thyme [39] oils. It has a herbaceous, phenolic odor [32]. (-)-Carvone has a herbal scent and is found in caraway seed oil; (+)-carvone with a spicy-minty odor can be found in spearmint oil [40]. 1,8-Cineole is obtained primarily by isolation from eucalyptus oil. It has a camphor odor [41].

2.2. Straight-chain compounds, not containing any side branches

This group contains only straight chain non-terpenoid hydrocarbons and their oxygen derivatives: alcohols, aldehydes, ketones, acids, ethers and esters. These hydrocarbons range from n-heptane, to compounds with 35 carbon atoms. Heptane content represented 3.8 and 36.8% of the wood volatile oils of *Pinus jeffreyi* and *Pinus sabiniana,* respectively [42]. The leaf alcohol (3(Z)-hexen-1-ol, **Figure 7**) and its esters are responsible for the intense grassy-green odor of freshly cut green grass and leaves via the octadecenoic pathway [43–45].

$$CH_3\text{-}CH_2\text{-}CH{=}CH\text{-}CH_2\text{-}CH_2\text{-}OH$$

Figure 7. Chemical structure of leaf alcohol.

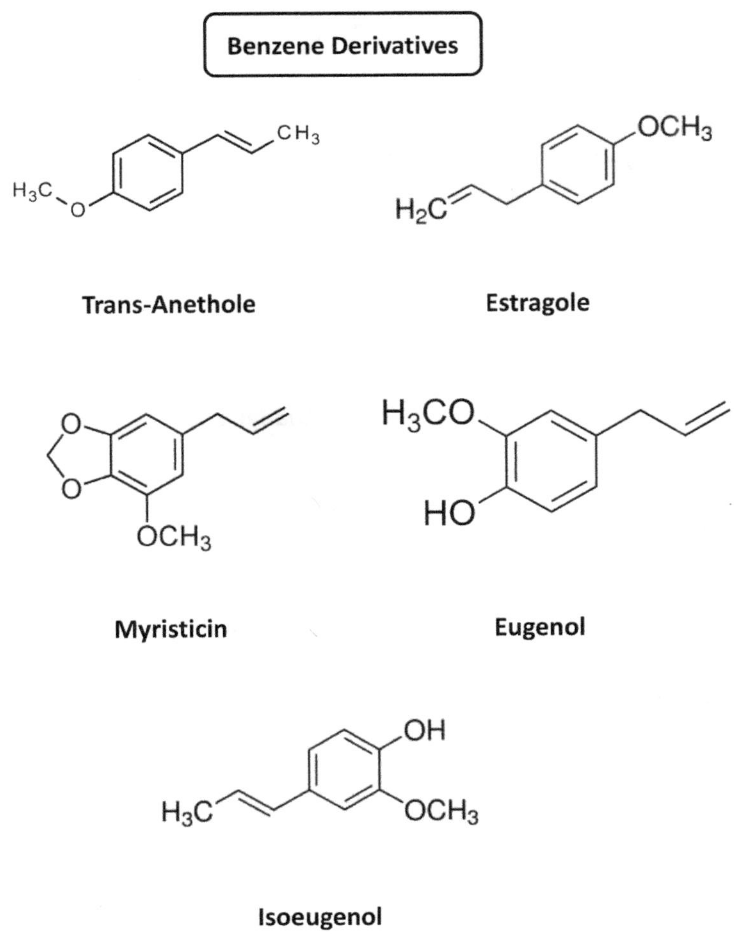

Figure 8. Chemical structures of phenylpropenes.

2.3. Phenylpropenes (benzene derivatives)

These aromatic compounds are an important group to flavor and fragrance industry though it constitutes a relatively small part of the essential oils. This non-terpenoid group comprises of constituents derived from n-propyl benzene. The aromatic ring may carry hydroxy, methoxy and methylene dioxy groups; the propyl side chain may contain hydroxyl or carboxyl group [25].

Phenylpropenes constitute a subfamily of phenylpropanoids that are synthesized from the amino acid phenylalanine and L-tyrosine via the shikimic acid pathway [46]. Examples of this group include trans-anethole, methyl chavicol, eugenol, isoeugenol, vanillin, safrole, myristicin and cinnamaldehyde [19, 47] (**Figure 8**).

2.4. Miscellaneous group (sulfur- and nitrogen-containing compounds)

The representatives of this group are the compounds, which are not included in the above mentioned three groups [25]. They are different degradation products originating from unsaturated fatty acids, lactones, terpenes, glycosides and sulfur- and nitrogen-containing compounds [48].

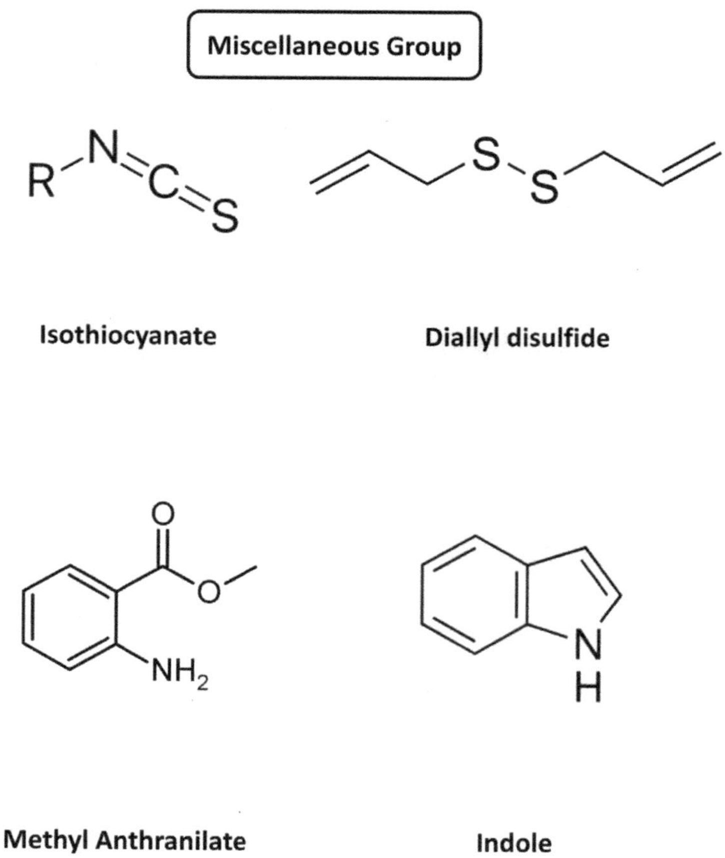

Figure 9. Chemical structures of sulfur- and nitrogen-containing compounds.

Sulfur- and nitrogen-containing compounds occur mainly as aglycones or glucosinolates, or their breakdown products, which include isothiocyanates [49]. The Brassicaceae is an important source of glucosinolates and isothiocyanates [50]. Garlic, onion, leek and shallots contain volatile sulfur compounds, namely allyl sulfide, dimethyl sulfide, diallyl disulfide and dimethylthiophene [51]. The sulfur compounds are responsible for the characteristic aroma and taste [52]. Cysteine sulfoxides including alliin predominate in mature, intact Allium spp., along with γ-glutamylcysteines [53]. Upon rupture, such as when chopped or pressed, the action of a class of enzymes known as alliinases catalyzes the conversion of cysteine sulfoxides into the volatile thiosulfinates [54] including allicin. Allicin makes up 70–80% of the thiosulfinates. Allicin and other thiosulfinates decompose diallyl sulfide, diallyl disulfide, diallyl trisulfide, dithiins and ajoene, while the γ-glutamylcysteines are converted to S-allyl cysteine through a non-alliin/allicin pathway [53]. Nitrogen-containing compounds are found in only a few essential oils. Examples include methyl anthranilate, indole, pyridine and pyrazine. Methyl anthranilate is present in orange, lemon and bergamot oils [35] and jasmine oil [55]. Indole occurs in neroli and some citrus fruit oils [32]. Pyridines and pyrazines occur in black pepper, sweet orange and vetiver oils [35] (**Figure 9**).

3. Quality indices of essential oils

The studies have shown that a differentiation in oil quality and volatile components is associated with climatic conditions, geographical location of collection sites and other ecological and genetic factors. The influence of those factors on the accumulation of distinct volatile compounds defines its chemotypes [56–58].

3.1. Black pepper oil

Black pepper oil is obtained from the dried unripe fruits of *Piper nigrum* [59]. The monoterpenes hydrocarbons (i.e., limonene, sabinene, β-pinene, 3-carene and phellandrene) to sesquiterpenes hydrocarbons (β-caryophyllene) ratio represents the quality of the oil and indicates the aroma value; the monoterpenes provide the body of the flavor, but the sesquiterpenes provide the spicy note. A lower value represents a higher quality of the essential oil [60, 61]. A high total monoterpenes content results in a strong "peppery" top-note and a predominantly pinene content of the terpene fraction gives a turpentine-like note, while a high caryophyllene content results in a sweet, flowery note, which is more desirable in the flavor industry [62]. In addition to the ratio of monoterpenes to sesquiterpenes, the oxygenated compounds are supposed to provide the heart of the aroma of pepper oil [63]. The pepper oil extracted with supercritical fluid carbon dioxide was found to have a higher content of caryophyllene and oxygenated sesquiterpene compounds. The volatile oil obtained under these conditions was considered superior to the steam-distilled oil, using aroma, taste and monoterpene to sesquiterpene hydrocarbons ratio as the criteria [64, 65]. Tipsrisukond et al. [66] reported that this ratio reached 3.02 and 0.95 in the steam distilled oil and supercritical fluid extract, respectively. On the other hand, this ratio was found to be 2.21 in the hydro-distilled oil while it was 1.66 in the supercritical fluid extract [67].

Storage of black pepper hammer milled powder for 6 months at 4°C, markedly increased monoterpene to sesquiterpene hydrocarbons ratio from 1.31 to 4.47. They attributed this increase to the degradation of some sesquiterpenes, as a result of oxidative decomposition during storage [68].

3.2. Cardamom oil

Cardamom oil is obtained from the dried ripe fruits of *Elettaria cardamomum* [59]. Salzer [60] reported that 1,8-cineole and α-terpinyl acetate together with the terpene alcohols are important for the evaluation of the aroma quality of cardamom. 1,8-Cineole is reported to contribute to pungency while terpinyl acetate is known for its desirable, pleasant flavor of cardamom [69, 70]. The higher level of α-terpinyl acetate compared to that of 1,8-cineole could be used as an indicator of the superior quality of cardamom essential oil [71, 72].

Monoterpenes hydrocarbons are less odoriferous than oxygenated monoterpenes [73]. Amma et al. [74] recorded superior flavor quality for the Malabar variety with the highest α-terpinyl acetate/1,8-cineole ratio (1.55) when compared with the Mysore variety (1.34). Morsy [75] found that this ratio exceeded 1.6 when ultrasound-assisted extraction (30 W, for 30 min) was used as a pretreatment for hydrodistillation (30 min) compared to 1.13 when hydrodistillation was conducted for 6 h. The presence of a low level of hydrocarbons in cardamom oil could be used as an indicator of its high quality [74].

3.3. Caraway essential oil

Caraway oil is obtained from the dried ripe fruits of *Carum carvi* [59]. The main components of caraway essential oil are carvone and limonene, whose mixture constituted from 97.69 to 98.62% of total oil composition [76]. The overall quality of fruits is considered to correlate with the content of essential oil and its carvone/limonene (C/L) ratio: the higher the ratio, the better the quality. C/L ratio varies from 0.90 to 2.74 [77, 78]. This ratio is variable during ripening. Limonene is of high level in green immature seeds [79]. Aćimović et al. [76] considered the quality of essential oil poor when C/L ratio recorded 0.47. The essential oil of biennial caraway varieties usually has a higher C/L ratio compared to that of the annual varieties [80, 81]. The C/L ratio decreased with the time of storage (70 days, at room temperature) of caraway seed samples [82].

3.4. Peppermint oil

Peppermint (*Mentha piperita*) has bright green leaves, with a fresh, slightly sweet, tangy, peppery and strong menthol notes [83]. The principal constituents of peppermint oil are menthol (30–55%), menthone, menthyl acetate and other esters [84]. The ratio of menthol/menthone is the major determinant of the flavoring quality of distilled essential oil [85]. For commercial purposes, a high oil yield with a ratio of menthol to menthone of 2:1 is desired [86]. In general, high-quality peppermint oil (i.e., high menthol/menthone ratio) develops during full bloom [87]. The English oil contains 60–70% of menthol, the Japanese oil contains 85% and the American only about 50%. The odor and taste afford a good indication of the quality of the oil.

3.5. Lavender oil

Lavender flowers (*Lavendula angustifolia*) have a strong perfumery odor with crusty woody undertones a camphor-like note. The leaves have herbaceous and more pronounced bitter notes [83]. Linalool and its ester form, linalyl acetate, are the most abundant monoterpenes in lavender varieties and are the most desired components of the lavender oil, while trace amounts of camphor generally contribute an undesirable odor, diminishing the quality of the oil [88–90]. The linalyl acetate to linalool ratio may change in different distillation times and may affect the final odor of the oil [91]. The oil samples that were obtained after 1 and 2 h of steam distillation had linalyl acetate to linalool ratio of 0.57 and 0.44, respectively. The ratio of linalyl acetate to linalool should be higher than one in high-quality lavender oil [92].

3.6. Rose oil

Rosa damascena is an ornamental plant. This plant is used for food flavoring as dried flowers, dried bud and dried petals [93]. The flavor compounds that contribute to the distinctive scent of rose oil are β-damascenone, β-damascone, β-ionone and rose oxide. Even though these compounds exist in <1% of rose oil, they make up for more than 90% of the odor content due to their low odor thresholds. The concentration of β-damascenone is considered as the marker for the quality of the rose oil [94, 95].

Citronellol/geraniol (C/G) ratio could be used for evaluating the quality of rose oil [96]. The finest quality rose oil has C/G ratio between 1.25 and 1.30 [97]. In the rose oil trade, the citronellol content should be higher than 35%. The oils from non-fermented petals generally contain citronellol lower than this level. Therefore, a short-term fermentation is conducted to increase the citronellol content. The C/G ratios were higher in the oils distilled from long-term fermented petals (e.g., 10.3 in 36 h fermentation) than non-fermented petals (0.56). Based on these results, rose oils distilled from long-term fermented petals are of poor quality [98].

3.7. Ginger oil

Ginger oil is obtained from the rhizomes of *Zingiber officinale* [59]. α-Zingiberene is the major sesquiterpene hydrocarbon of ginger oil [99]. Salzer [60] reported that citral, zingiberene, β-sesquiphellandrene and ar-curcumene could be used for evaluating the quality of the ginger oil. Govindarajan [100] reported that citral and citronellyl acetate are co-determinants of the odor of ginger oil, while zingiberene and β-sesquiphellandrene are the main components of the freshly prepared oil. ar-Curcumene increased with storage. A good quality oil has a ratio of zingiberene + β-sesquiphellandrene to ar-curcumene = 2:3.

The lemony note is attributed to citral together with α-terpineol, while nerolidol is responsible for the woody note. β-Sesquiphellandrene and ar-curcumene contribute to the characteristic ginger flavor [101].

3.8. Juniper oil

Juniper (*Juniperus communis*) has green and sharp leaves (needles) [102]. Juniper's odor is woody and astringent with sweet, lemon and pinelike overtones. It has a ginlike aroma. Its flavor is released when it is lightly crushed [83].

Butkienë et al. [103] identified 143 components in the juniper leaves essential oil. They found that monoterpenes (M)/sesquiterpenes (S) ratio ranged from 2:1 to 5:1 according to localities in Vilnius district, Lithuania. Sela et al. [104] found that M/S ratio ranged from 1:1 to 3:1 for leaves essential oil of Macedonian juniper, from different localities. Orav et al. [105] reported

(2.5:1). Pourmortazavi et al. [106] found that supercritical fluid extraction products from *J. communis* L. leaves using carbon dioxide were markedly different from the hydrodistilled oil. The hydrodistilled oil was characterized by a high concentration of β-phellanderene. The ratio of α-pinene to 3-carene in hydrodistilled oil was high (0.62) compared with that of the supercritical carbon dioxide extracts (0.04–0.065). Looman and Svendsen [107] reported that the average ratio of α-pinene:sabinene:limonene was generally 21:45:5 in the leaf essential oil of Norwegian mountain juniper (*Juniperus communis* L. var. saxatilis Pall).

3.9. Oregano, thyme and savory oils

Oregano, wild marjoram, *Origanum vulgare*, has dark green fresh leaves. Fresh oregano is available whole, chopped, or minced. The dried light green leaves are available whole, flaked, or ground [83]. The thyme plant, *Thymus vulgaris* L., is an evergreen herb that is used for its flavor [108]. Summer savory, *Satureja hortensis,* is often used as a culinary herb either as a fresh or dried herb [109].

In oregano essential oil, the total content of the thymol and carvacrol was the highest and amounted to 67.51%; in thyme essential oil, 47.47%; and in savory essential oil, 49.71%. The thymol and carvacrol types have sharp, warm and penetrating herbal (thyme type) odors, with woody, spicy and tobacco-like notes; thymol itself has a powerful, medicated and herbaceous odor while carvacrol itself has a tar-like odor [110]. The ratio of carvacrol to thymol in oregano, thyme and savory essential oils was 15:1, 1:19 and 1.8:1, respectively [111]. Oils containing predominantly thymol are generally considered of superior quality [112, 113].

3.10. Lemongrass oil

Lemongrass (*Cymbopogon* spp.) is a tall perennial C4 grass belonging to the family Poaceae (Gramineae), commonly known as the "sweet grass family" [114]. Lemongrass gives a refreshing lemon-lime-like taste with a tinge of mint and ginger. It has a citral odor with floral-like (rose) and a fresh, grassy aroma. Its flavor is found in the lower tender part of the stem. The root-end stalk gives the most flavor. The whole fresh stalk becomes aromatic when it is crushed or cut. The dried form has a very little aroma [83]. The quality of the lemongrass essential oil is measured by its citral content [115, 116]. Citral is a natural mixture of two monoterpene aldehydes, geranial (trans isomer) and neral (cis isomer). Supercritical fluid extraction was found to be a superior process than steam distillation, producing better quality lemongrass oil containing 90% citral [117]. The leaves yield aromatic oil, containing 70–90% citral. *C. flexuosus* has higher citral content than *C. citratus* [118, 119].

4. Bioactivities of essential oil constituents

Essential oils from different plant parts exhibit different biological activities [120]. Biological activities of essential oils include antioxidant, antimicrobial, antiviral, anti-mutagenic and anticancer [34]. Essential oils are complex mixtures of terpenoids and phenylpropanoids compounds extracted by distillation or solvent extraction [121]. Overall activity cannot be attributed to only one of the major constituents [122]. The inactive compounds might influence resorption, the rate of reactions and biological activity of the active compounds. The combination of the major and minor constituents modifies the activity to exert significant synergistic or antagonistic effect [123].

4.1. Antioxidant activity

Antioxidants are substances that protect cells from being oxidized by free radicals. Reactive oxygen species (ROS) are highly reactive toxic molecules. ROS induced oxidative diseases such as ageing, arteriosclerosis, cancer, Alzheimer's disease and Parkinson's disease [124]. Living cells possess scavenging activity to diminish excess ROS that induced cellular injury. These mechanisms become inefficient, with ageing and under external stress. Therefore, dietary supplementation of natural and synthetic antioxidants is required [125]. Some synthetic antioxidants cause liver damage and have carcinogenic effects. Natural antioxidants are preferred to synthetic ones [126].

The essential oil of lemon balm, containing neral/citral, citronellal, menthone and isomenthone, showed strong antioxidant activity [127].

The essential oils with good radical-scavenging activity could be arranged in the following order, clove > cinnamon > nutmeg > basil > oregano > thyme [128].

Misharina and Samusenko [129] stored a mixture of lemon, coriander and clove buds essential oils (1:1:1) at room temperature in the light for 145 days. They found that the mixture of the three essential oils increased the stability of limonene and γ-terpinene significantly higher than in the individual essential oils and inhibited oxidation of hexanal efficiently. It was shown that terpene hydrocarbons break free-radical chain reactions, which is accompanied by their irreversible oxidation into inert compounds, such as *p*-cymene. Therefore, terpene hydrocarbons do not exhibit the properties of prooxidants.

Wei and Shibamoto [130] proposed that terpenes and terpenoids that contribute to the antioxidant activity of essential oils include α-terpinene, β-terpinene and β-terpinolene in tea tree; 1,8-cineole in water mint, menthone and isomenthone in peppermint; thymol, eugenol and linalool in black cumin, cinnamon bark and ginger; and thymol and eugenol in thyme and clove leaf.

Eugenol, the major constituent of clove essential oil, was found to have an inhibitory activity against lipid peroxidation by interfering with chain reactions of free radicals. The inhibitory activity of eugenol was about fivefold higher than that observed for alpha-tocopherol [131]. Thymol and carvacrol the main constituents of thyme oil are shown to act as strong antioxidants [132]. The antioxidant activity of caraway oil may be due to the presence of linalool, carvacrol, anethole and estragole [133]. Marjoram and clove essential oils exerted a powerful antioxidant activity in beef burger prepared with sunflower oil during storage at -18°C for 3 months. The addition of marjoram oil at 250 mg/kg kept thiobarbituric acid value of the beef burger samples after 3 months of storage at a level not significantly different from that of control samples stored frozen for 1 month [134]. Flavoring refined corn oil with thyme increased its oxidative stability (induction time) from 4.36 to 6.48 h [135]. Blending cold-pressed oregano (*Origanum vulgare*) oil with sunflower oil at 10 and 20% levels increased its induction time from 3 to 6 h and 8 h, respectively. Assiri et al. [136] attributed the superior antioxidant activity of sunflower oil blends to the high levels of phenolic compounds in oregano oil.

4.2. Antibacterial activity

Essential oils display broad-spectrum inhibitory activities against various bacterial pathogens [137]. Essential oil is easily permeable through the cell wall and cell membrane due to its lipophilic characteristic. Interaction of essential oil components with polysaccharides, fatty acids and phospholipids causes loss of membrane integrity, leakage of the cellular contents, interference in proton pump activity and leads to cell death [124, 138–140]. Other important mechanisms of action include denaturation of cellular proteins [9, 34, 141]. Carvone partitioned in the lipid membrane [142], while terpinen-4-ol inhibits cellular respiration and both damage cell membrane function as a permeable barrier [143]. Carvacrol and *p*-cymene accumulate in the lipid phase of the membrane by causing expansion of the phospholipids bilayer and increasing spaces through which ion leakage might occur [144].

Sage essential oil is rich in antimicrobial agents [145]. The single layer wall of *S. aureus* is highly sensitive to essential oils with a high content of *p*-cymene [34]. Cold-pressed oregano (*Origanum vulgare*) oil exhibited antimicrobial activity against *Staphylococcus aureus, Escherichia coli, Salmonella enteritidis,* and *Listeria monocytogenes* with minimum lethal concentrations ranging between 160 and 320 μg/mL. The antimicrobial activity of the oregano oil could be due to the presence of phenolic constituents and the differences in the permeability of cell wall of those bacteria [136]. Ghabraie et al. [146] found that essential oils of Red bergamot (Flower top) and Chinese cinnamon (bark) inhibited *Escherichia coli, Listeria monocytogenes, Staphylococcus aureus* and *Salmonella Typhimurium*. The inhibition zone ranged from 20 to more than 70 mm depending on the target bacteria. Chinese cinnamon inhibited *S. aureus* and *E. coli* at minimum inhibition concentration of 470 ppm in microbroth dilution assay. Antibacterial activity of Red bergamot oil could be due to carvacrol and *p*-cymene, while trans-cinnamaldehyde is responsible for this effect in Chinese cinnamon oil. Radaelli et al. [147] studied the antimicrobial activities of basil, rosemary, marjoram, peppermint, thyme and anise essential oils against *Clostridium perfringens* strain A. They found that all oils showed bactericidal activity at their minimum inhibitory concentration, except anise oil, which displayed bacteriostatic effect.

4.3. Antifungal activity

Fungi are important causes of human infections [148]. Several crops are susceptible to fungal attack either in the field or during storage [149]. Fungicide residues are problems for the food industry [150]. Prevention of fungal growth is an effective way of impeding mycotoxin accumulation [151]. Essential oils have the ability to attack the life cycle of molds [152].

The high cost of essential oils production and the low concentration of active constituents limit their direct use in the control of fungal diseases of plants and animals. Therefore, investigation of antifungal compounds of the essential oils is considered important because of the possibility of synthesizing these compounds for the use in the control of fungal diseases [153].

Bouchra et al. [154] reported that the major essential oils constituents of Moroccan Labiatae *Origanum compactum* and *Thymus glandulosus* consisted of carvacrol, linalyl acetate and thymol. Both oils inhibited completely the growth of the mycelium of *Botrytis cinerea* at 100 ppm.

Serrano et al. [155] reduced the growth of yeasts and molds for stored cherries by developing active packaging materials containing eugenol, menthol, thymol and eucalyptol.

The essential oil of cinnamon had a high antifungal effect (very low minimum inhibitory concentration) against *Aspergillus flavus* [156, 157]. The antimycotic activity of *Cinnamomum zeylanicum* bark essential oil is due to the presence of cinnamaldehyde [158].

Carvacrol, the major active ingredient, of oregano oil was found to cause complete inhibition of *Saccharomyces cerevisiae* growth at 0.01%. Its potency was 1500 times that of the oregano oil. In contrast, the γ-terpinene, which is the biosynthetic precursor of carvacrol, was ineffective as a fungicide. Carvacrol interfered in the target of rapamycin signaling pathway, resulting in loss of viability. Eugenol, thymol and carvacrol affect Ca^{2+} and H^{+} homeostasis leading to loss of ions and inhibition of *Saccharomyces cerevisiae* [159]. Citral, citronellol, geraniol and geranyl acetate that are the major components of eucalyptus oil, tea tree oil and geranium oil possess cell cycle inhibitory activities against *Candida albicans* [160].

Sourmaghi et al. [161] found that hydrodistilled coriander essential oil had a potent antifungal activity against *Candida albicans*. Linalool was the major component in coriander oil. The essential oil of coriander had synergistic antimicrobial effect with amphotericin B [162].

Rahman et al. [153] reported that the hydrodistilled essential oil of the leaves of *Piper chaba* Hunter displayed potent antifungal activity against *Fusarium oxysporum, Phytophthora capsici, Colletotrichum capsici, Fusarium solani,* and *Rhizoctonia solani*. They attributed this activity to α-humulene, caryophyllene oxide, viridiflorol, globulol, β-selinene, spathulenol, (E)-nerolidol, linalool, 3-pentanol and *p*-cymene that present in the oil. At a concentration of 125 μg/mL, the fungicidal action of oil showed complete spore germination inhibition of *Phytophthora capsici.*

de Oliveira et al. [163] found that the essential oil of *Piper ilheusense* was active in combatting activity of *Candida albicans, Candida krusei,* and *Candida parapsilosis.* (E)-Caryophyllene and patchouli alcohol were the major components of the oil. γ-Cadinene, germacrene B and gleenol were found in significant quantities. Marino et al. [164] reported that the minor components might be involved in some type of synergism with the other active compounds.

4.4. Anticancer activity

Cancer is a multifactorial disease contributing towards the uncontrolled growth of the abnormal cells, leading to the formation of a tumor [165]. Carcinogenesis is a multistep process and oxidative damage that is linked to the formation of tumors. Secondary metabolites from different plants are capable of halting development of cancer [166]. Essential oil constituents have cytotoxic and antitumor activities. They play an important role in cancer prevention and treatment [18, 167]. Essential oils can be used in combination with cancer therapy to decrease the side effects of the drugs [168]. Cytotoxicity of essential oils is due to its action upon cellular integrity, leading to necrosis and apoptosis, cell cycle arrest and loss of key organelles function [169, 170]. Therefore, the evaluation of the anticancer activity of essential oils and their safety on normal cell lines are of great importance [171].

The essential oil of *Ricinus communis* leaves exhibited a moderate antiproliferative activity against cervical cancer line. The composition of the oil was predominantly by α-thujone and 1,8-cineole [172]. The *Eugenia caryophyllata* essential oil showed significant cytotoxic effects against HT29, A549 and Hep2 cancer cell lines. The cytotoxicity is likely due to the high concentrations of phenolic compounds, particularly eugenol [173].

Eugenol displayed cytotoxic action in a dose-dependent manner against human hepatoma cells HepG2 and colon cells Caco-2 [174], HL-60 leukemia cells [175] and osteoblastic cell line U2OS [176].

Terpenoids of essential oils prevent tumor cell proliferation [34]. Linalool and linalyl acetate represented the major constituents in lavender essential oil. They were more cytotoxic than the whole essential oil against 153BR, HNDF and HMEC-1 cancer cell lines [177]. Geraniol suppressed the growth of MCF-7 breast cancer cells [178] and PC-3 prostate cancer cells [179]. It was reported to interfere with membrane functions, ion homeostasis; inhibit DNA synthesis; and reduce the size of colon tumors [180]. β-Caryophyllene did not inhibit cell growth of MCF-7 breast cancer cell lines, but α-humulene was cytotoxic. However, β-caryophyllene potentiated the cytotoxicity of α-humulene [181]. Limonene and linalyl acetate had no effect on neuroblastoma cells. However, their combination induced apoptosis [182]. This synergic effect was consistent in several studies for antitumor properties [183].

Carvacrol is a major component of oregano and thyme essential oils. It inhibits tumor cell proliferation and induces apoptosis in human colon cancer cell lines, HCT116 and LoVo [184] and in human oral squamous cell carcinoma [185]. Perillyl alcohol decreases the growth of HCT116 cells [186].

5. Conclusion

The essential oils are multi-component systems, while their key components represent single component systems. Quality assurance of essential oils is imperative to ensure authenticity and product quality. The ratio of one special component or group of components to another is one of the quality indices of an essential oil as it affects its aroma.

Some of the essential oil constituents contribute to the essential oil antioxidant, antimicrobial and anticancer activities, regardless their concentration. They contribute by their synergistic effect to the property of the essential oil.

Author details

Nashwa Fathy Sayed Morsy

Address all correspondence to: nanafsm@yahoo.com

Food Science Department, Faculty of Agriculture, Cairo University, Giza, Egypt

References

[1] British Pharmacopoeia Commission. British pharmacopoeia (vol. II). London (GB): The Stationary Office; 2013.

[2] Burdock GA. Handbook of flavor ingredients. Fenaroli's handbook of flavor ingredients. 5th ed. New York: CRC Press; 2005.

[3] Sarac N, Ugur A. Antimicrobial activities of the essential oils of *Origanum onites* L., *Origanum vulgare* L. subspecies hirtum (Link) Ietswaart, *Satureja thymbra* L. and *Thymus cilicicus* Boiss. & Bal. growing wild in Turkey. Journal of Medicinal Food. 2008;11:568–573. doi:10.1089/jmf.2007.0520

[4] Mechergui K, Coelho JA, Serra MC, Lamine SB, Boukhchina S, Khouja ML. Essential oils of *Origanum vulgare* L. subsp. glandulosum (Desf.) Ietswaart from Tunisia: chemical composition and antioxidant activity. Journal of the Science of Food and Agriculture. 2010;90:1745–1749. doi:10.1002/jsfa.4011

[5] Hussaina AI, Anwar F, Sherazi STH, Przybylski R. Chemical composition, antioxidant and antimicrobial activities of basil (*Ocimum basilicum*) essential oils depends on seasonal variations. Food Chemistry. 2008;108:986–995. doi:10.1016/j.foodchem.2007.12.010

[6] Figueiredo AC, Barroso JG, Pedro LG, Scheffer JJC. Factors affecting secondary metabolite production in plants: volatile components and essential oils. Flavour and Fragrance Journal. 2008; 23:213–226. doi:10.1002/ffj.1875

[7] Taiz L, Zeiger E. Plant physiology, 5th ed. MA, USA: Sinauer Associates Inc., Publishers Sunderland; 2010. p. 782. doi:10.1086/658450

[8] Di Cesare LF, Forni E, Viscardi D, Nani RC. Changes in the chemical composition of basil caused by different drying procedures. Journal of Agricultural and Food Chemistry. 2003;51:3575–3581. doi:10.1021/jf021080o

[9] Burt S. Essential oils: their antibacterial properties and potential applications in foods—a review. International Journal of Food Microbiology. 2004;94:223–253. doi: 10.1016/j.ijfoodmicro.2004.03.022

[10] Karakaya S, El SN, Karagözlü N, Sahin S. Antioxidant and antimicrobial activities of essential oils obtained from oregano (*Origanum vulgare* spp. hirtum) by using different extraction methods. Journal of Medicinal Food. 2011;14:645–652. doi:10.1089/jmf.2010.0098

[11] Shahidi F, Zhong Y. Citrus oils and essences. In: Shahidi F. editor. Bailey's industrial oil and fat products. 6th ed. Wiley Interscience. Hoboken, NJ: John Wiley & Sons, Inc.; 2005. pp. 49–66. doi:10.1002/047167849X

[12] Başer KHC, Buchbauer G, editors. Handbook of essential oils science, technology and applications. 2nd ed. New York: CRC Press Taylor & Francis Group, LLC,; 2016. p. 1109. doi:10.1201/b19393

[13] Turek C, Stintzing FC. Stability of essential oils: a review. Comprehensive Reviews in Food Science and Food Safety. 2013;12:40–53. doi:10.1111/1541-4337.12006

[14] Reineccius G, editor. Source book of flavors. 2nd ed. Dordrecht: Springer Science +Business Media; 1994. 928 p. doi:10.1007/978-1-4615-7889-5

[15] Bassolé IH, Juliani HR. Essential oils in combination and their antimicrobial properties. Molecules. 2012;17:3989–4006. doi:10.3390/molecules17043989

[16] Iqbal T, Hussain AI, Chatha SAS, Naqvi SAR, Bokhari TH. Antioxidant activity and volatile and phenolic profiles of essential oil and different extracts of wild mint (*Mentha longifolia*) from the Pakistani Flora. Journal of Analytical Methods in Chemistry. 2013;536490. doi:10.1155/2013/536490

[17] Victoria FN, Lenardão EJ, Savegnago L, Perin G, Jacob RG, Alves D, da Silva WP, da Motta Ade S, Nascente Pda S. Essential oil of the leaves of *Eugenia uniflora* L.: antioxidant and antimicrobial properties. Food and Chemical Toxicology. 2012;50:2668–2674. doi: 10.1016/j.fct.2012.05.002

[18] Bhalla Y, Gupta VK, Jaitak V. Anticancer activity of essential oils: a review. Journal of the Science of Food and Agriculture. 2013;93:3643–3653. doi:10.1002/jsfa.6267

[19] Hyldgaard M, Mygind T, Meyer RL. Essential oils in food preservation: mode of action, synergies and interactions with food matrix components. Frontiers in Microbiology. 2012;3:1–24. doi:10.3389/fmicb.2012.00012

[20] Surburg H, Panten J. Common fragrance and flavor materials. Preparation, properties and uses. 6th ed. Germany: Wiley-VCH Verlag GmbH & Co.; 2016. pp. 84–85. doi: 10.1002/3527608214

[21] Ríos JL. Essential oils: what they are and how the terms are used and defined. In: Preedy VR, editors. Essential oils in food preservation, flavor and safety. New York: Academic Press; 2016. pp. 3–5.

[22] Tongnuanchan P, Benjakul S. Essential oils: extraction, bioactivities and their uses for food preservation. Journal of Food Science. 2014;79:1231–1249. doi:10.1111/1750-3841.12492

[23] Masango P. Cleaner production of essential oils by steam distillation. Journal of Cleaner Production. 2005;13:833–839. doi:10.1016/j.jclepro.2004.02.039

[24] Dima C, Dima S. Essential oils in foods: extraction, stabilization and toxicity. Current Opinion in Food Science. 2015;5:29–35. doi:10.1016/j.cofs.2015.07.003

[25] Shukla YM, Dhruve JJ, Patel NJ, Bhatnagar R, Talati JG, Kathiria KB. Plant secondary metabolites. New India Publishing Agency, New Delhi; 2009. p. 306.

[26] Schmidt E. Production of essential oils. In: Baser KHC, Buchbauer G, editors. Handbook of essential oils. Science, technology and applications. Taylor & Francis Group, New York; 2010. pp. 83–118.

[27] Mohamed AA, El-Emary GA, Ali HF. Influence of some citrus essential oils on cell viability, glutathione-s-transferase and lipid peroxidation in Ehrlich ascites carcinoma cells. Journal of American Science. 2010;6:820–826.

[28] Chizzola R. Regular monoterpenes and sesquiterpenes (essential oils). In: Ramawat KG, Mérillon JM, editors. Natural products. Berlin Heidelberg: Springer-Verlag; 2013. pp. 2973–3008. doi:10.1007/978-3-642-22144-6_130

[29] Croteau R, Kutchan TM, Lewis NG. Natural products (secondary metabolites). In: Buchanan B, Gruissem W, Jones R, editors. Biochemistry and molecular biology of plants. Rockville, MD, USA: American Society of Plant Biologists; 2000. pp. 1250–1268.

[30] Zuzarte M, Salgueiro L. Essential oils chemistry. In: de Sousa DP, Paraíba JP, editors. Bioactive essential oils and cancer. Switzerland: Springer International Publishing; 2015. pp. 19–28.. doi:10.1007/978-3-319-19144-7_2

[31] George, KW, Alonso-Gutierrez, J, Keasling JD, Lee TS. Isoprenoid drugs, biofuels and chemicals—artemisinin, farnesene and beyond. Advances in Biochemical Engineering/Biotechnology. 2015;148:355–389. doi:10.1007/10_2014_288

[32] Hunter M. Essential oils: art, agriculture, science, industry and entrepreneurship (a focus on the Asia-Pacific region). Agriculture issues and policies series. New York: Nova Science Publishers, Inc; 2009.

[33] Langenheim JH. Plant resins: chemistry, evolution, ecology and ethnobotany. Portland, OR, USA: Timber Press; 2003. p. 586.

[34] Bakkali F, Averbeck S, Averbeck D, Idaomar M. Biological effects of essential oils—a review. Food and Chemical Toxicology. 2008;46:446–475. doi: 10.1016/j.fct.2007.09.106

[35] Baser KHC, Demirci F. Chemistry of essential oils. In: Berger RG, editor. Flavours and fragrances—chemistry, bioprocessing and sustainability. Berlin: Springer; 2007. pp. 43–86. doi:10.1007/b136889

[36] Darjazi BB. A comparison of volatile components of flower of page mandarin obtained by ultrasound-assisted extraction and hydrodistillation. Journal of Medicinal Plants Research. 2011;5:2839–2847.

[37] Srividya N, Davis EM, Croteau RB, Lange BM. Functional analysis of (4S)-limonene synthase mutants reveals determinants of catalytic outcome in a model monoterpene synthase. Proceedings of the National Academy of Sciences. 2015;112:3332–3337. doi: 10.1073/pnas.1501203112

[38] Lafhal S, Vanloot P, Bombarda I, Kister J, Dupuy N. Identification of metabolomic markers of lavender and lavandin essential oils using mid-infrared spectroscopy. Vibrational Spectroscopy. 2016;85:79–90. doi:org/10.1016/j.vibspec.2016.04.004

[39] Siroli L, Patrignani F, Gardini F, Lanciotti R. Effects of sub-lethal concentrations of thyme and oregano essential oils, carvacrol, thymol, citral and trans-2-hexenal on membrane fatty acid composition and volatile molecule profile of *Listeria monocytogenes*, *Escherichia coli* and *Salmonella enteritidis*. Food Chemistry. 2015;182:185–192. doi:org/10.1016/j.foodchem.2015.02.136

[40] Nogoceke FP, Barcaro IMR, de Sousa DP andreatini R. Antimanic-like effects of (R)-(-)-carvone and (S)-(+)-carvone in mice. Neuroscience Letters. 2016;619:43–48. doi:org/10.1016/j.neulet.2016.03.013

[41] Navarro AM, García B, Hoyuelos FJ, Peñacoba IA, Leal J M. Preferential solvation and mixing behaviour of the essential oil 1,8-cineole with short-chain hydrocarbons. Fluid Phase Equilibria. 2016;429:127–136. doi: 10.1016/j.fluid.2016.08.035

[42] Adams RP, Wright JW. Alkanes and terpenes in wood and leaves of *Pinus jeffreyi* and *P. sabiniana*. The Journal of Essential Oil Research. 2012;24:435–440. doi:10.1080/10412905.2012.703512

[43] Hatanaka A, Kajiwara T, Matsui K. The biogeneration of green odour by green leaves and its physiological functions—past, present and future. Zeitschrift für Naturforschung. 1995;50:476–472. doi:10.1515/znc-1995-7-801

[44] Vasiliev AA, Cherkaev GV, Nikitina MA. Novel approach to fragrances with a green odour. Chemistry and Computational Simulation. Butlerov Communications. 2003; 4:33–43

[45] Gigot C, Ongena M, Fauconnier M-L, Wathelet J-P, Jardin PD, Thonart P. The lipoxygenase metabolic pathway in plants: potential for industrial production of natural green leaf volatiles. Biotechnology, Agronomy, Society and Environment. 2010;14:451–460.

[46] Vogt T. Phenylpropanoid biosynthesis. Molecular Plant. 2010;3:2–20. doi:10.1093/mp/ssp106

[47] Kfoury M, Sahraoui AL-H, Bourdon N, Laruelle F, Fontaine J, Auezova L, Greige-Gerges H, Fourmentin S. Solubility, photostability and antifungal activity of phenylpropanoids encapsulated in cyclodextrins. Food Chemistry.2016;196:518–525. doi: 10.1016/j.foodchem.2015.09.078

[48] Caballero B, Trugo LC, Finglas PM. Encyclopedia of food sciences and nutrition. Amsterdam: Academic Press; 2003. pp. 2169–2176. doi:10.1016/B0-12-227055-X/00424-7

[49] Mastelič J, Blažević I, Jerković I. Free and bound sulphur containing and other volatile compounds from evergreen candytuft (*Iberis sempervirens* L.). Croatica Chemica Acta. 2006;79:591–597.

[50] Fahey JW, Zalcmann AT, Talalay P. The chemical diversity and distribution of glucosinolates and isothiocyanates among plants. Phytochemistry. 2001;56:5–51. doi:10.1016/S0031–9422(00)00316–2

[51] Iranshahi M. A review of volatile sulfur-containing compounds from terrestrial plants: biosynthesis, distribution and analytical methods. The Journal of Essential Oil Research. 2012;24:393–434. doi:10.1080/10412905.2012.692918

[52] Stajner D, Milić N, Canadanović-Brunet J, Kapor A, Stajner M, Popović BM. Exploring Allium species as a source of potential medicinal agents. Phytotherapy Research. 2006;20:581–584. doi:10.1002/ptr.1917

[53] Amagase H, Petesch BL, Matsuura H, Kasuga S, Itakura Y. Intake of garlic and its bioactive components. The Journal of Nutrition. 2001;131:955S–962S.

[54] Tellez MR, Khan IA, Kobaisy M, Schrader KK, Dayan FE, Osbrink W. Composition of the essential oil of *Lepidium meyenii* (Walp.). Phytochemistry. 2002;61:149–155. doi: 10.1016/S0031-9422(02)00208-X

[55] Rath CC, Devi S, Dash SK, Mishra RK. Antibacterial potential assessment of jasmine essential oil against *E. coli*. Indian Journal of Pharmaceutical Sciences. 2008;70:238–241. doi:10.4103/0250-474X.41465

[56] Alma MH, Mavi A, Yildirim A, Digrak M, Hirata T. Screening chemical composition and in vitro antioxidant and antimicrobial activities of the essential oils from *Origanum*

syriacum L. growing in Turkey. Biological and Pharmaceutical Bulletin. 2003;26:1725–1729. doi:10.1248/bpb.26.1725.

[57] Başer KHC, Kürkcüoğlu M, Demirci B, Özek T. The essential oil of *Origanum syriacum* L. var. sinaicum (Boiss.) letswaart. Flavour and Fragrance Journal. 2003;18:98–99. doi: 10.1002/ffj.1169.

[58] Loizzo MR, Menichini F, Conforti F, Tundis R, Bonesi M, Saab AM, Statti GA, de Cindio B, Houghton PJ, Menichini F, Frega NG. Chemical analysis antioxidant antiinflammatory and anticholinesterase activities of *Origanum ehrenbergii* Boiss and *Origanum syriacum* L. essential oils. Food Chemistry. 2009;117:174–180. doi:10.1016/j.foodchem.2009.03.095

[59] Bhattacharya, S. Culitvation of essential oils. In: Preedy, VR, editor. Essential oils in food preservation, flavor and safety. London, UK: Academic Press, Elsevier; 2016. pp. 25–28.

[60] Salzer U-J. Analytical evaluation of seasoning extracts (oleoresins) and essential oils from seasonings. I. International Flavours Food Additives. 1975;6:151–157 (II. Ibid. 6, 206–210. III. Ibid. 6, 253–258).

[61] Salzer UJ, Furia TE. The analysis of essential oils and extracts (oleoresins) from seasonings—a critical review. Critical Reviews in Food Science and Nutrition. 1977;9:345–373.

[62] Salzer U. Analytical evaluation of seasoning extracts: oleoresins and essential oils from seasonings. Critical Reviews in Food Science and Nutrition. 1977;9:242–269.

[63] Govindarajan VS. Pepper-chemistry, technology and quality evaluation. CRC Critical Reviews in Food Science and Nutrition. 1977;9:115–125. doi:10.1080/10408397709527233

[64] Sankar KU. Studies on the physicochemical characteristics of volatile oil from pepper (*Piper nigrum*) extracted by supercritical carbon dioxide. Journal of the Science of Food and Agriculture 1989;48:483–493. doi:10.1002/jsfa.2740480411

[65] Kumoro AC, Hassan M, Singh H. Extraction of Sarawak black pepper essential oil using supercritical carbon dioxide. Arabian Journal for Science and Engineering. 2010;35:7–16

[66] Tipsrisukond N, Fernando LN, Clarke AD. Antioxidant effects of essential oil and oleoresin of black pepper from supercritical carbon dioxide extractions in ground pork. Journal of Agricultural and Food Chemistry. 1998;46:4329–4333. doi:10.1021/jf9802880

[67] Perakis C, Louli V, Magoulas K. Supercritical fluid extraction of black pepper oil. Journal of Food Engineering 2005;71:386–393. doi:10.1016/j.jfoodeng.2004.10.049

[68] Liu H, Zeng F, Wang Q, Ou S, Tan L, Gu F. The effect of cryogenic grinding and hammer milling on the flavour quality of ground pepper (*Piper nigrum* L.). Food Chemistry. 2013;141:3402–3408. doi:10.1016/j.foodchem.2013.06.052

[69] Karibasappa GS. Postharvest studies in large cardamom (*Amomum subulatum* Roxb.). Journal of Plantation Crops. 1987;15:63–64.

[70] Zacharia TJ, Gopalam A. Nature, production and quality of essential oils of pepper, ginger, turmeric, cardamom and tree spices. Indian Perfumer 1987;31:188–205.

[71] Pillai OGN, Mathulla T, George KM, Balakrishnan KV, Verghese J. Studies in cardamom 2. An appraisal of the excellence of Indian cardamom (*Elettaria cardamomum* Maton). Indian Spices. 1984;21:17–25.

[72] Korikanthimath VS, Ravindra M, John ZT. Variation in yield and quality characters of cardamom clones. Journal of Medicinal and Aromatic Plant Sciences. 1997;19:1024–1027.

[73] Ferhat MA, Meklati BY, Smadja J, Chemat F. An improved microwave clevenger apparatus for distillation of essential oils from orange peel. Journal of Chromatography A. 2006;1112:121–126. doi:10.1016/j.chroma.2005.12.030

[74] Amma, KPP, Sasidharan I, Sreekumar, MM, Sumathykutty MA, Arumughan C. Total antioxidant capacity and change in phytochemicals of four major varieties of cardamom oils during decortication. International Journal of Food Properties. 2015;18:1317–1325. doi:10.1080/10942912.2011.587621

[75] Morsy NFS. A short extraction time of high quality hydrodistilled cardamom (*Elettaria cardamomum* L. Maton) essential oil using ultrasound as a pretreatment. Industrial Crops and Products 2015;65:287–292. doi:10.1016/j.indcrop.2014.12.012

[76] Aćimović MG, Oljača SI, Tešević VV, Todosijević MM, Djisalov JN. Evaluation of caraway essential oil from different production areas of Serbia. Horticultural Science (Prague). 2014;41:122–130.

[77] Kallio H, Kerrola K, Alhonmaki P. Carvone and limonene in caraway fruits (*Carum carvi* L.) analyzed by supercritical carbon dioxide extraction-gas chromatography. Journal of Agricultural and Food Chemistry. 1994;42:2478–2485. doi:10.1021/jf00047a021

[78] Sedláková J, Kocourková B, Lojková L, Kubáň V. Determination of essential oil content in caraway (*Carum carvi* L.) species by means of supercritical fluid extraction. Plant, Soil and Environment. 2003;49:277–282.

[79] Chizolla R. Composition of the essential oil of the wild grown caraway in meadows of the Vienna region (Austria). Natural Product Comunications. 2014;9:581–582.

[80] Bouwmeester HJ, Kuijpers A-M. Relationship between assimilate supply and essential oil accumulation in annual and biennial caraway (*Carum carvi* L.). Journal of Essential Oil Research. 1993;5:143–152. doi:10.1080/10412905.1993.9698193

[81] Bouwmeester HJ, Davies JAR, Smid HG, Welten RSA. Physiological limitations to carvone yield in caraway (*Carum carvi* L.). Industrial Crops and Products. 1995;4:39–51. doi:10.1016/0926-6690(95)00009-2

[82] Sedláková J, Kocourková B, Kubán V. Determination of essential oils content and composition in caraway (*Carum carvi* L.). Czech Journal of Food Sciences. 2001;19:31–36

[83] Raghavan, S. Handbook of spices, seasonings and flavorings. 2nd ed. New York: CRC Press, Taylor & Francis Group; 2007. p. 330.

[84] Barceloux DG. Medical toxicology of natural substances. Foods, fungi, medicinal herbs, plants and venomous animals. Hoboken, New Jersey: John Wiley & Sons, Inc.; 2008. p. 1200. doi:10.1002/9780470330319.

[85] Singhal RS, Kulkarni PR, Rege DV, editors. Spices, flavourants and condiments (Chapter 8). In: Handbook of indices of food quality and authenticity. Abington Hall, Abington, Cambridge, England: Woodhead Publishing Limited; 1997. pp. 386–437.

[86] Lawrence BM. Peppermint oil. Perfumer and flavorist. 1984;9:92–94.

[87] Rohloff J, Dragland S, Mordal R, Iversen T-H. Effect of harvest time and drying method on biomass production, essential oil yield and quality of peppermint (*Mentha x piperita* L.). Journal of Agricultural and Food Chemistry. 2005;53:4143–4148. doi:10.1021/jf047998s

[88] Mosandl, A. Lavender oil. In: Berger RG, editor. Flavours and fragrances. Chemistry, bioprocessing and sustainability. New York: Springer; 2007. pp. 400–403. doi:10.1007/b136889

[89] d'Acampora Zellner B, Casilli A, Dugo P, Dugo G, Mondello L. Odour fingerprint acquisition by means of comprehensive two-dimensional gas chromatography-olfactometry and comprehensive two-dimensional gas chromatography/mass spectrometry. Journal of Chromatography A. 2007;1141:279–286. doi:10.1016/j.chroma.2006.12.035

[90] Lane A, Boecklemann A, Woronuk GN, Sarker L, Mahmoud SS. A genomic resource for investigating regulation of essential oil production in *Lavandula angustifolia*. Planta 2010;231:835–845. doi:10.1007/s00425-009-1090-4

[91] Bowles EJ. The chemistry of aromatherapeutic oils. 3rd ed. Allen & Unwin, Crows Nest, Australia; 2003. pp.164–165.

[92] Porter NG, Shaw ML, Hurndell LC. Preliminary studies of lavender as an essential oil crop for New Zeland. New Zealand Journal of Agricultural Research. 1982;25:389–394. doi:10.1080/00288233.1982.10417902

[93] Nasery M, Hassanzadeh MK, Najaran ZT, Emami SA. Rose (*Rosa* × *damascena* Mill.) essential oils. In: Preedy VR, editor. Essential oils in food preservation, flavor and safety. London, UK: Academic Press, Elsevier; 2016. pp. 659–665.

[94] Gupta LM, Raina R. Side effects of some medicinal plants. Current Science. 1998; 75(9): 897–900.

[95] David F, De Clercq C, Sandra P. GC/MS/MS analysis of β-damascenone in rose oil. GC/MS Varian App. Note 2006;52:1–3.

[96] Kováts E. Composition of essential oils. Part 7. Bulgarian oil of rose (*Rosa damascena* Mill). Journal of Chromatography A. 1987;406:185–222. doi:10.1016/S0021-9673(00)94030-5

[97] Baser KHC. Turkish rose oil. Perfumer Flavorist. 1992;17:45–52.

[98] Baydar H., Baydar NG. The effects of harvest date, fermentation duration and Tween 20 treatment on essential oil content and composition of industrial oil rose (*Rosa damascena* Mill.). Industrial Crops and Products. 2005;21:251–255. doi:10.1016/j.indcrop.2004.04.004

[99] Parthasarathy VA, Chempakam B, Zachariah TJ, editors. Chemistry of spices. Oxfordshire, UK: CABI Head Office.. 2008. p. 445.

[100] Govindarajan VS. Ginger—chemistry, technology and quality evaluation: part 1. CRC Critical Reviews in Food Science and Nutrition. 1982; 17:1–96. doi:10.1080/10408398209527343

[101] Zachariah TJ. Ginger. In: Parthasarathy VA, Chempakam B, Zachariah TJ, editors. Chemistry of spices. Oxfordshire, UK: CABI Head Office; 2008. pp. 70–96. doi:10.1079/9781845934057.0000

[102] Ložiene K, Venskutonis PR. Juniper (*Juniperus communis* L.) oils. In: Preedy, VR, editor. Essential oils in food preservation, flavor and safety. London, UK: Academic Press, Elsevier; 2016. pp. 495–499.

[103] Butkienë R, Nivinskienë O, Mockutë D. α-Pinene chemotype of leaf (needle) essential oils of *Juniperus communis* L. growing wild in Vilnius district. Chemija. 2005;16:53–60.

[104] Sela F, Karapandzova M, Stefkov G, Cvetkovikj I, Trajkovska-Dokik E, Kaftandzieva A, Kulevanova S. Chemical composition and antimicrobial activity of leaves essential oil of *Juniperus communis* (Cupressaceae) grown in Republic of Macedonia. Macedonian Pharmaceutical Bulletin. 2013;59:23–32.

[105] Orav A, Kailas T, Müürisepp M. Chemical investigation of the essential oil from berries and needles of common juniper (*Juniperus communis* L.) growing wild in Estonia. Natural Product Research. 2010;24:1789–1799. doi:10.1080/14786411003752037

[106] Pourmortazavi SM, Baghaee P, Mirhosseini MA. Extraction of volatile compounds from *Juniperus communis* L. leaves with supercritical fluid carbon dioxide: comparison with hydrodistillation. Flavour and Fragrance Journal. 2004;19:417–420. doi:10.1002/ffj.1327

[107] Looman A, Svendsen AB. The needle essential oil of Norwegian mountain juniper, *Juniperus communis* L. var. saxatilis Pall. Flavour and Fragrance Journal. 1992;7:23–26. doi:10.1002/ffj.2730070106

[108] Mandal S, DebMandal M. Thyme (*Thymus vulgaris* L.) oils. In: Preedy, VR, editor. Essential oils in food preservation, flavor and safety. London, UK, Academic Press, Elsevier; 2016. pp. 825–832.

[109] Hassanzadeh MK, Najaran ZT, Nasery M, Emami SA. Summer savory (*Satureja hortensis* L.) oils. In: Preedy, VR, editor. Essential oils in food preservation, flavor and safety. London, UK: Academic Press, Elsevier; 2016. pp. 757–763.

[110] Rhind JP. Aromatherapeutic blending: essential oils in synergy. London: Singing Dragon. 2016. p. 338.

[111] Alinkina ES, Misharina TA, Fatkullina LD. Antiradical properties of oregano, thyme and savory essential oils. Applied Biochemistry and Microbiology. 2013;49: 73–78. doi: 10.1134/S000368381301002X

[112] Panda H. Essential oils handbook. Chap. 110, 1st ed. New Delhi: National Institute of Industrial Research; 2003. p. 625.

[113] Pirbalouti AG, Hashemi M, Ghahfarokhi FT. Essential oil and chemical compositions of wild and cultivated *Thymus daenensis* Celak and *Thymus vulgaris* L. Industrial Crops and Products 2013;48:43–48. doi:10.1016/j.indcrop.2013.04.004

[114] Abdulazeez MA, Abdullahi AS, James BD. Lemongrass (Cymbopogon spp.) oils. In: Preedy, VR, editor. Essential oils in food preservation, flavor and safety. London, UK: Academic Press, Elsevier; 2016. pp. 509–515.

[115] Chisowa EH, Hall DR, Farman DI. Volatile constituents of the essential oil of *Cymbopogon citratus* Stapf grown in Zambia. Flavour and Fragrance Journal. 1998;13:29–30. doi:10.1002/(SICI)1099-1026(199801/02)13:1<29

[116] Desai MA, Parikh J, De AK. Modelling and optimization studies on extraction of lemongrass oil from *Cymbopogon flexuosus* (Steud.) wats. Chemical Engineering Research and Design 2014;92:793–803. doi:10.1016/j.cherd.2013.08.011

[117] Ha HKP, Maridable J, Gaspillo P, Hasika M, Malaluan R, Kawasaki J. Essential oil from lemongrass extracted by supercritical carbon dioxide and steam distillation. The Philippine Agricultural Scientist. 2008;91:36–41

[118] Weiss EA, editor. Essential oil crops. Wallingford, UK: CAB International; 1997. p. 600.

[119] Taskinen J, Mathela DK, Mathela CS. Composition of the essential oil of *Cymbopogon flexuosus*. Journal of Chromatography A. 1983;262:364–366. doi:10.1016/S0021-9673(01)88121-8

[120] Cowan MM. Plant products as antimicrobial agents. Clinical Microbiology Reviews. 1999;12:564–582.

[121] Nakatsu T, Lupo AT, Chinn JW, Kang RKL. Biological activity of essential oils and their constituents. Studies in Natural Products Chemistry. 2000;21:571–631. doi:10.1016/S1572–5995(00)80014-9

[122] Isman MB, Wilson JA, Bradbury R. Insecticidal activities of commercial rosemary oils (*Rosmarinus officinalis*) against larvae of *Pseudaletia unipuncta* and *Trichoplusia ni* in relation to their chemical compositions. Pharmaceutical Biology. 2008;46:82–87. doi:10.1080/13880200701734661

[123] Pandey AK, Singh P, Tripathi NN. Chemistry and bioactivities of essential oils of some Ocimum species: an overview. Asian Pacific Journal of Tropical Biomedicine. 2014;4:682-694. doi:10.12980/APJTB.4.2014C77

[124] Edris AE. Pharmaceutical and therapeutic potentials of essential oils and their individual volatile constituents: a review. Phytotherapy Research. 2007;21:308–323. doi:10.1002/ptr.2072

[125] Halliwell B. Antioxidants and human disease: a general introduction. Nutrition Reviews. 1997; 55:49–52. doi:10.1111/j.1753-4887.1997.tb06100.x

[126] Wanasundara UN, Shahidi F. Antioxidant and pro-oxidant activity of green tea extracts in marine oils. Food Chemistry. 1998;63:335–342. doi:10.1016/S0308-8146(98)00025-9

[127] Mimica-Dukic N, Bozin B, Sokovic M, Simin N. Antimicrobial and antioxidant activities of *Melissa officinalis* L. (Lamiaceae) essential oil. Journal of Agricultural and Food Chemistry. 2004;52:2485–2489. doi:10.1021/jf030698a

[128] Tomaino A, Cimino F, Zimbalatti V, Venuti V, Sulfaro V, De Pasquale A, Saija A. Influence of heating on antioxidant activity and the chemical composition of some spice essential oils. Food Chemistry. 2005;89:549–554. doi:10.1016/j.foodchem.2004.03.011

[129] Misharina TA, Samusenko AL. Antioxidant properties of essential oils from lemon, grapefruit, coriander, clove and their mixtures. Applied Biochemistry and Microbiology. 2008;45:438–442. doi:10.1134/S0003683808040182

[130] Wei A, Shibamoto T. Antioxidant/lipoxygenase inhibitory activities and chemical compositions of selected essential oils. Journal of Agricultural and Food Chemistry. 2010;58:7218–7225. doi:10.1021/jf101077s

[131] Nagababu E, Rifkind JM, Boindala S, Nakka L. Assessment of antioxidant activity of eugenol in vitro and in vivo. Methods in Molecular Biology. 2010;610:165–180. doi: 10.1007/978-1-60327-029-8_10

[132] Miguel MG. Antioxidant and anti-inflammatory activities of essential oils: a short review. Molecules. 2010;15:9252–9287. doi:10.3390/molecules15129252

[133] Johri RK. *Cuminum cyminum* and *Carum carvi*: an update. Pharmacognosy Review. 2011;5:63–72. doi:10.4103/0973-7847.79101

[134] Abdel-Aziz ME, Morsy NFS. Keeping quality of frozen beef patties by marjoram and clove essential oils. Journal of Food Processing and Preservation. 2015;39:956–965. doi: 10.1111/jfpp.12309

[135] Karoui IJ, Dhifi W, Jemia MB, Marzouk B. Thermal stability of corn oil flavoured with *Thymus capitatus* under heating and deep-frying conditions. Journal of the Science of Food and Agriculture. 2011;91:927–933. doi:10.1002/jsfa.4267

[136] Assiri AMA, Elbanna K, Al-Thubiani A, Ramadan MF. Cold-pressed oregano (*Origanum vulgare*) oil: a rich source of bioactive lipids with novel antioxidant and antimicrobial properties. European Food Research and Technology. 2016;242:1013–1023. doi:10.1007/s00217-015-2607-7

[137] Teixeira B, Marques A, Ramos C, Neng NR, Nogueira JMF, Saraiva JA, Nunes ML. Chemical composition and antibacterial and antioxidant properties of commercial essential oils. Industrial Crops and Products. 2013;43:587–595. doi:10.1016/j.indcrop.2012.07.069

[138] Oussalah M, Caillet S, Lacroix M. Mechanism of action of Spanish oregano, Chinese cinnamon and savory essential oils against cell membranes and walls of *Escherichia coli* O157:H7 and *Listeria monocytogenes*. Journal of Food Protection. 2006;69:1046–1055.

[139] Di Pasqua R, Betts G, Hoskins N, Edwards M, Ercolini D, Mauriello G. Membrane toxicity of antimicrobial compounds from essential oils. Journal of Agricultural and Food Chemistry. 2007;55:4863–4870. doi:10.1021/jf0636465

[140] Saad NY, Muller CD, Lobstein A. Major bioactivities and mechanism of action of essential oils and their components. Flavour and Fragrance Journal. 2013;28:269–279. doi:10.1002/ffj.3165

[141] Gustafson JE, Liew YC, Chew S, Markham J, Bell HC, Wyllie SG, Warmington JR. Effects of tea tree oil on *Escherichia coli*. Letters in Applied Microbiology. 1998;26:194–198. doi: 10.1046/j.1472-765X.1998.00317.x

[142] Oosterhaven K, Poolman B, Smid EJ. S-Carvone as a natural potato sprout inhibiting, fungistatic and bacteriostatic compound. Industrial Crops and Products. 1995;4:23–31. doi:10.1016/0926-6690(95)00007-Y

[143] Cox SD, Mann CM, Markham JL, Bell HC, Gustafson JE, Warmington JR, Wyllie SG. The mode of antimicrobial action of the essential oil of *Melaleuca alternifolia* (tea tree oil). Journal of Applied Microbiology. 2000;88:170–175.

[144] Ultee A, Bennik MHJ, Moezelaar R. The phenolic hydroxyl group of carvacrol is essential for action against the food-borne pathogen *Bacillus cereus*. Applied and Environmental Microbiology. 2002;68:1561–1568. doi:10.1128/AEM.68.4.1561-1568. 2002

[145] Jassbi AR, Asadollahi M, Masroor M, Schuman MC, Mehdizadeh Z, Soleimani M, Miri R. Chemical classification of the essential oils of the Iranian Salvia species in comparison with their botanical taxonomy. Chemistry and Biodiversity. 2012;9:1254–1271. doi: 10.1002/cbdv.201100209.

[146] Ghabraie M, Vu, KD, Tata L, Salmieri S, Lacroix M. Antimicrobial effect of essential oils in combinations against five bacteria and their effect on sensorial quality of ground meat. LWT-Food Science and Technology. 2016;66:332–339. doi:10.1016/j.lwt.2015. 10.055

[147] Radaelli, M, da Silva B P, Weidlich L, Hoehne L, Flach A, da Costa, LA, Ethur EM. Antimicrobial activities of six essential oils commonly used as condiments in Brazil against *Clostridium perfringens*. Brazilian Journal of Microbiology. 2016;47:424–430. doi: 10.1016/j.bjm.2015.10.001

[148] Cavaleiro C, Pinto E, Gonçalves M, Salgueiro L. Antifungal activity of Juniperus essential oils against dermatophyte, Aspergillus and Candida strains. Journal of Applied Microbiology. 2006;100:1333–1338. doi:10.1111/j.1365-2672.2006.02862.x

[149] Reyes-Jurado F, Franco-Vega A, Ramírez-Corona N, Palou E, López-Malo A. Essential oils: antimicrobial activities, extraction methods and their modeling. Food Engineering Reviews. 2015;7:275–297. doi:10.1007/s12393-014-9099-2

[150] Will F, Krüger E. Fungicide residues in strawberry processing. Journal of Agricultural Food Chemistry. 1999;47:858–61. doi:10.1021/jf980830k

[151] Varga J, Kocsubé S, Péteri Z, Vágvölgyi C, Tóth B. Chemical, physical and biological approaches to prevent ochratoxin induced toxicoses in humans and animals. Toxins (Basel). 2010;2:1718–1750. doi:10.3390/toxins2071718

[152] Sridhar SR, Rajagopal RV, Rajavel R., Masilamani S, Narasimhan S. Antifungal activity of some essential oils. Journal of Agricultural Food Chemistry. 2003;51: 7596–7599. doi: 10.1021/jf0344082

[153] Rahman A, Al-Reza SM, Kang SC. Antifungal activity of essential oil and extracts of *Piper chaba* hunter against phytopathogenic fungi. Journal of the American Oil Chemists' Society. 2011;88:573–579. doi:10.1007/s11746-010-1698-3

[154] Bouchra C, Achouri M, Idrissi Hassani LM, Hmamouchi M. Chemical composition and anti-fungal activity of essential oils of seven Moroccan Labiatae against *Botrytis cinerea*

Pers:Fr. Journal of Ethnopharmacology. 2003;89:165–169. doi:10.1016/S0378-8741(03)00275-7

[155] Serrano M, Martínez-Romero D, Castillo S, Guillén F, Valero D. The use of natural antifungal compounds improves the beneficial effect of MAP in sweet cherry storage. Innovative Food Science and Emerging Technologies. 2005;6:115–123. doi:10.1016/j.ifset.2004.09.001

[156] López P, Sanchez C, Batlle R, Nerín C. Vapor-phase activities of cinnamon, thyme and oregano essential oils and key constituents against food borne microorganisms. Journal of Agricultural Food Chemistry. 2007;55:4348–4356. doi:10.1021/jf063295u

[157] Nasir M, Tafess K, Abate D. Antimicrobial potential of the Ethiopian *Thymus schimperi* essential oil in comparison with others against certain fungal and bacterial species. BMC Complementary and Alternative Medicine. 2015;15:260–264. doi:10.1186/s12906-015-0784-3

[158] Rota MC, Herrera A, Martínez RM, Sotomayor JA, Jordán MJ. Antimicrobial activity and chemical composition of *Thymus vulgaris*, *Thymus zygis* and *Thymus hyemalis* essential oils. Food Control. 2008;19(7):7681–687. doi:10.1016/j.foodcont.2007.07.007

[159] Rao A, Zhang Y, Muend S, Rao R. Mechanism of antifungal activity of terpenoid phenols resembles calcium stress and inhibition of the TOR pathway. Antimicrobial Agents and Chemotherapy. 2010;54:5062–5069. doi:10.1128/AAC.01050-10

[160] Zore GB, Thakre AD, Jadhav S, Karuppayil SM. Terpenoids inhibit *Candida albicans* growth by affecting membrane integrity and arrest of cell cycle. Phytomedicine 2011;18:1181–1190. doi:10.1016/j.phymed.2011.03.008

[161] Sourmaghi MHS, Kiaee G, Golfakhrabadi F, Jamalifar H, Khanavi M. Comparison of essential oil composition and antimicrobial activity of *Coriandrum sativum* L. extracted by hydrodistillation and microwave-assisted hydrodistillation. Journal of Food Science and Technology. 2015;52:2452–2457. doi:10.1007/s13197-014-1286-x

[162] Silva F, Ferreira S, Duarte A, Mendonça DI, Domingues FC. Antifungal activity of *Coriandrum sativum* essential oil, its mode of action against *Candida* species and potential synergism with amphotericin B. Phytomedicine. 2011;19:42–47. doi:10.1016/j.phymed.2011.06.033

[163] de Oliveira RA, de Assis AMAD, da Silva LAM andrioli JL, de Oliveira FF. Chemical profile and antimicrobial activity of essential oil of *Piper ilheusense*. Chemistry of Natural Compounds. 2016; 52:331–333. doi:10.1007/s10600-016-1634-3

[164] Marino M, Bersani C, Comi G. Impedance measurements to study the antimicrobial activity of essential oils from Lamiaceae and Compositae. International Journal of Food Microbiology. 2001;67:187–195. doi:10.1016/S0168–1605(01)00447-0

[165] Pavet V, Portal MM, Moulin JC, Herbrecht R, Gronemeyer H. Towards novel paradigms for cancer therapy. Oncogene. 2011;30:1–20. doi:10.1038/onc

[166] Rajput S, Mandal M. Antitumor promoting potential of selected phytochemicals derived from spices: a review. European Journal of Cancer Prevention. 2012;21:205–215. doi:10.1097/CEJ.0b013e32834a7f0c

[167] Magalhães HIF, de Sousa ÉBV. Antitumor essential oils. In: de Sousa DP, editor, Bioactive essential oils and cancer. Switzerland: Springer International Publishing; 2015. pp. 135–174. doi:10.1007/978-3-319-19144-7_7

[168] Hadfield N. The role of aromatherapy massage in reducing anxiety in patients with malignant brain tumours. International Journal of Palliative Nursing. 2001;7:279–285. doi:10.12968/ijpn.2001.7.6.9025

[169] Bhardwaj P, Alok U, Khanna A. In vitro cytotoxicity of essential oils: a review. International Journal of Research in Pharmacy and Chemistry. 2013;3:675–681.

[170] Russo R, Corasaniti MT, Bagetta G, Morrone LA. Exploitation of cytotoxicity of some essential oils for translation in cancer therapy. Evidence-Based Complementary and Alternative Medicine. 2015. doi:10.1155/2015/397821

[171] Sieniawska E, Świątek Ł, Rajtar B, Kozioł E, Polz-Dacewicz M, Skalicka-Wózniak K. Carrot seed essential oil—source of carotol and cytotoxicity study. Industrial Crops and Products. 2016;92:109–115. doi:10.1016/j.indcrop.2016.08.001

[172] Zarai Z, Ben Chobba I, Ben Mansour R, Békir A, Gharsallah N, Kadri A. Essential oil of the leaves of *Ricinus communis* L.: in vitro cytotoxicity and antimicrobial properties. Lipids in health and disease. 2012;11:102–108. doi:10.1186/1476-511X-11-102

[173] Kouidhi B, Zmantar T, Bakhrouf A. Anticariogenic and cytotoxic activity of clove essential oil (*Eugenia caryophyllata*) against a large number of oral pathogens. Annals of Microbiology. 2010;60:599–604. doi:10.1007/s13213-010-0092-6

[174] Yoo CB, Han KT, Cho KS, Ha J, Park HJ, Nam JH, Kil UH, Lee KT. Eugenol isolated from the essential oil of *Eugenia caryophyllata* induces a reactive oxygen species-mediated apoptosis in HL-60 human promyelocytic leukemia cells. Cancer Letters. 2005;225:41–52. doi:10.1016/j.canlet.2004.11.018

[175] Okada N, Hirata A, Murakami Y, Shoji M, Sakagami H, Fujisawa S. Induction of cytotoxicity and apoptosis and inhibition of cyclooxygenase-2 gene expression by eugenol-related compounds. Anticancer Research. 2005;25:3263–3269.

[176] Ho, YC. Huang FM, Chang YC. Mechanisms of cytotoxicity of eugenol in human osteoblastic cells in vitro. International Endodontic Journal. 2006;39:389–393. doi: 10.1111/j.1365-2591.2006.01091.x

[177] Prashar A, Locke IC, Evans CS. Cytotoxicity of lavender oil and its major components to human skin cells. Cell Proliferation. 2004;37:221–229. doi:10.1111/j.1365-2184.2004.00307.x

[178] Duncan RE, Lau D, El-Sohemy A, Archer MC. Geraniol and beta-ionone inhibit proliferation, cell cycle progression and cyclin-dependent kinase 2 activity in MCF-7

breast cancer cells independent of effects on HMG-CoA reductase activity. Biochemical Pharmacology. 2004;68:1739–1747. doi:10.1016/j.bcp.2004.06.022

[179] Kim SH, Park EJ, Lee CR, Chun JN, Cho NH, Kim IG, Lee S, Kim TW, Park HH, So I, Jeon JH. Geraniol induces cooperative interaction of apoptosis and autophagy to elicit cell death in PC-3 prostate cancer cells. International Journal of Oncology. 2012;40:1683–1690. doi:10.3892/ijo.2011.1318

[180] Carnesecchi S, Bras-Gonçalves R, Bradaia A, Zeisel M, Gossé F, Poupon MF, Raul F. Geraniol, a component of plant essential oils, modulates DNA synthesis and potentiates 5-fluorouracil efficacy on human colon tumor xenografts. Cancer Letters. 2004;215:53–59. doi:10.1016/j.canlet.2004.06.019

[181] Legault J, Pichette A. Potentiating effect of beta-caryophyllene on anticancer activity of alpha-humulene, isocaryophyllene and paclitaxel. Journal of Pharmacy and Pharmacology. 2007;59:1643–7. doi:10.1211/jpp.59.12.0005

[182] Russo R, Ciociaro A, Berliocchi L, Cassiano MG, RombolÃ L, Ragusa S, Bagetta G, Blandini F, Corasaniti MT. Implication of limonene and linalyl acetate in cytotoxicity induced by bergamot essential oil in human neuroblastoma cells. Fitoterapia. 2013;89:48–57. doi:10.1016/j.fitote.2013.05.014

[183] El-Shemy HA, Aboul-Enein KM, Lightfoot DA. Predicting in silico which mixtures of the natural products of plants might most effectively kill human leukemia cells? Evidence-Based Complementary and Alternative Medicine. 2013;801501. doi:10.1155/2013/801501

[184] Fan K, Li X, Cao Y, Qi H, Li L, Zhang Q, Sun H. Carvacrol inhibits proliferation and induces apoptosis in human colon cancer cells. Anticancer Drugs. 2015;26:813–823. doi:10.1097/CAD.0000000000000263

[185] Dai W, Sun C, Huang S, Zhou Q. Carvacrol suppresses proliferation and invasion in human oral squamous cell carcinoma. Journal of OncoTargets and Therapy. 2016;9:2297–2304. doi:10.2147/OTT.S98875

[186] Ma J, Li J, Wang KS, Mi C, Piao LX, Xu GH, Li X, Lee JJ, Jin X. Perillyl alcohol efficiently scavenges activity of cellular ROS and inhibits the translational expression of hypoxia-inducible factor-1α via mTOR/4E-BP1 signaling pathways. International Immunopharmacology. 2016;39:1–9. doi:10.1016/j.intimp.2016.06.034.

Permissions

All chapters in this book were first published in AIAMP, by InTech Open; hereby published with permission under the Creative Commons Attribution License or equivalent. Every chapter published in this book has been scrutinized by our experts. Their significance has been extensively debated. The topics covered herein carry significant findings which will fuel the growth of the discipline. They may even be implemented as practical applications or may be referred to as a beginning point for another development.

The contributors of this book come from diverse backgrounds, making this book a truly international effort. This book will bring forth new frontiers with its revolutionizing research information and detailed analysis of the nascent developments around the world.

We would like to thank all the contributing authors for lending their expertise to make the book truly unique. They have played a crucial role in the development of this book. Without their invaluable contributions this book wouldn't have been possible. They have made vital efforts to compile up to date information on the varied aspects of this subject to make this book a valuable addition to the collection of many professionals and students.

This book was conceptualized with the vision of imparting up-to-date information and advanced data in this field. To ensure the same, a matchless editorial board was set up. Every individual on the board went through rigorous rounds of assessment to prove their worth. After which they invested a large part of their time researching and compiling the most relevant data for our readers.

The editorial board has been involved in producing this book since its inception. They have spent rigorous hours researching and exploring the diverse topics which have resulted in the successful publishing of this book. They have passed on their knowledge of decades through this book. To expedite this challenging task, the publisher supported the team at every step. A small team of assistant editors was also appointed to further simplify the editing procedure and attain best results for the readers.

Apart from the editorial board, the designing team has also invested a significant amount of their time in understanding the subject and creating the most relevant covers. They scrutinized every image to scout for the most suitable representation of the subject and create an appropriate cover for the book.

The publishing team has been an ardent support to the editorial, designing and production team. Their endless efforts to recruit the best for this project, has resulted in the accomplishment of this book. They are a veteran in the field of academics and their pool of knowledge is as vast as their experience in printing. Their expertise and guidance has proved useful at every step. Their uncompromising quality standards have made this book an exceptional effort. Their encouragement from time to time has been an inspiration for everyone.

The publisher and the editorial board hope that this book will prove to be a valuable piece of knowledge for researchers, students, practitioners and scholars across the globe.

List of Contributors

Eduardo Lozano Guzmán and Francisco Javier Moreno Cruz
Faculty of Chemistry, Juarez University of the State of Durango, Durango, Dgo, Mexico

Ana M. Džamić
Faculty of Biology, Institute of Botany and Botanical Garden "Jevremovac", University of Belgrade, Belgrade, Serbia

Jelena S. Matejić
Faculty of Medicine, University of Niš, Niš, Serbia

Peiman Zandi
Institute of Crop Science, Chinese Academy of Agricultural Sciences, Beijing, P. R. China

Saikat Kumar Basu
Department of Biological Sciences, University of Lethbridge, Lethbridge, AB, Canada

William Cetzal-Ix
Instituto Tecnológico de Chiná, Colonia Centro Chiná, Campeche, México

Mojtaba Kordrostami
Department of Biotechnology, Faculty of Agricultural Sciences, University of Guilan, Rasht, Iran

Shahram Khademi Chalaras
Department of Agronomy and Plant Breeding, Rasht branch, Islamic Azad University, Rasht, Iran

Leila Bazrkar Khatibai
Department of Plant Breeding, Faculty of Agriculture, Zabol University, Zabol, Iran

Nontokozo Z. Msomi and Mthokozisi. B. C Simelane
Department of Biochemistry, School of Life Science, University of KwaZulu-Natal, Pietermaritzburg, South Africa

Angela Cerempei
Faculty of Textiles, Leather and Industrial Management, Department of Chemical Engineering in Textile and Leather, "Gheorghe Asachi" Technical University, Iasi, Romania

Sanghamitra Samantaray and Umakanta Ngangkham
ICAR-National Rice Research Institute, Cuttack, Odisha, India

Alma Delia Alarcon-Rojo and Ana Renteria-Monterrubio
Autonomous University of Chihuahua, Chihuahua, Mexico

Hector Janacua-Vidales
Autonomous University of Ciudad Juarez, Ciudad Juarez, Mexico

Christel Brunschwig
Integrated Study of Secondary Metabolites (EIMS), Research Unit UMR 241 Insular Ocean Ecosystems (EIO), University of French Polynesia, Faaa, Tahiti, French Polynesia
Research and Development Department, Institute "Vanille de Tahiti", Raiatea, French Polynesia

François-Xavier Collard and Sandra Lepers-Andrzejewski
Research and Development Department, Institute "Vanille de Tahiti", Raiatea, French Polynesia

Phila Raharivelomanana
Integrated Study of Secondary Metabolites (EIMS), Research Unit UMR 241 Insular Ocean Ecosystems (EIO), University of French Polynesia, Faaa, Tahiti, French Polynesia

Gema Nieto and Gaspar Ros
Department of Food Technology and Science and Human Nutrition, Veterinary Faculty, University of Murcia, Espinardo, Murcia, Spain

Nayara Vieira de Lima, Daniela Granja Arakaki, Paula F. Saldanha Tschinkel, Anderson Fernandes da Silva, Rita de Cássia Avellaneda Guimarães, Priscila Aiko Hiane and Valter Aragão do Nascimento
Post Graduation Program in Health and Development in the Middle West Region, Federal University of Mato Grosso do Sul—UFMS, Campo Grande, MS, Brazil

Fernanda Leal and Manuela Matos
Genetics and Biotechnology Department, University of Trás-os-Montes and Alto Douro (UTAD), Vila Real, Portugal

BioISI—Biosystems & Integrative Sciences Institute, Faculty of Sciences University of Lisboa, Lisboa, Portugal

Meriem Taghouti and Amélia Silva
Centre for Research and Technology of Agro-Environmental and Biological Sciences (CITAB, UTAD), Vila Real, Portugal

Fernando Nunes
CQ-VR Chemistry Research Center, UTAD, Vila Real, Portugal

Ana Cláudia Coelho
Animal and Veterinary Research Centre (CECAV), UTAD, Vila Real, Portugal

Saaya Minematsu
Environmental Chemistry, Fukuoka Technical High School Fukuoka, Japan

Xing-Zheng Wu
Department of Life, Environment and Materials Science, Fukuoka Institute of Technology Fukuoka, Japan

Pozi Milow, Sorayya Malek and Raznan Mohd. Ramli
Institute of Biological Sciences, University of Malaya, Kuala Lumpur, Malaysia

Xiujuan Lei, Zhiqing Wang, Juan Song, Shao Liang, Lina Yao, Zhifang Hou and Yingping Wang
Institute of Special Wild Economic Animal and Plant Science of Chinese Academy of Agricultural Sciences, Changchun, P. R. China

Nashwa Fathy Sayed Morsy
Food Science Department, Faculty of Agriculture, Cairo University, Giza, Egypt

Index

www.ingramcontent.com/pod-product-compliance
Lightning Source LLC
LaVergne TN
LVHW080925210926
848485LV00004B/731